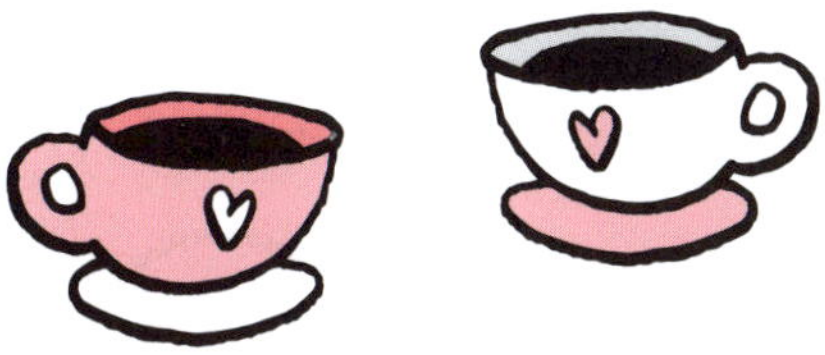

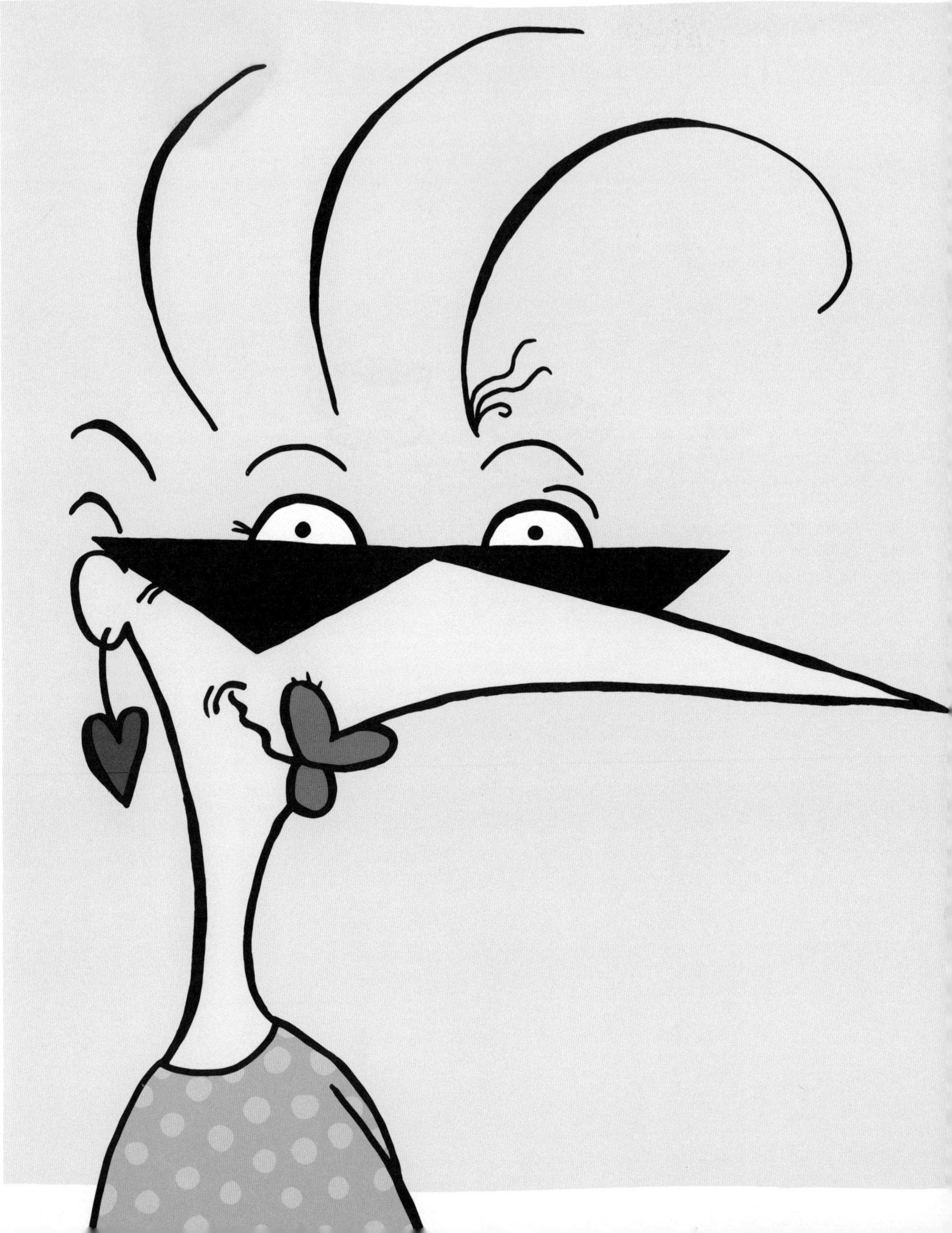

KAZ COOKE

IT'S THE MENOPAUSE

what you need to know in your 40s, 50s and beyond

VIKING
an imprint of
PENGUIN BOOKS

Contents

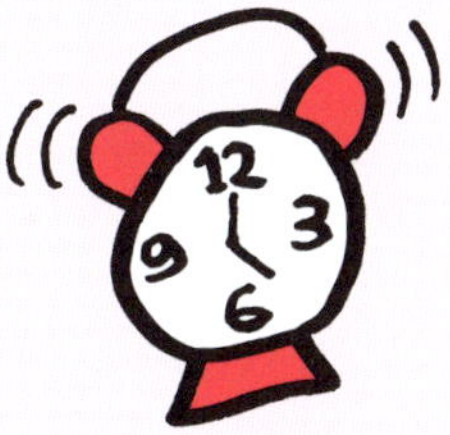

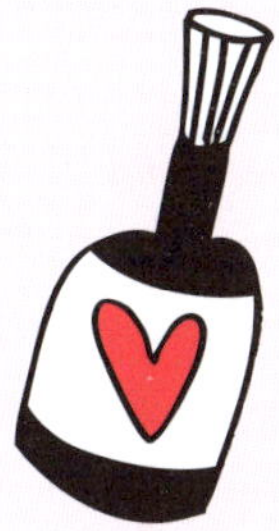

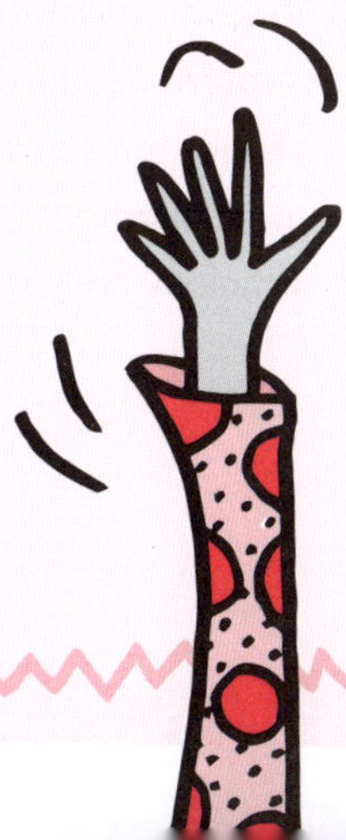

Definitions

Perimenopause (pronounced perry-menno-pause): 'Around' the time of menopause, usually meaning leading up to it.

Menopause: The medical definition is when your last period was at least a year ago.

Menopause symptoms: Often used to mean symptoms experienced during the perimenopause, or in menopause.

Post-menopause: Some people use this to mean the rest of your life after you stop having periods; doctors usually call it menopause.

MHT (Menopause Hormone Therapy): The newer accepted name for hormone medication used to relieve menopause symptoms (previously known as HRT).

HRT (Hormone Replacement Therapy): The older term for menopause medication.

A note on spelling

Doctors and scientists worldwide disagree on spelling for medical words, often because they're Team Latin or Team Greek, or one side of an 'American' versus 'English and Australian' debate, even when the so-called American spelling was originally the English one.

So, this book spells it estrogen, not oestrogen, for the same reason I use the spelling fetus not foetus. It's easier, it's more sensible, and I'm not keen on arguing about it.

When searching online, you may need to vary spellings of keywords to cast a wider net for info.

Some organisations in Australia and England use the American spelling 'organization' on their sites because they want US and South American online search result traffic. UK and Australian searches for 'organisation' usually include results for 'organization', but US searches for 'organization' don't usually include 'organisation'. So, in this book, that spelling varies as to what organisations officially call themselves.

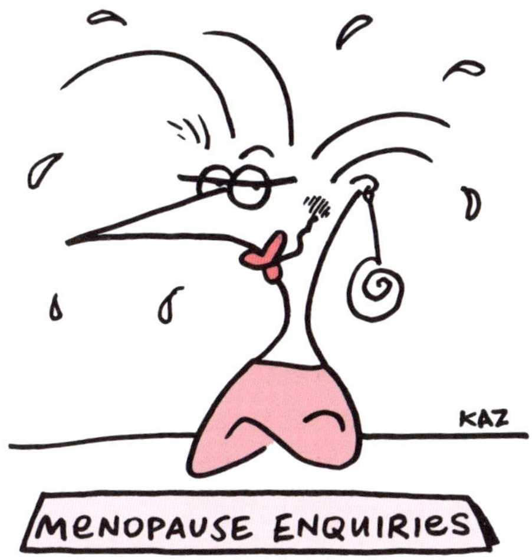

Intro

When people find out you're writing a Menopause Book, everyone has something to say. The most common response from any woman over 40 was to grab me by both biceps and shout into my face, 'HURRY UP!'. Unnerving, but understandable.

After a lot of thinking and researching, and interviewing medical experts, and reading more than 75,000 answers from nearly 9000 mostly confused and furious women . . . here, at last, is the book.

Another thing some people did when they heard I was writing it was to make a wincing face when they heard the word 'menopause'. I suspect they'd like a book saying, 'I've found a way to abolish the menopause. We shall never speak of it again, let alone go through it.'

Most of us don't know the perimenopause (pronounced perry-menno-pause, the first signs that menopause is coming) will probably start in our early to mid-40s – possibly with invisible symptoms we mistake for going bonkers. And some of us experience complete menopause before we turn 40 when our ovaries stop producing the levels of hormones they used to, for unknown reasons or because of surgery or medication side effects. ('What even is it?', I hear you ask, with a resting shriek-face, reaching for my biceps. See Chapter 1, What Even Is The Menopause?)

Before we get there, most of us of don't know there are more than 35 full-on symptoms that perimenopause and menopause can throw at us (there's a list on pages 36–37), with varying degrees of awfulness. We're rarely told how it's hardly noticeable for some, and life-changing and derailing for others.

We hadn't anticipated that hormonal causes need a hormonal solution and that suddenly we'd be at the mercy of predatory marketing for menopause-related sexual products and procedures that don't work, and 'wellness' supplement products with misleading ads that can't affect our hormones in a useful way. ('Which bloody hormones, and how and what and when?' I hear you hiss through clenched teeth. See Chapter 2, It's Your Hormones.)

This book is for all of us approaching or in perimenopause or menopause, whether we dread it or think it's the greatest idea since banana toasties. Whether it's over the horizon, on the horizon, in the rear-view mirror or a cyclone all around us.

Some of us have a uterus, some do not. Some of us don't have ovaries; some of us do have ovaries, probably gearing down or sputtering along, heading towards the end of their hormone production. Some have no sex life, some are rarely off the chandelier with a sailor; some have a male partner, and some a girlfriend or wife. Some are mothers, some aren't. Some of us need to take medical hormones, some don't, and some can't, for all sorts of reasons.

We do know a lot more than we used to about the menopause, and I've been very lucky to have so many specialist experts talk to me about the latest that's known about menopause, and to help us through. I'm a very convincing lowest common denominator so this book dispenses with medical jargon, while recognising info doesn't have to be dumbed down for us. Luckily, there's a big gap between loose talk of follicular mass and gonadotropins, and, 'It's your hormones, dear.'

It grips different women in different ways and is an essential part of the sisterhood – where we can share wisdom, support, and love. Tania, 53

If you've been the one who has always used contraception, the one who had babies, the one who was the primary carer of those children, it's your time to put yourself first. Educate boys and men about our hormonal life. Sisters: listen, laugh, cry, support each other. Di, 51

Having your say

It made me emotional to read the tens of thousands of answers to questions in the Menopause Survey I conducted online for this book; as I said, almost 9000 women did the survey and 75,000 answers were in words rather than checking a box. Not everyone answered every question – sometimes more than 7000 women answered the same question, in one case it was less than 100 and there were some yes/no answers – but thousands of people poured out their feelings in whole paragraphs.

As I scrolled through all those responses, I laughed, I gasped, I said things like 'Oh, no' or 'Oh my God', and sometimes I felt the prickle of tears. Thousands said they thought menopause only happened to old women; they had no knowledge of any symptoms of perimenopause except hot flushes; and they didn't realise they were experiencing perimenopausal symptoms until they read the Survey.

So many surprising things came out of the Survey: more women identify mental issues, heavy periods and lower self-esteem as their main perimenopause symptom rather than hot flushes. (Chapter 4, It's Your Mind, and Chapter 5, It's Your Body, cover mental and physical symptoms.) While website articles bang on about libido, most women sidled up to say the problem is more that sex starts to hurt, a lot.

So many women had been suffering mental and physical symptoms for years with no end in sight and had given up on getting help. Older women, all the way through and on the other side, shared their struggles and what they'd learned or regretted.

> I honestly don't feel it is taken very seriously by younger women, the medical profession and workplaces. Melissa, 44

Women talked about being blindsided by symptoms that up-ended their personal and professional lives: they lost relationships, jobs, confidence and faith in themselves and the medical profession. We were by turns furious, curious, sweary, sweaty, frightened, angry, determined to tough it out and desperate for information. Thankfully, thousands of us also had positive attitudes and suggestions to share.

The Survey isn't a scientific study; it was an online survey that women opted in to, so the statistics shouldn't be viewed as scientific, peer-reviewed information. But it's the biggest collection of data so far in Australia showing women's thoughts, feelings and experiences of perimenopause and menopause. It's about what women want to share, or investigate, or shout about.

I'm so grateful to you all. (More thanks to everyone who helped with the book, including medical and other experts, are in the Acknowledgements.)

You were aged from your 40s to your 90s, most in your 50s, closely followed by your late 40s: peak perimenopause and menopause times.

You told me about having cancer, and what you're afraid of. You told me your worries. You told me private things about your sex life; your vagina; things you've never told anyone else. You told me what makes you feel stronger; you told me you wanted other women to be informed of what you'd found out. Thank you.

Many of us expected our periods to just stop one day with no further ado, and then we had our lives turned upside down by a shitload of ado. Lots of us didn't know there were hormonal reasons for feeling awful about ourselves, and sudden, bewildering mental health problems. Some of us had firm expectations of perimenopause based on a mother's experience or our philosophy of medical or natural approaches, only to have those expectations totally exploded by the real thing.

Thousands said their GP (general practitioner doctor) had dismissed their concerns, failed to recognise symptoms as perimenopausal, wrongly told them they were too young in their 40s to be experiencing perimenopause, suggested they 'suck it up' and even laughed at their concerns. Others talked of the great relief of finding an understanding, knowledgeable GP.

Common themes included the assumption that menopause didn't happen until you were an old woman. Many people thought the symptoms lasted for 5 years, perhaps an easy number to remember or a mix-up with outdated advice on how long you can stay on hormone medication.

Already ambushed by symptoms, a lot of us were sad and freaked out about how much they affected our relationships with our kids, partners and at work. Some of us were so unprepared – didn't know about the higher risk of dark thoughts and self-harm in the perimenopause years that can be reversed with help and medication.

Thousands of women said they tried natural therapies, or medical ones, or were scared of HRT (now known as MHT, explained coming up). Chapter 2, It's Your Hormones, has all you need to know about hormone medication and Chapter 3, It's Your Approach, talks about self-help including exercise and eating.

Women talked wistfully or triumphantly about becoming invisible, 'losing their looks', horrified that the new weight around their middle was unshiftable, bamboozled by what to do about losing hair, or their greying hair, or chin hair, or whether their wardrobe was supposed to be fancypants or elastic pants. (See Chapter 7, It's How You Look.)

I asked questions about all sorts of things: experiences of expected or early perimenopause and menopause, how easy or horrible the mental and physical symptoms were from sneezy weeing and workplace adjustments to sleep difficulties, medications and other treatments, attitudes, what you knew about menopause before you got to it, what you felt you needed, and positive messages to share.

There are hundreds of voices in this book. The Survey statistics are startling and helpful enough, but the quotes are the backbone of this book: they told me how you felt, what you'd been through, how you thought things could be made easier for other women. The most emblematic ones are scattered throughout the book. The most common opening word of the answers to 'What do you want to know about menopause?' was 'Everything!'

It was fascinating to see in the Survey how most women recognised a change in alcohol habits during perimenopause: most found it didn't agree with them anymore, but lots of women found they drank more to try to self-medicate. It was also clear that there is a huge, secret problem affecting so many women: leaking and unexpected weeing.

Every woman's experience of perimenopause and menopause is different, but there are so many shared elements. I want this book to be like a big discussion among us all, with trusted info from experts. Of course, medical advice can change and be different for everyone, and that's why what's presented here is about a buffet spread of choices. I avoid the brand names of medication because that's what's most likely to change: and a book is no substitute for individual medical advice.

It's the devil's work! It is way more than the glossy articles portray it as. It affects every part of your body from thinning hair to arthritic, aching toes. It's a thing that society goes silent on. Caroline, 55

Occasional hot spells are nothing! No more periods!!! No more PMT!!! Fantastic sex, ready to go. Fitter and healthier than I have been for years. THIS is the prime of my life. Jayne, 53

Perhaps menopause isn't the beginning of the end of our lives but the end of the beginning of our lives. Cait, 45

Your suit of armour

It's the Menopause will arm you with the information you need to better understand what you might be going through, and how and where to get help from reliable sources – not the advertisers who are getting to know the symptoms of perimenopause and adjust their marketing accordingly, targeting you for the greatest miseries: interrupted sleep, anxiety, weight migrating to your middle, flyaway hair and painful sex. It includes a list of questions to ask your GP, and Who's Who lists of which medical practitioners do what, and which qualifications they should have.

The Survey also showed that many women wanted a 'natural' solution to menopause symptoms but weren't sure if there was any evidence. Many had tried one and found it didn't work for them, or were absolutely convinced it helped, or wondered if it was a placebo effect or their symptoms coincidentally dissipated. It was notable that nobody who said they had severe, difficult or debilitating symptoms reported success with a 'natural' treatment. Still, lots of non-medical approaches have also eased the way for many of us.

There was a lot of talk in the Survey results from women who said perimenopause or menopause means they no longer care what people think about them. Literally thousands of answers started with, 'I don't care' or 'Not caring anymore about . . .' And goodness, there was a lot of serious swearing and people who said they swore more since experiencing perimenopause.

There were thousands who said they didn't give a fuck, had no fucks left, or estimated their amount of fucks to give at zero, none or no more. One woman could not give two fucks. What other women said they had none included: stuffs, shits, and tosses.

Cassandra, 50, replied to a question about whether she'd had any menopause symptoms: 'I have done none of these things. Good God, what is the matter with people? This isn't a goddamn illness, it's just what is happening now.' And added for good measure: 'This Survey Was Too FUCKING LONG'. So no rage or irritability, then. In answer to another question, 'Do you have a motto or philosophy on menopause?' Cassandra wrote: BURN IT ALL DOWN.'

It is a transformative experience. I love that my mood is much more even now. I love not bleeding each month. I loved having sex and rediscovering my body after a long break. **Sharon, 49**

More women said they felt wholly negative about menopause (they came to the Survey because they wanted to share, so that's no surprise), but lots of women also said getting through perimenopause to the other side, enduring menopause, was a totally positive experience. Thousands said they truly thought they were going crazy; hundreds more talked about the relief in no longer being prey to street or other sexual harassment; hundreds said they'd gained wisdom or used a variation of 'I know myself now'. So many felt they'd moved to a better to place of knowledge, experience, wisdom and freedom.

Some Survey respondents didn't give their age, and some used their own pseudonym, which is reflected in the quotes throughout.

Please choose the bits of the book that are relevant and helpful for you. This book is about having the emotional and practical tools and solutions to get you through. Everyone I know who's approaching perimenopause, in perimenopause, or in menopause will benefit from knowing the stuff in this book:

1. Know what's happening to you.
2. Manage what's happening to you.
3. Skip off into the distance singing la la la, having kicked the arse of menopause.*

You might not want to read this book through in the way you do a novel. If you do, you may see safety info repeated in a couple of places. You can make friends with the index at the back of the book to find what you need.

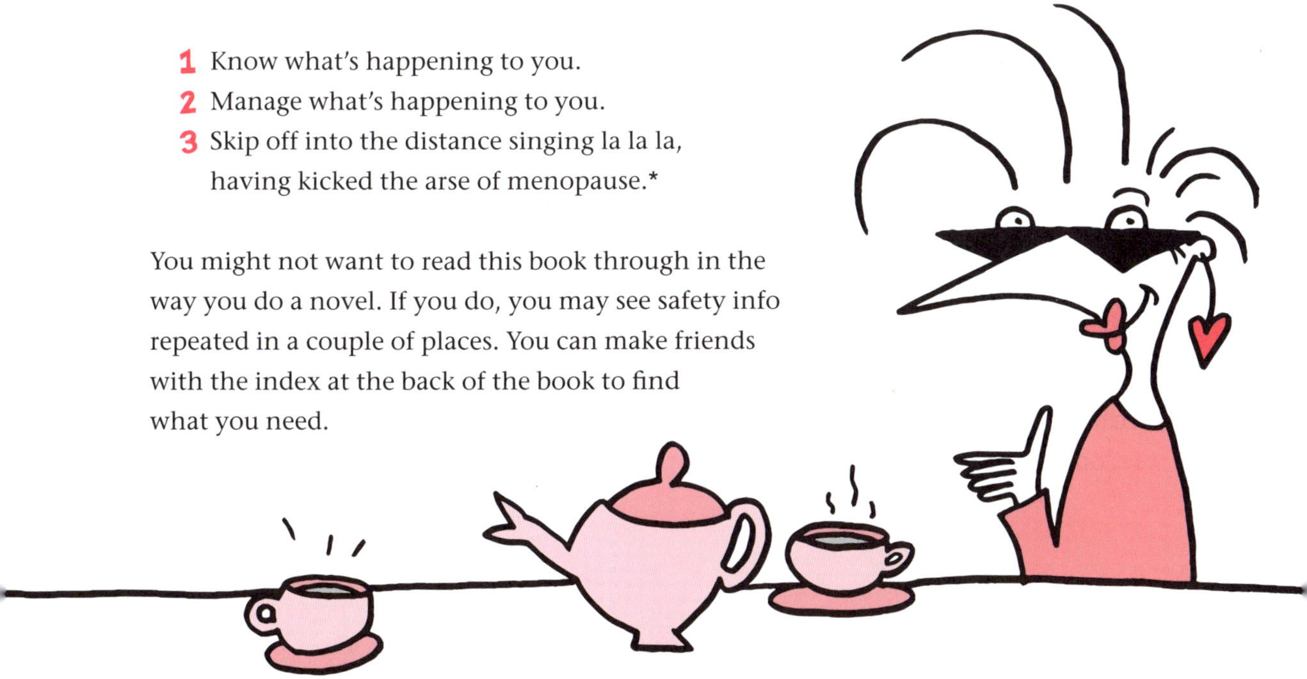

* There is not an actual Arse of Menopause, but if you need a name for your thrash-metal band, you're welcome.

Your brain turns to mush and fighting it will only make you sad. Be open with the people around you about what is happening and let them help. Ness, 51

Blood, sweat and tears: menopause has it all. Luckily, nobody gets absolutely all of them in a way that makes them miserable, and they don't all happen at once. I don't know if this is comforting or horrifying, but for some unlucky souls, the symptoms can last more than a decade, and even 15 years or more.

This book can't tell you how to avoid the menopause. If we're lucky to live long enough, we'll all eventually, naturally stop having periods, and need to deal with any side effects that come with it. And even if you take medication forever and get into lifestyle changes that make things easier, you'll still technically be in menopause.

A visit from the Menopause Fairy

I can't tell you how much I wish I knew all of this myself before I plummeted into perimenopause. In many ways I was the textbook example of clueless perimenopausal woman, flailing around for years. Women are told we can expect menopause at the average age of 50, and yet it's totally average and normal for menopause to happen any time from age 45, with mental and other symptoms happening up to 5 years earlier. That immediately changes the timeline of when we should suspect the possibility of perimenopause symptoms.

I reckon I wasn't just visited by the Menopause Fairy but a flying squadron of 'em. Like the winged monkeys in *The Wizard of Oz*, or a murmuration of sparrows with arrows. First they came for my self-esteem, and my 8 hours' sleep. Later, they took hair from my eyebrows and legs and put them on my chin and my top lip. And then, night sweats and oddly misbehaving periods, and weirdly itching skin I had no idea was a menopause symptom.

It really affects your mood, I got so angry very quickly over the simplest of things. I felt the family tiptoed around me. Susan, 57

Surely the Dept of Health can inform women when they turn 40 of what their bodies are going to do to them? Elouise, 43

It is truly fucked up. Simone, 49

I was by turns plummeted into feelings of anxiety, depression, bewilderment and rage. I couldn't concentrate or find the right words when I was writing. I had brain fog, lack of mojo; once I stayed awake all night. I had random heart rate changes, sore finger joints, and the return of tendon conditions dormant for 30 years. More defyingly, I wee'd a little bit if I coughed suddenly. It was frightening and inexplicable.

My GP at the time prescribed me antidepressants in a 10-minute conversation with no mention of perimenopause. Looking back, I'm sure I was experiencing the first hidden signs of it, and had I been prescribed hormone medication that targeted the reason for my problems, I might have had a much easier time and known which symptoms were likely to be hormone-related: weird anxiety spikes that were hot flushes, recurring vaginal infections and the rest. Instead, I thought they were all unrelated and I was falling apart.

Doctors should do more than shrug and say, 'It's just menopause.' Get fucked.
Vanessa, 45

Just as an estrogen patch picks up fluff on its edges, the menopause attracts connotations of the messy, the unglamorous, the unattractive, the over-sharing, and hairy bits in the 'wrong' places.

I used to take estrogen pills but then another doctor told me it was safer to use a patch or gel; it carries a lower risk of blood clots. Every morning I smear one or two pumps of estrogen hormone gel (a bit like aloe vera) on my arms and wait for it to dry before I cover it with clothes. It's cold in winter and annoying on the days I forget and then have to get undressed and dressed again, after waiting for it to dry. I tried estrogen patches, but the brand prescribed was constantly 'out of stock' that year, and when I could get them, each one would roll up off my skin at one corner.

I also take a daily progesterone tablet to make my hormone medication as safe as possible because I still have a uterus. (See Chapter 2, It's Your Hormones, for why.) And I take another pill prescribed by a dermatologist that combines a hormone and a hair loss medication to stop the genetic, galloping receding lady's hairline of my dad's side of the family, accompanied by a front-phouff situation. Turns out, the hair loss marked a bridge-too-far in what I could accept as 'natural'.

I do pelvic floor exercises . . . when I remember.

There's a Mirena intrauterine device (IUD) in my uterus (best place for it), also quietly dispatching progesterone.

Two or three times a week I use a plastic plunger to deliver a small amount of estrogen cream to the top of my vagina. I originally wrote a typo in that sentence and it read, 'I use a plumber to deliver estrogen cream to the top of my vagina', and honestly, that would involve marginally more palaver and expense. (It's tremendously edifying to read 'vag cream $29' on a pharmacy receipt.)

I've been suffering for 16 years with no end in sight. I feel like this is me for the rest of my life. Jo, 54

The estrogen cream is so that I don't have to deal with Mysteriously Irritable Vulva (see Chapter 5, It's Your Body) or the characteristically menopausal vaginal 'good' bacteria imbalance, which can cause a romantically termed 'discharge' (don't you love the words doctors invented? I mean, *discharge* from the vagina, the same word used in the 19th century to describe a rifle going orrf).

It feels embarrassing for me to write about my own experience here, where anyone might read it, even though I'm not ashamed of being menopausal. It's just we're so trained to be ashamed of what's natural, and real, and out of our control. As if it were a weakness, or a confession. The details seem so wrongly intimate, TMI, and it goes hard against my journalism training to even mention my own experience. Despite a grown-up lifetime of writing books for women, I'd not anticipated ever writing the phrase 'top of my vagina', except perhaps as a jaunty morning greeting.

But what is the point of pretending I am one of the lucky few who experienced no troublesome perimenopause symptoms? Or that, like a lot of women, it took me years to recognise that what had been happening to me was perimenopause, and years more to work out how to manage it? To hide that truth doesn't make me better or braver, or more useful to others.

It just made me shooshier. And we should all stop being shooshier. Years after that first GP misstep, after finding new doctors and researching for this book, I find myself a lot more informed, and with symptoms much more manageable in ways that work for me (but may not be in your preferred buffet).

I honestly thought I had early-onset dementia. Stacey, 47

It costs me between $800 and $1500 a year for various hormonal and other medications. And more for haircuts and colour to cover the grey. My moisturiser is a pretty cheap pump-pack, and that's because I know some secrets (see Chapter 7, It's How You Look). I want to acknowledge that many of the suggested medical and even self-help solutions in this book are too expensive for many of us, but I hope the info will afford you shortcuts and hints on how not to waste time or money finding what works for you.

Some of the things I share with you in this book, backed by the kind advice and fact-checking from a host of Australia's globally respected top medical experts in menopause, won't last as good advice forever. There'll be much more research, and long-term data. And that will yield more information and better treatments. The info in this copy of the book will become outdated, so I'll update it every couple of years in new reprints for future readers. Please don't lend, borrow or buy second-hand books with medical information.

Sell, sell, sell

This book is also a warning to resist the hard-sell marketers that are coming for us all. My social media and internet use is now splattered with ads for mechanical chairs to whizz me upstairs, and hideous shoes with zips – partly because I always tell the internet I'm 87 and live somewhere called Bentleigh, which isn't true. 'Bentleigh woman horrified by lip wrinkles!' I am often told. 'Bentleigh woman fixes ugly stomach fat' makes a regular appearance, and my favourite is 'Depressed in Bentleigh?' Well, could you blame me?

And this bombardment happens at a time when we feel as vulnerable as we ever have, faced with inexplicable plummeting self-esteem about our looks, our feelings, our work performance, our love life, and our cracking heels. The other day I got four messages to buy a 'Seniors Love Relief Sock', without quite knowing what that was, I began regularly erasing my search histories.

Two main groups have emerged as the loudest ones in menopause media and marketing: the 'menopause is natural, not a hormone deficiency and there's a scare campaign to make you take medication for its symptoms which are mild' group versus 'menopause symptoms are a berloody nightmare, and you have to take hormone medication forever to stop going mad and weeing on the bus'.

Depending on your philosophy, your severity of symptoms, and access to trustworthy advice, your approach can be at either end of that spectrum or somewhere in between, taking from both ends as needed.

> Any positive aphorisms are rubbish. Menopause is shit. Don't go through it alone!
> **Lenore, 51**

WHY? WHY?? WHHHHYYYYYYYY??? **Kit, 50**

See Chapter 3, It's Your Approach, for all the lowdown on what might fit with your philosophy, and what else might help.

I complain in this book that there hasn't been enough research into perimenopause and menopause, or even hormones themselves that, I kid you not a jot, doctors didn't even *know* existed until less than 100 years ago. But menopause-related research is happening more and more, in gynaecology, psychiatry, neurology, bone health, exercise physiology, the blood systems – carried out by many wonderful leading Australian and global specialists, and scientific researchers, and specialist doctors. I love them.

Women have been told to ignore their perimenopausal symptoms and menopause health risks for centuries. Imagine a man who goes to the doctor and says, 'I've put on 10 kilos while eating the same as I always did; I fly into rages; I think I'm a failure; I can't concentrate, sleep or remember anything at work. I bleed so much without warning it soaks through my clothes; I have heart palpitations; I can't sleep to the point of feeling demented; my penis is itchy all the time and it hurts to have sex. My fingernails are breaking off; I have unexplained fevers; and I want to leave my family and live in a bucket.'

Do you reckon the doctor would say, 'Well, you'll just have to put up with it'?

Please stop thinking you have to go it alone or try to be perfect, even at menopause. With the best available knowledge right now to make your own choices, you can concentrate on just being you, and on making the most of the rest of your life (see Chapter 8, It's Your Future).

And now, on with the shitshow.

Don't google and don't listen to relatives. (My gynaecologist.)

I feel like I don't know what's wrong with me. Or I try and list my symptoms to the doctor and they are repeatedly dismissed. Mandy, 44

I felt a little out of control because of mood swings, fear of heavy periods leaking in public, and the sweats were awful. However, conversely, I felt quite a strong sense of sisterhood with like-aged and older women. Merilyn, 56

I feel like I've been hit by a truck. That I'm not the person I thought I was. My brain is so fogged at times I can't even make a sandwich. I'm now anxious all the time. Fiona, 50

My mother told me that menopause was no bother to her. But she also told me that childbirth doesn't hurt, so I'm a bit suspicious. Jen, 52

I felt 'me' disappearing. I felt invisible, useless, unattractive and became a fumbling flutter-head. I wanted to be 'me' again. Angie P, 57

I feel more alive, mostly. So I've had a lot of anger, but also a lot of joy. Rachel, 50

My mother and both my sisters sailed through with zero symptoms. I assumed I would too! I was so very wrong. Catherine, 60

If men suffered this, there'd be menopause clinics on every corner. Jane, 58

It affects you in ways that you won't even put down to menopause until that little missing piece of information lands in your lap. Bridget, 53

Advocate for your own health. If it doesn't feel right, then get a second opinion. Kanga, 49

It makes women go crazy, wee and sweat. Nat, 46

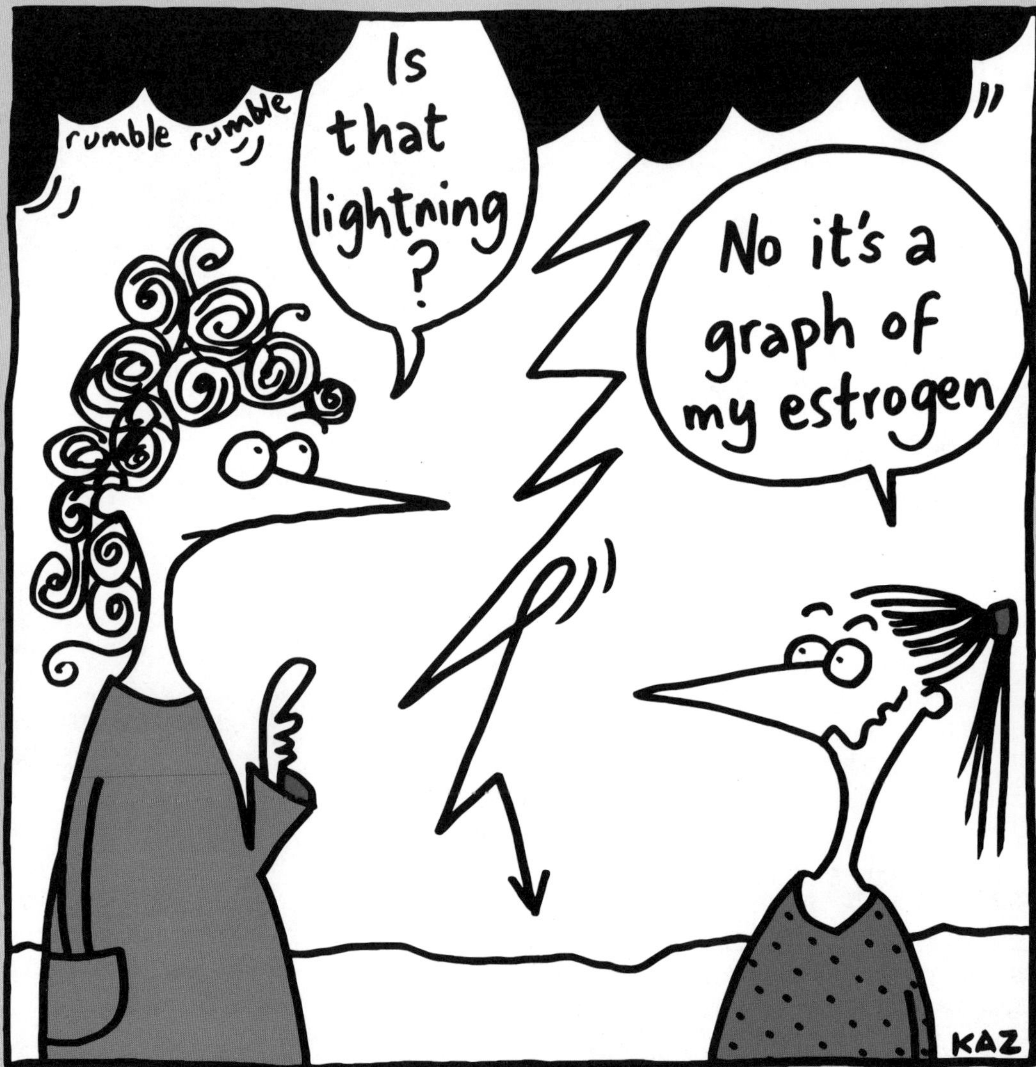
rumble rumble
Is that lightning?
No it's a graph of my estrogen
KAZ

1

What Even Is The Menopause?

Menopause is when you'll go totally mad, and fall into a pit of despair and bite people in the street and quit your job, isn't it? And it's when you can't sleep and start looking like a real witch from a fairytale. No, wait, it's an almost hallucinogenic explosion of life-changing freedom, right?

Or menopause means it's compulsory to take at least six magic supplements plus hormone medication and do an hour and a half of elite-level exercise every day or your bones will turn to icing sugar. And it's when your vagina turns into a dried apricot, you sweat like a football oval sprinkler and you'd rather floss than have sex.

Except it isn't.

Everyone's experience is different, and causes varied symptoms that can range from unnoticeable to unbearable, even though the reason for menopause is the same. In simple terms, your ovaries will stop producing the stable levels of hormones that in the past probably ran your monthly-ish cycle in order to ovulate, have periods, and perhaps be able to get pregnant.

When the ovaries stop making enough of the hormones to keep doing this (mostly estrogen and progesterone, but others too), your hormone levels start to drop. This rarely happens suddenly and forever; more often it staggers on erratically over months or years as your brain and ovaries do their best to valiantly carry on, causing zig-zag levels of hormone production.

This gradual fall, or wild ride of upsy-downsy hormone levels, sometimes changes over hours, days, weeks, months and years, and is experienced differently by each individual woman.

Some women hardly even notice the eventual or sudden transition to settled, lower hormone levels; others will have a mix of no periods, light periods and full-on heavy periods and other symptoms all without warning.

There's a list of more than 30 other possible symptoms coming up on pages 36–37, and they affect every part of you, from hot flushes to jaunty chin hair, from sneezy weeing to fizzy-feeling bosoms, from all-over itchiness to sudden rage; affecting your mind, your skin, your sleep patterns and your heart.

You won't necessarily get all the symptoms, or get them at the same time, or experience the most severe effects: it's more like an unlucky dip.

An increasingly popular explanation is that menopause is 'puberty in reverse'. Yeah but nah. Unless your bosoms disappear, all your bones halve in length, your pubic hair vanishes and you start sitting in the back of the car whingeing, 'Are we there yet?'

Menopause often coincides with the onset of autoimmune disorders or other conditions: similar symptoms can be experienced with a thyroid problem or coeliac disease and bleeding changes can have other dangerous causes, so a good GP is important when sorting out a possible diagnosis. Nobody should be told they can't be in perimenopause because they're 'too young': investigation and consideration of symptoms is crucial. See Chapter 3, It's Your Approach, for more on getting the most out of your doctor(s).

[I feel] acceptance rather than fighting it, gratitude that I will never have another period. Brunhilda, 53

I just thought life was making me more anxious, and the flooding and other annoying symptoms were a drag but unrelated to my anxiety. Amanda, 52

Some rough stats: of more than 7400 women who responded to the question about their experience of menopause symptoms in the Survey for this book, nearly 40 per cent said it went on for a long, annoying time, and nearly 20 per cent said it was a long, terrible time. One in five said it was annoying but brief, a few said it was truly awful but brief. Almost 45 per cent said it was unpredictable, about 7 per cent said it was a relief and just over 5 per cent said it was positive or enjoyable.

About a third said they didn't realise that the symptoms they experienced were related to hormones.

There was such a huge range in when people noticed the symptoms, and whether they were recognised as hormone-related. A lot of women said mental and physical changes came on at about the same time; others nominated mental first or physical first, and the gap between was put at anything from 6 months to more than 5 years.

About 46 per cent of Survey respondents said they were technically in menopause (hadn't had a period for more than a year) and just over 40 per cent said they were in perimenopause with symptoms. Almost 7 per cent said they had experienced some form of early menopause due to surgery or medication side effects, but only 1 per cent said they'd been diagnosed with some form of early menopause.

More than a third of women said they hadn't had a period for more than a year but still had recognisable perimenopause symptoms. About 5 per cent said they were in menopause and didn't get any symptoms.

The medical definition of menopause

Being in a same-sex relationship, I can share more with my partner on the topic, as she has already been through it. Helen, 52

You're officially given a medical diagnosis of being in menopause if it's been more than a year since your last ever period. The official time of your menopause has to be backdated to that last period and a doctor might note FMP (Final Menstrual Period) on your file.

Of course there are lots of reasons why periods can stop, including pregnancy and breastfeeding, intense stress or exercise and not eating enough healthy food, and a bunch of hormone-altering medical conditions. Doctors call not getting any periods amenorrhoea (pronounced ay-men-oh-rear).

I just hope I get out of this on the other side and maybe have a laugh at how crazy it was. I honestly wouldn't wish this on my worst enemy. **Candice, 47**

If you're older than 45, and you're experiencing classic menopausal symptoms you or your doctor recognise, you can probably assume you're in perimenopause, the time leading up to and around the official medical time of menopause. If you're under 45 it's still well worth investigating or thinking about.

Some women hit menopause suddenly because of side effects of surgery, or cancer treatment, and their hormone levels plummet suddenly as a result. Some have an 'early menopause' when their ovaries stop doing their thing before they turn 45, or the medically termed 'premature menopause' if it's before 40. (See the section 'Early menopause', coming up.)

I had a child at 43, so going through menopause as a single parent with a 9-year-old in my care at home has its challenges. My adult son is a big help. **Jordana, 52**

There are a bunch of people walking around with radically different ideas of what the menopause is. If you ask a woman in her 40s or 50s, she's more likely to say it's the annoying symptoms of perimenopause, not the anniversary of her last period or the rest of her life after that. For something that happens to all women who live long enough to experience it, what we know and think about it is a total schemozzle.

It becomes even more confusing when we're told we're post-menopausal, which feels like it means we're beyond and past the thing called menopause, when in fact we're *in* the state of menopause – 'menopausal', according to doctors – and will be for the rest of our lives. Another complication is that, for many people, their perimenopausal symptoms may continue for several years, all through the time that's described as perimenopausal, and then years beyond the technical point of menopause.

At 40 I was experiencing what I thought were perimenopause symptoms. Went to my GP, who did a blood test, and it came back that I was type 2 diabetic instead. **Ngaire, 44**

Eighteen months after my last period (i.e. just over a year ago) I had what looked and felt like a period. I had a few tests and some exploratory surgery, and it turned out I had a rare type of ovarian cancer. **Lynda**

It's all part of our life journey: some of us get a raw deal and others get a free ride – most of us are somewhere in between! **Christina, 52**

Different experiences of perimenopause & menopause

We all react differently to different levels and combination levels of hormones. Hormone levels can jump up and down during the perimenopause in strange ways: not like a graph heading down in a straight line on an angle, or even like a zig-zag. It can look like a relief map of the Andes or a vortex of scribble.

Say five women are sitting on the same bus one morning. And let's say, in a wild coincidence at this moment, each of them has exactly the same percentage level of hormones in her body: of estrogen, progesterone, testosterone, and brain chemicals.

Of the five:

Aisha is 43, and is having a fierce hot flush. Michelle, 47, is plagued by a weird feeling of low self-esteem and concentration problems that have affected her work, and has just come back from the GP, who prescribed her antidepressants. At 52, Tarni's just started a weirdly heavy period even though she had a light one two weeks ago. Kim, 51, is suffering with every perimenopausal symptom known to womankind and wants to lie down on the floor. She's worried she's heading for a heart attack because of an erratic heartbeat that seems to strike most nights while she's watching TV: or is that only because that's when she's sitting still and notices it?

Penny, 56, sitting perkily in the front seat, stopped having periods recently but hasn't noticed, and she'll never have another one. (At the next stop, all the other women are going to throw Penny out of the window.)

If they all get on another bus in the afternoon to go home, everyone's hormone levels will have

I started to feel anxious and unlovable, depressed, and didn't realise it had anything to do with menopause. How would I know? No one talks about it. Ros, 55

Shitty, bored attitudes by doctors did not help. I felt as if they thought I was being a whinger, as I had so many issues and nothing seemed to work. Leanne, 59

A sense of freedom, a loss of vanity, much appreciation for survival so far and the survival of friends – a weird kind of acceptance. Madame, 71

Can't believe my periods stopped when I was 48. No menopausal issues or anything. Jane, 57

A friend's mother advised how she never complained or spoke about her symptoms with others. At the time I thought this was sage advice, however now I feel you need to chat to fellow menopausers. Nicole, 53

changed – and a bunch of symptoms will be jumbled up and distributed between them. Each woman experiences varying symptoms herself – depending on her hormone levels compared to yesterday, next week, or at half past four. Like periods, menopause can be no big deal, or a nightmare.

What happens to ovaries & eggs in perimenopause

Most of us have a 20–30 year period of ovulating about every month – we release an egg from our ovaries. And every time we do that, progesterone production increases from our ovaries. We're all born with one to two million eggs in our baby ovaries, most of which are reabsorbed over our lifetime. Depending on whether we get pregnant, breastfeed, or take continuous hormone contraceptives or medication, we may have up to about 400 menstrual cycles during which we release an egg.

But you'll be developing less (okay, fewer) eggs in perimenopause as your estrogen levels fall and jitter about.

As your estrogen and progesterone levels eventually become erratic or generally fall, your ovaries will try to respond to your brain's messages telling them it's time to make another egg and dispatch it down a fallopian tube to the uterus to await possible fertilisation by a sperm. In a heroic effort, an ovary might pop out two eggs in a month, none for 2 months then one more, and stagger on like that for a few months or even years.

What happens to ovaries & eggs in menopause

Eventually, we simply run out of useful eggs to be released. Your ovaries shrink in size, and any leftover eggs reabsorb into your body.

Perimenopause

Perimenopausal symptoms can start in your early to mid-40s and cause symptoms you don't recognise as hormone-related, including brain fog, headaches, tender-feeling breasts and period changes (see the big list on pages 36–37).

Doctors now understand that a lot of us have mental health symptoms caused by estrogen drop, perhaps up to 5 years before we have something as obvious as a physical symptom of menopause, such as a hot flush. So perimenopause can start ten or so

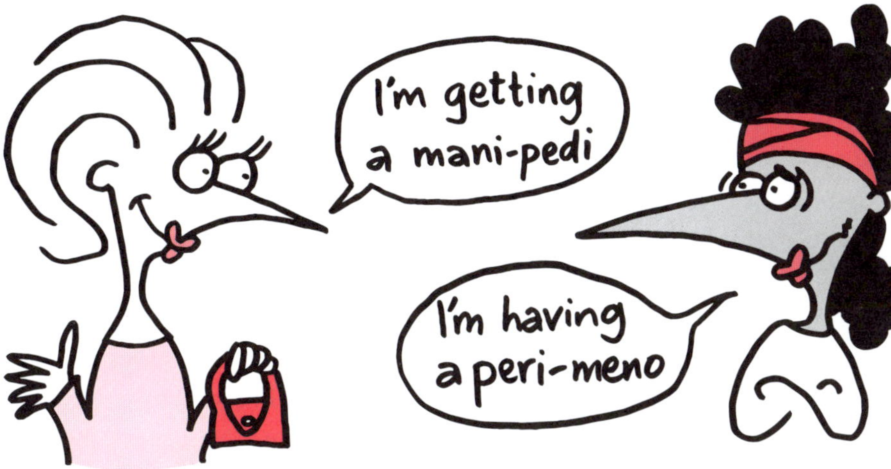

years before menopause, and the annoying symptoms associated with perimenopause and menopause can last just as long, or longer afterwards. (See Chapter 2, It's Your Hormones, for why.)

Menarche (which rhymes with malarkey) is the medical term for your first period when you're a girl, and menopause is the word for having had your last period at least a year ago.

The time around the official medical menopause is officially diagnosed by changes in your period cycle (changed length between periods, some too heavy, and eventually getting lighter). But doctors will very often factor in your experience of other known perimenopausal symptoms. Although many people believe it means 'leading up to' the menopause, it also means afterwards. 'Peri' means 'around' in ancient Greek; it has nowt to do with piri piri or peri-peri chicken recipes based on African-Portuguese words for chillies and peppers, or the heat of hot flushes.

Perimenopause started for me at 43. The symptoms were so bad over the last 4 years that I've given up work. **Elizabeth, 48**

I did heaps of research when I was pregnant but have done almost none about menopause. **Ruth, 58**

Every doctor gives slightly different advice. Friends have provided more info, once I bring it up, but no one really discusses it, like it's shameful. **Jenny, 45**

I hit puberty very early so expected to hit menopause early too but didn't. **Sarah, 49**

Menopause

As we've already heard, official menopause is backdated – you're medically menopausal if you're over 45 and haven't had a period for at least a year, if pregnancy and other possible reasons are ruled out.

Once you've reached this official technical diagnosis of menopause you might be told you're 'in menopause', 'menopausal', 'hitting menopause' or 'post-menopause', whether or not you still have symptoms, including hot flushes. In the Survey for this book, hundreds of women said that during perimenopause they had gaps of up to 11 months and up to 2 years or more between periods, so had to keep resetting the possible date of official menopause. Any bleeding after a long period of none must be investigated by a doctor, in case it's a symptoms of something else, BTW.

I thought it only happened to old women! I was wrong. I was 33! Heather, 64

The reason doctors backdate their definition of menopause to an arbitrary one year of no periods is because not many women have their regular periods for decades then suddenly stop. Most of us don't have periods that peter out gradually in a sedate fashion: in other words, it's a recognition of a normal, common, long period of perimenopause.

But for most of us, the date of official menopause is pretty irrelevant. What matters is what symptoms we have, whether they're making us miserable, and what we can do about them.

As well as the usual noticeable perimenopause symptoms, there are also associated ongoing risk factors in menopause, such as more brittle bones, heart disease and stroke. Risks and benefits of medication for these symptoms vary according to the type of medication and your individual circumstances.

My mum, she was real old school, just said, 'It's when you are no longer a woman.' Please! What a crock of shit that was. Ruth, 58

Early menopause

You can have an official diagnosis of premature menopause before the age of 40, caused by medication, surgery, or what doctors call Premature Ovarian Insufficiency (POI). Others experience menopause at the earlier end of the normal scale. It's hard to hear people deny the possibility or reality: 'You're too young.'

Many women under 40 don't want their situation called menopause. The experience of a POI diagnosis or surgical inevitability and its implications for health and fertility can be really confronting and difficult. But there's lots of help and medication available for symptoms and risk factors (there's a whole section on early menopause coming up in this chapter).

Menopausal

Menopausal is a word doctors often use to mean the rest of your life after the anniversary date of your last ever period. But many of us say, 'I'm menopausal' to explain that we're experiencing menopausal symptoms. Menopausal symptoms can refer to all the symptoms associated with perimenopause, as well as the symptoms of ongoing menopause.

> Twelve months without a period and the symptoms are huge in range and intensity, and women who don't suffer them should be burned at the stake – just kidding. Kinda.
> Sally, 49

Post-menopausal

Many people use the word post-menopause, or 'been through the menopause', to mean their known menopausal symptoms have stopped, because their hormones are no longer erratic and have settled down to consistently low levels. Many doctors call this menopausal.

> The best thing about menopause is you forgive yourself faster and more often. You give yourself more permission to be yourself in all situations. 'Martian', 56

> Post-menopause is the best! I feel great, able, self-assured and more confident than ever! Highly recommend!
> Kaye, 62

The average age of perimenopause

About 47 is said to be the average age women notice or report typical known perimenopause symptoms such as hot flushes and insomnia. In fact, the average age of perimenopause might be more like 44 or 45, if we count in mental symptoms like estrogen-related blues and brain fog that can happen years before any period carry-on. For some women, with certain cultural or racial heritage, it can be earlier, although shamefully – you'll be hearing this a lot in this book – there isn't enough solid research on this.

The average age of menopause

Fifty-one is the average age of official menopause, a year after your final ever period. Most of us will get there earlier, or later, so a better way to express the average age is 47 to 53.

When will you become menopausal?

Menopause before the age of 40 is known to run in some families. But doctors say the timing of expected menopause has nothing to do with when it happened to your grandmothers or mother. Certainly, heaps of women in the Survey said they expected their mother's experience and got the opposite, in terms of timing as well as severe or mild symptoms.

> My mother and sister went through it a bit early (47?) and are actually hostile that at 51 I'm still not done and don't have hot flushes. Lainie, 51

There's no recognised general difference in time of onset between women who had children, and women who didn't, and women with different diets or exercise programs. There's no research that suggests it's triggered by previous medical conditions, stress or attitude.

> My mum was in disbelief, as she went through menopause at 60 and I'm so much younger. Vikki, 49

Some people who started their first period at the earlier end of the normal range also start perimenopause earlier, but lots don't. As far as we know, it's individual and random. The time that menopause starts has nothing to do with how long you'll live.

The average time span of symptoms

There's no way to predict how long your symptoms will last. Mothers and daughters differ; sisters differ; everyone differs. An often-quoted average for perimenopause symptoms is 7 years. Another is 4 or 5 years. One study led to the statement that some women experience it for up to 12 years; a gynaecologist told me that's only because the study survey offered 11 years as a top range.

Menopausal symptoms will stop eventually, as hormone levels settle at levels too low to generate fluctuating symptoms. There are outliers: a woman in this book's Survey reported that her mum had hot flushes from perimenopause until she was 89.

Research is jumbled on this, and most of it's on white women in richer countries. Japanese women growing up in Japan eating a traditional soy-rich diet may tend to have less severe symptoms at the shorter end of the time-span range, and Black women in the US are known to have it tougher for longer.

I wish there were a visible clock so I could see where I'm at on the journey. Jennifer, 47

The ongoing history of substandard medical care and outcomes for Aboriginal and Torres Strait Islander women, and the lack of useful research on their health experiences, is a deplorable combination. Aboriginal women know they're at higher statistical risk of heart problems and diabetes, so menopause symptoms can be more frightening or sinister for them unless they get a proper diagnosis and care.

When will the symptoms be over? I've been going 8 years now? Joan, 60

The average age of first period and menopause is older in the modern era and well-fed countries. Australian women of African and South Asian heritage, with smaller body frames, may tend to have an earlier average age of menopause but we don't have the reliable research.

Fifteen years and symptoms still going. Jo, 47

Obviously, a woman who has non-annoying symptoms for 10 years will have a better time of menopause than someone who's staggering under a burden of ghastly insomnia and fierce unpredictable hot flushes for 'only' 2 years.

According to one reliable Australian study, at least 42 per cent of women still have menopausal symptoms when they're aged between 60 and 65. Some symptoms and changes, like drier skin and vagina, and declining bone strength will be indefinite: but can be treated and improved, or managed with medication.

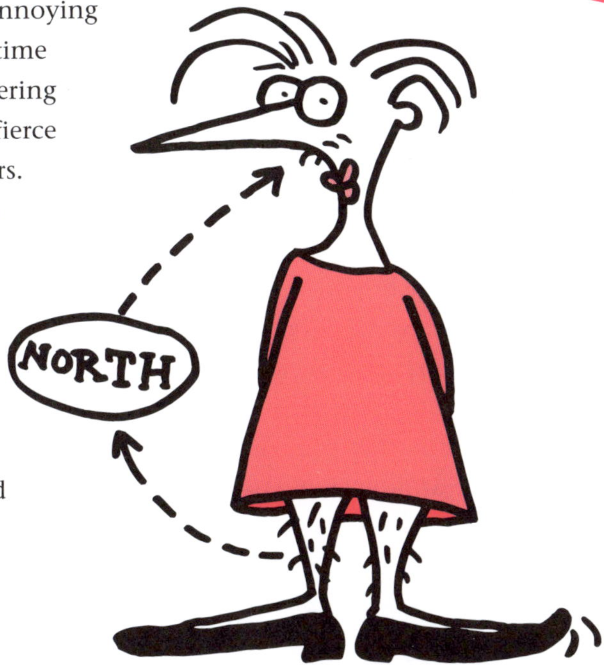

Migratory pattern of menopausal body hair.

Some women taking Menopause Hormone Therapy (MHT, formerly known as HRT) will want to stop when perimenopause symptoms are no longer a problem; others choose to stay on it indefinitely to help with ongoing effects of lower estrogen, including bone loss and pelvic floor changes. (See Chapter 2, It's Your Hormones, for all the palaver you need to know about MHT.)

Not a day goes by that I don't thank the universe for what I have. I think it makes me able to cope with the rotten symptoms of menopause, by looking at the bigger picture. I try to find something positive every day. Wanda, 50

Technically menopause is never over, because you're in it for the rest of your life.

Can you avoid the menopause?

No. You can impose more hormone balance and higher levels of relevant hormones, and avoid some perimenopausal symptoms, but you'll still eventually, technically be in menopause, even if you stay on medication forever.

The combined Pill has much higher hormone levels than MHT. It takes over from your body's hormone production, and imposes a fixed level of estrogen and progesterone. It will stop you bleeding each month if you take it every day, continuously. When you stop taking it, you'll have a 'bleed' that's experienced as a period, until you start taking it again.

Traditionally, the Pill is more likely to be prescribed for women experiencing menopause symptoms before the age of 45; newer combinations include a Mirena IUD (which emits a progestogen – much more on progestogens coming up, brace yourself) and an estrogen patch or gel, or a form of MHT: again, see Chapter 2 for all the guff on hormones and medication.

MHT has levels of estrogen and a progestogen close to the levels your body used to make, whereas the Pill contains higher doses to make sure contraception is covered. MHT tops up whatever residual hormone production your body is still making. If you stay on MHT indefinitely, you may not have to go through many perimenopausal symptoms, but you will eventually be in menopause a year after your ovaries stop making enough estrogen to run your periods cycle.

I had a Mirena in till this year so didn't have periods. When it came out I still didn't get periods, so I must be post-menopausal. Erin, 55

I thought HRT was only for hot flushes. Still don't know what else it's used for. Heather, 57

Menopause stigma & silence

Heaps of online and media stories say in their first paragraph that menopause is a subject nobody talks about – and then they go on to talk about it for 1500 words. And yet many women still stay silent about menopause because of cultural tradition, or it was a forbidden subject in their family, or they don't even think their feelings and physical symptoms are related to it, or they feel shame about being older, or afraid of being labelled as old or cranky at home or at work.

So while some of us are banging on about it all the time, even arguing all over social media about the best approach, some women and non-binary folk don't talk about it with their doctor, or friends.

In the 19th century, various tonics and pills and herbal palaver for the mortifying menopause were sold using code-words such as 'women's ailments', 'nervous complaints', and 'stoppages' (pregnancy or menopause). In lots of ways they were very similar to most of the supplements and even the same homeopathic and 'essence' liquids today, which could only work as a placebo. At least these days you're far less likely to find lead or mercury in your potion, as long as you stick to reputable pharmaceutical-grade products. (See Chapter 3, It's Your Approach, for more on the use and dangers of some products.)

My symptoms have affected my relationship with my husband; I'm now on HRT and I feel I'm improving. I've had him come to counselling, but he still doesn't get what's going on for me. I'm afraid we'll separate and I'll be far worse off in my later years. **BP, 46**

Talking to others helps to break down the stigma. **Edie, 44**

I was even abused on Facebook for writing about my experience with perimenopause on my own feed. **Rosemary, 48**

I dislike the way menopause is spoken of, as though it's a disease that has to be fixed. I don't want to fight it, I just want to understand it. **Polly, 66**

I took the risk and emailed 12 friends around the same age, told them what was happening to me and asked if they were going through anything similar and wanted to talk about it. Ten of them said, 'YES PLEASE!!!!' **Lenore, 51**

Am I letting the side down even mentioning it? I'm sure everyone is going through it, but why am I the only one who feels comfortable talking about it? **MW, 50**

What was menopause called in the past?

It was first called La Ménopause by a French dude in the 1820s who at least didn't name it after himself, as his first name was Charles-Pierre-Louis. He combined a French word related to the monthly cycle of the moon, to indicate a monthly event and pause, meaning stopped (periods, in this case). (Reputable, large studies have shown that women don't synch their periods to the moon, or to each other.)

Menopause was variously thought to be a kind of madness or illness brought on by alcohol, soft beds, spicy foods, gambling, lewd books, nudey paintings and racy conversations, says author Alison Downham Moore in her eyebrow-hoisting book *The French Invention of Menopause and the Medicalisation of Women's Ageing: A History*. Such pronouncements about nympho-meno women were made by the same doltish medical men who said sex after menopause caused cancer, corsets caused vaginal infections and stopped periods could be cured by hot pokers or leeches on the cervix. (Permission to shriek.)

Johnson's dictionary of 1755 doesn't seem to list any of the possible words of the time for menopause, but he did find room for crone, which probably meant a 36-year-old. Older texts, whether Greek, Roman, biblical or medieval, pretty much ignored menopause because they were almost exclusively written by men who really couldn't have been less interested, and besides, many women didn't live long enough to experience menopause and most didn't have the ability to write anything down.

Up until only 100 years or so ago, the unlearned brethren of male doctors didn't even know what a hormone was, and told us that periods made us weak, unable to learn or read, able to poison trees by walking past them and make penises corrode away on contact. You'd think, then, that menopause would make those doctors think we'd come good. Oh ho, no. Instead, menopause was pretty much ignored, said to be another sort of toxicity, or otherwise dismissed in sexist terms.

A grab bag of phrases that have been used for menopause includes Hysteria (that old thing), cessation of catamenia, the End of Women's Hell, Aged Greensickness, the Turn of Age,

I do remember my mother going to her GP to tell him she was 'nervy'. He told her she needed a psychiatrist! She was about 56. Jan, 63

It's not that long ago that women were committed for 'senile' behaviour we now know was due to menopause symptoms! I'm grateful every day for HRT. Kerri, 58

your all-purpose Women's Trouble, a derangement of the uterus, the Great Climacteric (meaning climax, not climate), the Critical Age, failed menstrous eruptions, That Time of Life, a Nervous Breakdown, The Change, and an illness called the Dodge, or Dodging.

Recognised symptoms were irregular or stopped periods, headaches, 'pursiness at stomack', fevers and 'flushings' (hot flushes) and 'rebellious distempers' i.e. being a crankypants. A man I once worked with referred to this book when it was commissioned as 'The Old Chooks Book'. Consequently there arose within me a bloody rebellious distemper, I can tell you.

Positive words for the menopause

None of the suggested modern terms for the menopause seem to have caught on at all, from The Go Time, The Leap Forward, Becoming a Queenager, The Ripening and The Bloom, to Thank Christ That's Over, The M Word, and The Partypause. No less an endocrinology expert than hard-sell celebrity supplements-spruiker Gwyneth Paltrow on her shop website has called for a rebranding of menopause, so perhaps we could go with The Marketing Opportunity. And I do like the way The Dodge makes it sound like a cool dance craze.

What should *we* call it?

Most people now just call it the menopause, so that's what this book does.

Is the menopause natural?

Yes. Menopause, like age-related failing eyesight and hearing, is normal and natural but that doesn't always make it something you have to accept the difficulties of, if they're awful or get in the way of your life.

Is menopause a hormone deficiency?

Some doctors say it is, and that's why the original name for hormone medication for menopause symptoms was called Hormone *Replacement* Therapy (now known as Menopause Hormonal Therapy, or MHT). Other doctors object strongly to the idea that a natural state everyone will go through could be called a deficiency, or that hormone medication is necessary for everyone – they also insist on the word therapy instead of medication, which they believe wrongly suggests an illness.

> I thought it was something that happened to old women. **Jude, 48**

How to tell if you're perimenopausal or menopausal

Hormone tests aren't usually helpful if you're in the average age range of being perimenopausal. They can be a waste of money: see Chapter 2, It's Your Hormones, to find out why.

Working out that you're perimenopausal is usually just a matter of realising that's the most likely reason for suspicious symptoms you're having. (See the list on pages 36–37.) If you're younger than 40 and have menopause symptoms, you could have Premature Ovarian Insufficiency: see the 'Early menopause' section coming up in this chapter. Hormone tests are more useful for diagnosing that.

If you need confirmation, a pelvic ultrasound may also show that your ovaries have gracefully retired and there are no more eggs trying to dress themselves up for a last fandango down the fallopians.

Is menopause terrible or no big deal?

Menopause is presented variously as a looming disaster, a mental maelstrom of triggered traumas, a desperate need for sleep, an endurance trial of endless intense hot flushes and the end of a decent sex life, so you must take all sorts of medication and not bother with lifestyle changes. OR, it's said to be a calm, gradual transition that heralds a beautiful confidence and freedom from periods and obligations, protected by natural supplements and a positive attitude because medication is always bad.

Neither of those extremes will happen to most of us, and neither of those approaches will work for everyone.

It's not helpful to feel forced to choose either extreme end of attitudes to menopause, which represent polarised positions in what seems like an increasingly polarised world. Most of us are in the middle for good reason.

You can't predict your menopause experience, although many people who had an awful time with hormones and their periods (e.g. premenstrual dysphoric disorder) report they've also had tough menopause symptoms. Menopause symptoms are harder to deal with if you have extra financial, health or other stressful problems.

Whatever happens to you as you approach and go into menopause, you won't get every symptom, and you won't be alone. You're still in charge of your health, and equipped with options to choose from. You can also choose different approaches at different times.

Thinking about menopause can feel like it's part of the slide towards your elderly self and a giddy whirl of orthotics, night-time bite-guards and having to moisturise your extremities with a spatula. But being in your 40s or 50s isn't old. Your best ally in this will be your own positive attitude, finding a good treatment team if you need one and an ability to ignore the traditional view that older women should settle for looking respectable and being ignored. (See Chapter 3, It's Your Approach, for a list of Who's Who on your treatment team, explaining the qualifications of doctors and therapists.)

The random apportionment of when menopause happens and whether you have a meh time or a bad time has nothing to do with how much yoga you do, or your medical–natural philosophy, but can be associated with some genetic, cultural and racial differences. Medication *and* self-help strategies can contribute to an easier time.

The idea of being able to redefine myself as I move into this new stage of life is actually quite exciting, although it's traumatic at times. It makes sense, though, that a massive identity shift would happen at this time. **Annie, 49**

Seriously? A natural part of life and to most of us a feeling of freedom. **Felicity, 70**

It's a beautiful rite of passage. We need to celebrate the new women we are becoming and mourn the loss of our old selves. We absolutely shouldn't have to hide this away with shame or guilt. **Jessica, 41**

I no longer have any fucks to give. I love being 50. My rage is righteous and my laughter is raucous. **Janne, 50**

This time of my life was a train wreck of hideousness. I am stunned I survived. **Kit, 50**

I am living it and I have a great doctor, so I am lucky and feel informed. **Clare, 54**

Cultural menopause attitudes

In some cultures, especially Indigenous cultures, older women are more likely to be respected and revered, seen as sources of wisdom both cultural and practical, teachers and sages, so becoming menopausal is the opposite of a stigma.

Elsewhere it's been traditionally seen more as a decline into unattractiveness to men and therefore relevance and status, and the symptoms a barrier to respect at home and at work.

It's making me more of a senior person, you know . . . more respect from the younger people. (A 55-year-old Aboriginal lady quoted in *Exploring Australian Aboriginal Women's Experiences of Menopause: a descriptive study*, University of WA, 2014.)

Catholic background – fearful and secret subject.
Sue, 54

Brought up in an Italian household. Anything about the body wasn't spoken about.
Angie, 47

We are Italian – we spoke about EVERYTHING related to women. I miss my mum and my aunties terribly.
Maria, 54

WTF? How can I be 49 and not know this stuff?
Zoe, 49

I am from an Anglo background where I feel the overwhelming emphasis is on looking and staying young.
Robyn, 52

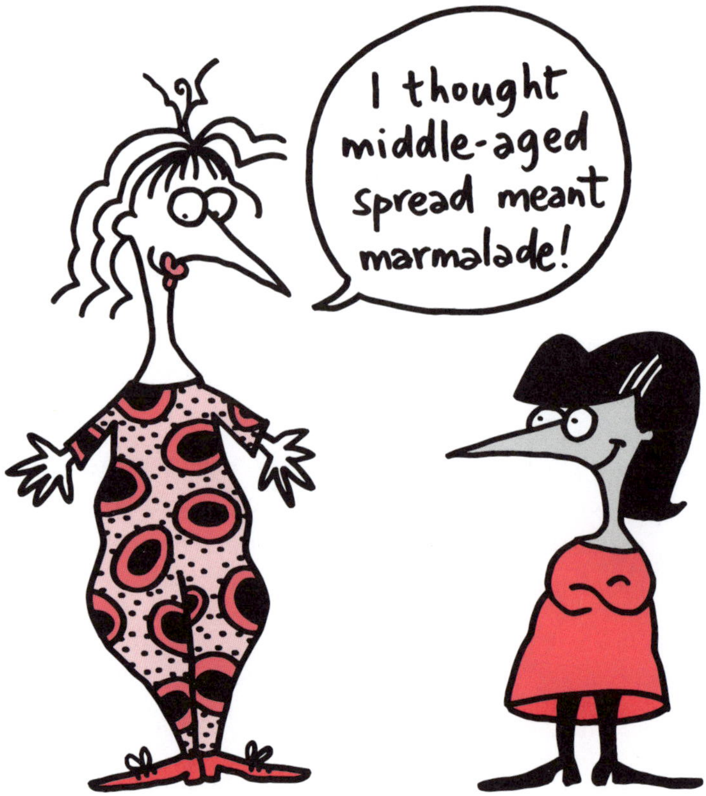

Some cultures don't have a word that bundles menopause symptoms together, just words for individual ones. Menopause is well known as a phenomenon globally, but means different things according to cultural ideas of responsibilities and roles in an extended family and community.

We need to be careful of assumptions that women in some cultures don't experience menopause symptoms. Women have rarely been asked at all, or asked in culturally appropriate and safe ways, to talk about their medical experiences. Many women have good reason not to trust a medical system and society built on racism, still perpetuating stupid ideas such as it's easier for Indigenous women to give birth, or that Black women don't feel pain in the same way as white women.

We don't know enough about menopause

More has been discovered in the last 20 years about menopause than was known about it in the 500 years before that. As I rudely scoffed in my book *You're Doing It Wrong: A History of Bad & Bonkers Advice to Women*, we used to be told periods stopped because our uteruses wandered off around our body, and I think you'll find menopause can be caused by the glance of a witch.

Until the very recent past, most doctors in training were given virtually no instruction on the range of menopausal symptoms or how to talk to or help menopausal women. There are many GPs working today who had less than an hour of training and lecturing about menopause at medical school, if they turned up for it. If doctors haven't kept up with new knowledge, their patients are at a disadvantage.

It wasn't until the 1920s and 1930s that the medical and scientific profession discovered what hormones even are, and began to work out how to make pharmaceutical and compounded recipes for hormone products. The first medical societies and conferences about menopause didn't happen until the 1970s. That's why they don't have Royal in their name, unlike the earlier-established British and Australian colonial-hangover medical colleges and medical membership organisations.

There's some good research now being done by extremely smart, informed people who've made this area of medicine their life's work, and that will influence future understanding and medical treatments . . . but we'll also no doubt have to put up with online tabloid reporting of a study funded by a miracle menopause bra company that asked 117 women in Nova Scotia if taking progesterone made them want to wear a bustière with propellers on. (Well, who doesn't?)

Why do we go through menopause?

Because most of us now live longer than the cyclical function of our ovaries. Various anthropological theories have been suggested, including: it's so grandmothers can help look after children, because that's the way whale pods operate, or it's to control the population so more babies survive and more children get fed. Other mammals have evolved without a menopause; elephants and cats, for example. Maybe humans are just surviving longer than we used to and some societies value women more than they used to.

So often our female elders are described in the media as grandmothers. It's as if society has no other way to picture older women. Kay, 65

Fair play to those doing research on anthropological theories. But not all women want to have children, or do have them, and not all grandmothers want to look after their grandchildren. None of us are whales. We don't have to have to justify staying alive after our years of possible baby-making by being useful to men, society, or anyone.

Telling a partner about menopause

Show your partner the list of possible symptoms over the page: especially if they're a man, they may have rarely thought about menopause, or known about women's brains and bodies being different except for the idea that most women can get pregnant and bad jokes about women being annoyed when they have their periods.

You can explain that your body is shutting down most hormone production over time and this can cause erratic, mild or severe symptoms. If it helps, tell any male partner that your body is like an old Renault: it's unpredictable and hard to get the parts.

> Doctors only asked about night sweats, hot flushes and bad moods. Nobody mentioned anxiety.
> Jo, 56

> I thought people who complained about menopause were sooks till I started it myself.
> Marlene, 72

> I work in a male-dominated workplace; the men now come to me with their crazy wife stories asking, 'Is she going through menopause?' It is actually good to hear it from their side too. Fiona, 44

Trans & non-binary experiences of menopause

This book welcomes all LGBTQIA+ readers including non-binary folk and trans people.

Most trans and non-binary folk are already taking gender-affirming medication, so when they reach a menopausal-ish age, they just truck on through, and don't have a classic menopause. If they don't take hormone therapy, most trans and non-binary folk who were assigned female at birth will experience menopause. Trans men who don't take hormone therapy or who transition after menopause will experience it, too.

Some trans and non-binary people assigned female at birth take testosterone for its masculinising effects such as a deeper voice, increase in facial and body hair and body-shape changes.

Non-binary folk and trans women assigned male at birth may be taking continuous estrogen and medication to block testosterone. Whether trans women should take progesterone is controversial. Like some cis women, they don't have a uterus, so don't need progestogens for the protective effects. Some people believe progesterone can boost breast growth; others don't. Research continues. If estrogen therapy is stopped or levels fluctuate, some trans and non-binary folk can have peri-menopause type symptoms.

Most trans and non-binary people, like an increasing number of cis women, are likely to stay on hormone medication for the rest of their lives to maintain levels consistent with good physical and mental results. Testosterone does a magic trick and converts some of itself into an estrogen hormone in the body, so a trans man on full doses of testosterone therapy will have relatively high levels of testosterone and estrogen compared to a cis woman who isn't taking hormone medication. This can help protect a trans chap's bones as he ages.

There's very little research about older trans people, but some suggests that they may have a higher risk of heart attack; and trans women may have a higher risk of stroke and blood clots, too. The best advice for a trans person navigating getting older is to find a specialist GP or endocrinologist who's respectful and knowledgeable about hormones and gender-affirming treatment.

The words 'woman' and 'women' are used throughout the book, not always followed by 'and many non-binary folk and perhaps some trans people'. I refer to 'us' to include anyone who might benefit from the info at hand. I want to be as inclusive as possible.

This is as good a place as any to say that millions of women don't have a uterus because it was removed for medical reasons, or wasn't formed when they were born. Having a uterus isn't relevant to whether you're a woman. We're all different, with varying experiences and needs, and we're all in this together.

I find myself knowing more about HRT than all of my cis women friends, and advising them how to break their GP's incorrect assumptions. Most don't know I'm trans. Doctors aren't well versed in HRT because it's only needed for a minority. A minority of 50 per cent!
Ashley, 58

Because I've gone through it earlier than a lot of my friends, I've been able to share my experiences and what helped me. They've told me that has helped them, and they've shared that with others, who are feeling better too.
Karen, 52

Possible symptoms of perimenopause & menopause

Most women will get some of these symptoms in perimenopause and menopause. You won't get all of them all at once. Some might come and go. Some might arrive years before you realise the connection. Some are caused by low estrogen and other hormone changes that can be treated with MHT. Other symptoms don't have a simple one-size-fits-all treatment.

Brain bizzo

'Brain fog'
Concentration & memory lapses
Being irritable
Rage
Anxiety
Depression
Lack of enthusiasm
Self-esteem loss
Feeling tired
Feeling unmotivated

New or resurfacing:

Anxiety/Depression
Obsessive-compulsive disorder (OCD)
Trauma processing
Eating disorders
Addiction behaviours

Period changes

Irregular & unexpected periods
Heavy or flooding periods
Spotty, light periods
Extra cramps
No more periods

Blood-flow & temperature ('Vasomotor symptoms')

Hot flushes
Night sweats

Otherwise blood-vessel related

Headaches
Migraines
Heart rate changes

Weeing issues

Needing to wee more
Sudden urges to wee
Accidental weeing
Sneezy wee
Coughing wee
Jumping wee (I could go on)
Getting more urinary tract infections

Itchiness & dryness

All-over itches
Crawling sensation under the skin
Itches on extremities: feet & hands
Drier eyes, nostrils & mouth
Drier skin all over
Body dandruff
Brittle nails
Cracked heels

Sleep
Trouble falling asleep
Waking up in the night
Insomnia
Fatigue

Bosom oddness
Full/tight/sore feeling
Stabby/fizzy feeling

Vaginal & vulva palaver
Dry-feeling vagina
Painful friction during sex
Vaginal bacteria imbalance
Vaginal infections
Feelings of prolapsed organs into vagina
Smaller vulva & clitoris
Vagina & vulva itch or burning

Libido
More interest in sex
Declining interest in sex
Erratic interest in sex

Bones
Osteoporosis
Unexpected fractures

Connecty bits
Joint pain
Muscle soreness
Tendon weakness

Mouth carry-on
Mouth itch & dryness, gum problems
Strange taste in the mouth

Unlucky dip
More sensitive to smells
Higher cholesterol
Acid reflux
Slower metabolism
New intolerance/allergies
Digestion problems
Fartiness
Constipation

Weight & body image
Extra weight around middle

Skin (aside from dryness)
Loss of collagen and padding in face
Skin sagging
More skin tags
More different-shade patches
More wrinkles
More visible veins

Hair bizzo
Hair loss
Thinning head hair
Front phouff
Fewer leg, underarm, lash & eyebrow hairs
More chin, upper lip, ear & nose hairs

Some symptoms that can happen around the same time are not caused by hormones, including greying head and pubic hair, general weight gain, yelling at the goddamn patriarchy, feeling overwhelmed, etc.

MORE INFO on menopause & perimenopause

See the specific recommendations in the 'More info' sections throughout this book, but in general here's what you need to know about the best expert trustworthy, non-profit and independent health sources for menopause, and then the . . . erm . . . less recommended ones. These tippety-top websites are independent and usually fact-checked, with the latest info and research:

Australasian Menopause Society
menopause.org.au
Founded and maintained by the best independent medical and scientific experts in the country, with evidence-based info for us as well as doctors, nurses, and researchers. Contains fact sheets and videos out the wazoo and how to find a specialist doctor. Search a symptom or click on 'Consumer information'.

thewomens.org.au
Search 'menopause' on this premier women's hospital and health info site for fact sheets.

North American Menopause Society
menopause.org
The US organisation for medical and scientific experts. Choose 'For Women'. Any public health advice or medication brand names are probably only relevant in the US. Its app, called MenoPro, is only suited for the US.

Endocrine Society of the USA
endocrine.org
The Society explains women's sex hormones, thyroid issues and diabetes.

Jean Hailes for Women's Health
jeanhailes.org.au
Independent, non-profit organisation with evidence-based info on physical, mental and emotional health. Has fact sheets, videos and a question-answering service. Dr Hailes founded Australia's first women's health and menopause clinic. Part-funded by Australian governments.

British Menopause Society
thebms.org.uk
Any public health advice, lobbying info and medication brand names may only be relevant in the UK. A sister website, **womens-health-concern.org**, has more.

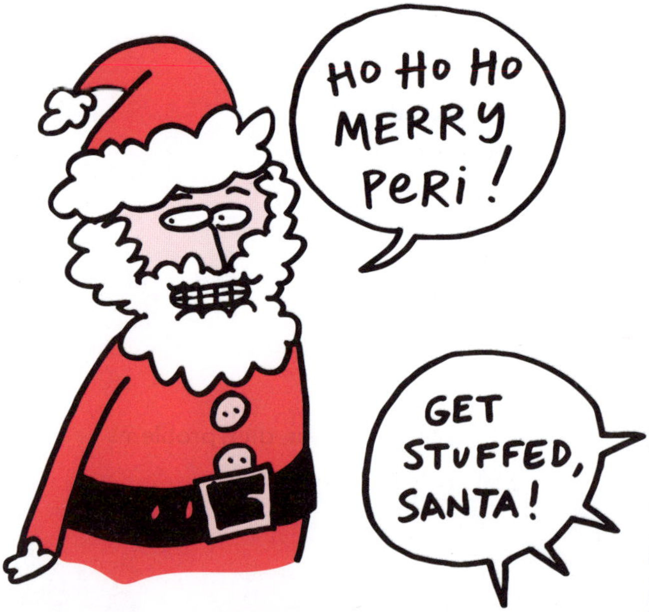

Best menopause websites

Most of the first online search results to come up are ads for sites boosting their company, charity, clinics, products, and apps. Yesterday I searched 'menopause symptom relief'; of about 4 million results, the first four and most of the rest were ads or articles about supplements with no reliable evidence. Independent, evidence-based local sites were items five through nine. Today I searched 'Australian menopause' and the first search result was from a private 'centre' run by somebody I wouldn't trust in a gerzillion years.

All sorts of people give advice about menopause-related products: some have medical qualifications, others have faith-based, 'natural' advice, and/or are maybe trying to enhance their profits, reputations and social media following.

See Chapter 3, It's Your Approach, for a Who's Who of doctors and other health practitioners, and which medical specialties are useful for menopause advice.

Other menopause websites Most menopause-related websites are marketing. Some sites run by a single clinic or doctor, charity and lobby groups may be well-intentioned, but can carry outdated and wrong info. With the caveat that advice can become outdated, you can check out experts' menopause info at **noon.org.uk** and Australian site **mamamia**'s articles, interviews and events, and also its **veryperisummit.com** site.

I'd avoid listening uncritically to anyone who is directly profiting from selling menopause-related products or whose info is on a site that also sells menopause-related products. Online shops, chain pharmacies and giant supplement corporations know you're worried about your menopause, your appearance, and your sex life. They pay to get their products into the top search results, and then target you with unsolicited ads, and sponsored posts that mention the known worrying symptoms of perimenopause.

Online selling & ad websites As I write there's a 'menopause bus' travelling around England sponsored by a morning TV show, plastered with ads for a giant pharmacy chain. Among the first menopause-related products on its website are vaginal douches (don't) and 'skin-tightening creams', which do nothing of the sort. Is there a commercial sponsor, or are you on a giant selling website? Get sceptical, or at least vigilant.

Menopause books

Books reflect the philosophies of their authors, from gynaecologist Dr Jen Gunter, who busts scams and shares evidence-based commonsense advice in *The Menopause Manifesto* (also at **vajenda.substack.com**), to *What Fresh Hell Is This?*, an anthology of essays on menopause edited by non-binary feminist and sex-educator activist Heather Corrinna. Some naturopaths have written books with information that contradicts medically accepted public health advice.

Most big-selling books are much more relevant to Britain or the US than Australia. Always get the latest reprint version (like my other books with medical info, this one will be updated and reprinted regularly).

Menopause apps

Many period and menopause symptom-tracking apps sell data, including private medical info, to Facebook and other marketing companies. An app can be launched or reconfigured with an update to use your data. If you want to be the only one who sees when you last got your period, and what menopause symptoms you may have, you can use your own phone or tablet, or a physical journal or diary. Or just write arrrrghhh on a brown paper bag.

Medical info on these apps may not be updated. Many menopause apps are just thinly disguised weight-loss prompters, with recipes and exercise suggestions.

There are useful anti–brain fog organiser and reminder diary apps, and ones that help with meditation, calming strategies and sleep. The warning on data privacy applies to all apps.

Menopause podcasts

They can be months or years old, which can affect the quality of info: no substitute for medical advice. They may be supportive and have interviews with clever experts. Overseas-based podcast info on medication supply, brands, health insurance and other details will be irrelevant.

Search 'menopause' in available podcasts and make your own decision about how local or useful it is.

Australian rules on who can dispense medical info can be thwarted by overseas-originating books, websites and podcasts. One global podcast is run by a woman calling herself a 'Doctor . . . in functional endocrinology and . . . medicine' – she's a chiropractor with no medical qualifications. Some podcasts are run by nutritionists and others who aren't qualified to give individual medical or dietary advice in menopause or otherwise. (See the 'Eating & weight' section in Chapter 3, It's Your Approach.)

Social media & online

Some menopause-related social media accounts and influencers are fronts for a company or post sponsored ads for supplements. Some online sites boast a supportive community of members sharing stories, but this is mainly for marketing, including testimonials for their products (some of which can't be true!). Even if somebody truly believes something worked for them or will work for you, some supplements can interfere with other medication, not work or even be harmful.

Menopause advice I'd avoid

Once you've told the internet's algorithms what you're interested in by searching, you'll get links and opinions and old news articles, even from respected sources, with wrong medical info and disproven cancer scares. Oblivious or time-starved writers on other sites search the same key words and repeat old, wrong info in their newer articles.

I'm not a fan of menopause info from:

* Celebrities who write books heavy on personal opinions and suggestions, mostly around appearance and weight but often disguised as 'wellness' and self-care, who promote their own or a friend's supplements and even homeopathy, which can't work.
* Famous people selling their own expensive, branded products. There's no reliable scientific evidence or regulated requirement on doses that suggest those specific 'natural' formulations have any effect.
* Gwyneth Paltrow's online mega-shop Goop has some curious opinions about menopause. It sells expensive handful-o-pills supplement packets 'designed to help' for sleep, libido, and to 'help smooth the menopausal transition by providing nutritional support' with no evidence of specific effects.
* Christiane Northrup, now-unregistered US doctor and menopause advisor, has been banned from social media platforms for wackadoodle posts about conspiracy theories and saying vaccines are murder weapons. She reckons hot flushes might be caused by unexpressed shame and anger. They are not.
* The late Louise Hay, whose books and branded products still sell, preached that medical symptoms are caused by your thoughts. (Menopause, she'd have you know, can be caused by not feeling wanted, whereas burping is caused by fear. Or, you know, boiled egg sandwiches.)

Early menopause & premature menopause

Millions of women are confronted with a medical diagnosis that means menopause has come to them years, even decades, earlier than expected. Technically, you're diagnosed with early menopause if it's before the age of 45; and if it happens before you're 40, the diagnosis is Premature Ovarian Insufficiency. (In US resources it's often called Primary Ovarian Insufficiency.)

This can happen as an effect of surgery or medication, or just seemingly for no reason at all. There's no medical reason why the line between definitions of early, earlyish, and expected menopause timing is set at 40 or 45; it's just that they had to put it somewhere.

It's not rare for menopause to happen before 45, it's just more unusual than the norm. Although it varies for many reasons across the world, it's thought to happen to four in 100 women under 40, one in 10,000 women under 30, and one in 10,000 under 20. In a small number of cases, some specific genes are suspected. Research is ongoing.

An age-expected menopause is sometimes called a usual, or natural-age menopause, whereas a menopause caused by medication or surgery might be called secondary menopause. 'Idiopathic' is a scary word you might hear doctors use: it just means they don't know the reason for something.

Some GPs and specialists can use early and premature menopause terms interchangeably, or use words that a patient prefers. Many younger women don't feel 'early menopause' describes their experience. In the past it used to be called something jargon-y like 'cessation of menses', or the usual insensitive ye olde doctory palaver such as Ovarian Failure.

I'm glad to have had the opportunity to have a surgery that could save my life, and early menopause was a small price to pay.
Jo, 45

I sought help from a doctor who said it wasn't menopause, as I was too young. I reached over his desk and grabbed him by his jacket lapels and said, 'Give me back my life; this one is f@#*ng shitful.' He wrote me a script for [a heavy sedative]. Next day I rang [a women's health centre]. Proper help and medication gave me back myself.
Glynnis, 64

An early menopause diagnosis for any reason can be devastating for those who thought they'd have more time to get pregnant. It can also tip women suddenly into severe, awful menopausal symptoms such as fierce hot flushes and vaginal dryness, and creates an early and ongoing, cumulative risk to their bone and heart health: so being offered protective hormone medication and/or alternatives is important.

> My mum stopped getting her period at the age of 26, and so she never knowingly went through menopause. However, looking back at her mental and physical struggles, I now think that she probably went into menopause then; the doctors never made a diagnosis.
> Toni, 55

Factors associated with earlier menopause

These things don't always cause earlier menopause, but are associated with it:

- family history of early menopause on either side of family
- starting your first period much earlier than average
- smoking
- being born a twin or triplet, especially from one egg
- having not yet had a pregnancy
- a childhood experience of food deprivation
- being in a lower weight range
- some autoimmune and thyroid disorders
- a grab-bag of other serious conditions including mumps, cytomegalovirus, tuberculosis and malaria
- some genetic conditions, including Turner syndrome
- living at a very high altitude.

What doesn't cause earlier menopause

These things:

- the Pill
- pregnancy termination
- IVF
- psychological reasons
- stress
- anything to do with sexuality.

> I knew I was experiencing early menopause, but it took 5 years to convince doctors. I was diagnosed with [bone density loss] at 35.
> Jo, 47

Menopause caused by medication or surgery

Many women are tumbled into menopause symptoms because of cancer treatment which affects their ovaries – usually chemotherapy and radiation of the whole body or pelvic region, but not if you've had radiation for breast cancer. Or it happens because of the deceptively fun-sounding oophorectomy, meaning surgical removal of ovaries, which can happen at the same time as a hysterectomy (which removes the uterus).

Doctors often now talk of 'preserving', or leaving ovaries inside you whenever possible if a hysterectomy is needed, so you can continue making your own estrogen. They should also be better these days at warning women who are at risk of menopause symptoms hitting hard and suddenly.

Some women may go into menopause temporarily or indefinitely because they need to take medication for another condition that prevents their ovaries producing estrogen. There are also medications that can cause symptoms that look like early menopause, including some treatments for endometriosis and breast cancer. Those women will need help with menopause symptoms, too, and should be offered them by doctors, perhaps especially if they are distracted with other aspects of their healthcare.

Also ask your surgeon, gynaecologist or endocrinologist about other associations with early menopause to look out for, including a higher risk of heart problems and brittle bones. According to women's experiences, other conditions may also appear after menopause or surgery that they weren't warned about, including tendon and joint problems and orgasm differences. Studies continue.

Symptoms of earlier menopause

Most symptoms are from the same unlucky-dip as menopause at any other time: disappearing periods, hot flushes, brain fog, self-esteem plummet, sleep interruption, irritability or rage, vaginal dryness: see the double-page spread of possibilities, back on pages 36–37.

I had a hysterectomy five weeks ago (with ovaries removed) and made sure I had a HRT script before I left hospital. Frances, 52

I was staggered by how little I knew and understood. I thought I was psychologically robust but early meno thrust me into a big episode of anxiety. Roberta, 51

I started perimenopause around 39 years old, and by 41 I was done and dusted. Patty, 54

Getting a diagnosis of early menopause

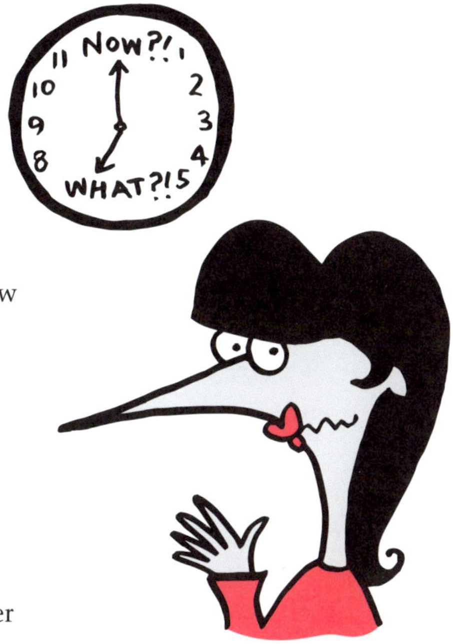

Often, the first symptoms are assumed to be something else – erratic periods are pretty normal and won't be obvious if you take the Pill continuously so as not to have bleeding. Lots of us who experience having foggy brain or a dry vagina or painful sex are too embarrassed to even mention it to a doctor or didn't know it was relevant to their hormones.

If you get bland reassurances from a GP, and you're getting perimenopausal symptoms, especially stopped periods, brain fog, hot flushes and dry vagina, insist on a referral to an endocrinologist (hormones specialist) or gynaecologist (women's 'reproductive' health specialist). Likewise, you may be getting no other perimenopausal symptoms except a stopped period: you still need a proper diagnosis.

Quite often, women delay seeing a doctor when their periods are erratic or stop and there are no other symptoms. Sometimes, being on the Pill means they don't know they're not ovulating. It can take a long time to get a diagnosis because patients and some doctors don't consider it a possibility at a younger age. See Chapter 3, It's Your Approach, for proactive strategies with doctors.

To make a diagnosis of Premature Ovarian Insufficiency, if your ovaries have given up producing enough hormones, doctors must combine the knowledge that you're not yet 40, you haven't had a period for at least 4–6 months, and that it's not caused by pregnancy or any other condition. They will also order some blood test results.

Blood tests must be done at least a month apart, and can inform the diagnosis if they show very low levels in the blood of estrogen but high levels of the hormone that is trying to signal the development and release of an egg, called follicle stimulating hormone (FSH).

I found out I was perimenopausal and too far along to undergo further fertility treatment after a failed IVF. I was 36.
Ellie, 54

Early menopause can be really tough – particularly if it results in no kids when these were deeply wished for. Reach out for help; there are others of us who have walked this path.
Edie, 44

Effects of early menopause

> My mother, her sister, my maternal grandmother and her sisters all had hysterectomies in their early 40s, due to severe bleeding and period cramping, so they all went into early menopause. Karen, 52

For women who are confronted with this much earlier than expected, it can have all sorts of extra emotional difficulties: perhaps coming to terms with the grief of unexpected infertility, dealing with what feels like ageing symptoms in your 20s and 30s; feelings of failure even though it absolutely *isn't your fault*; working out who to tell and who not to tell; needing a strategy to protect yourself in the decades to come, against higher risks of heart problems and more fragile bones.

Lower levels of estrogen give us a much higher risk of bone weakness, osteoporosis and heart disease: having this happen earlier in your life gives you the risk earlier, and more years in which to experience it. (On the plus side, Premature Ovarian Insufficiency lowers the statistical risk of breast cancer.)

If you don't want to be pregnant, you'll still need to take contraception, because if your ovaries are unpredictable and your hormone levels are still fluctuating at a lower level, you could release an egg without warning, leading to an unwanted pregnancy. Sadly for women who want to be pregnant, ovulating after a diagnosis is rare: perhaps 5 per cent of women with Premature Ovarian Insufficiency may be able to conceive.

Treatment for early menopause

Everyone with a diagnosis of early menopause should be offered hormone medication, or alternatives if that is not recommended. The Pill or Menopausal Hormone Therapy (MHT) will protect you in early menopause from the typical annoying menopausal symptoms and, crucially, protect you from what would otherwise be a much higher risk of heart disease, and bone weakness and osteoporosis in the future.

Most doctors should and will probably offer the Pill to be taken continuously without an imposed break to bleed: that's important because you need continuous

> I remember thinking 'Jeeeze hot flushes can't be that bad – toughen up a bit, it's only menopause'. How wrong I was. I had no idea what menopause actually does to a person. Tina, 53

> My ex-husband used to joke about when I hit menopause that I'd better not go crazy like his mum. I found that very upsetting. Minerva, 53

estrogen to protect your bones. Or they'll offer some form of MHT. Whichever it is, the recommendation is for you to take it at least until the average known cultural age of menopause. That's 52 for white Australian women, maybe 48 for some other cultural groups but again, shamefully not enough research, obvs.

Many will then switch to MHT or continue on it, weighing up the different risks and benefits of staying on. See Chapter 2, It's Your Hormones, for more on medication, and Chapters 4, 5 and 6 for the lowdown on mental, physical and sexual symptoms and solutions.

Early menopause & fertility

Many women and non-binary folk choose to have some of their eggs frozen and stored in an in-vitro fertilisation (IVF) assisted fertility clinic before surgery or, say, a course of chemotherapy that will cause early menopause. It's important not to be misled, and it's hard to hear that the rate of successful IVF pregnancies on the first attempt, or at all, is lower for frozen eggs; and very much lower if you're over 35 or you don't have many eggs in storage.

Many women who experience early menopause try to become pregnant using donor eggs or embryos: again, sadly, there are no guarantees. The storage of eggs can cost hundreds of dollars a year, IVF can cost tens of thousands: check your Medicare and health fund entitlements and waiting periods.

Research continues on how different combinations or levels of hormone medication might help to kickstart ovaries to make and release eggs again.

Doctors have developed a way to remove, preserve and freeze some ovary tissue from a patient's body while they're undergoing chemotherapy and radiation and then re-implant it afterwards, leading to a successful pregnancy at rates of up to 30 per cent. The procedure is still in its early days, and is probably most useful for younger women.

No so-called natural herbal, powdered food supplements or pills claiming to support or boost fertility, nor acupuncture, nor chiropracty will reverse an early (or later) menopause, no matter what the hard-sell ads, websites and social media posts claim.

> I held myself in a strong space of never-ending self-compassion around the premature ovarian failure/insufficiency, and always felt my absolute strength in my ability to support myself through that whenever I tuned in to my internal experience of grief around my early menopause and infertility. **Edie, 44**

The heartbreak and fierce hope felt by many women in this situation can make them vulnerable. When they hear 'unproven' they can think 'it might work', when often the opposite is true. A qualified psychologist experienced in fertility issues can help anyone in a couple or family struggling with fertility issues.

MORE INFO on early menopause & Premature Ovarian Insufficiency (POI)

askearlymenopause.org
Ask Early Menopause app
Independent info and reassurance from some of Australia's top professors, doctors and researchers in women's health, backed by Monash University; plus real life stories.

healthtalkaustralia.org
This is a website related to the app above, a trusted experts' site: search 'early menopause' for articles on feelings, relationships and sex life. Supported by the work of Australia's top independent health researchers and backed by the Australian Government, peak physical and mental health organisations and the National Medical Research Council.

menopause.org.au
The Australasian Menopause Society has fact sheets on menopause before 40, and Spontaneous Premature Ovarian Insufficiency. Click on 'Consumer information' and scroll down for fact sheets.

jeanhailes.org.au
Search 'Premature and early menopause' for compassionate and comprehensive info from this women's health site.

varta.org.au
The Victorian Assisted Reproductive Treatment Authority has lots of fact sheets about IVF, surrogacy, egg freezing and other info not influenced by IVF clinic marketing.

My husband sat the teenagers down in front of the computer and googled all the symptoms of menopause – sadness, depression, mood changes – and said, 'Yep, this is what we're all going to be dealing with – dry vagina, you two at least won't have to deal with one!' It was hilarious and stopped me crying, but Jesus . . . Kay, 52

I joke about it calling it 'the paws' with a sudden, claw-like double hand gesture. Takes the taboo out of it. A taboo which is ridiculous. Verity, 54

(This gesture was first used by Kim, at Kath, in the 'fillum' Kath & Kimderella, written by Gina Riley and Jane Turner.)

The takeaway on perimenopause & menopause

Whatever the official definitions, perimenopause and menopause are a combo of your own individual symptoms, your own timing, your own knowledge. We're all experimenting with what will work for us, at the same time that research and treatments are evolving.

Look for evidence-based information sources, and choose who to share stories and experiences with. Despite the social stigmas of the past (and sadly, last Thursday and probably next week), you're not doing it wrong, and you're not alone.

We're in this together.

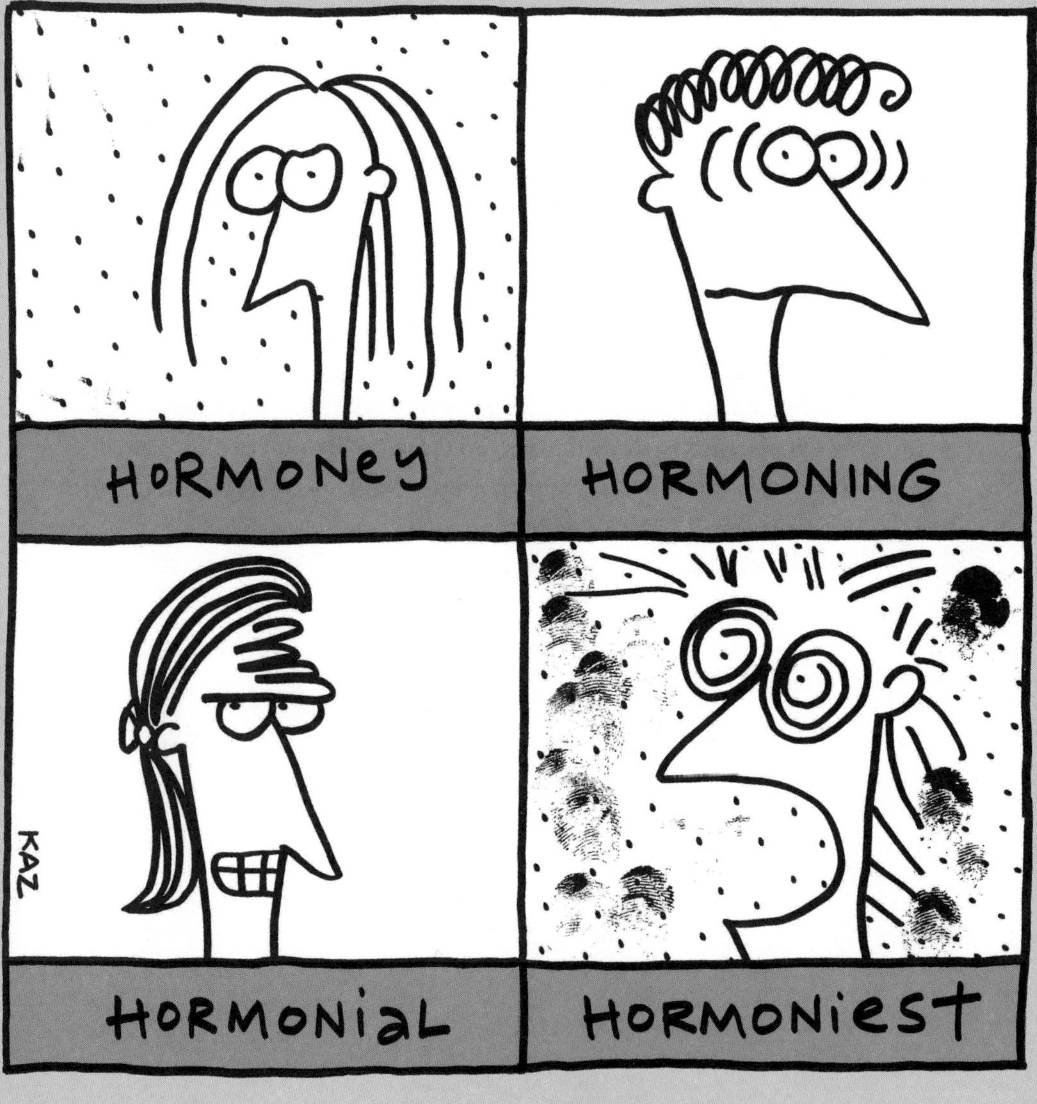
HORMONEY
HORMONING
KAZ
HORMONIAL
HORMONIEST

2

It's Your Hormones

Hormones are powerful. They can calm you down, send you crazy, turn your bosoms into milk sprinklers, alter the shape of your body, give you cramps, cheer you up, make you sick, give you an alibi, help change your gender, grow you a beard, create empathy, mask pain, spike your body temperature, keep you awake, get you pregnant, stop you getting pregnant, spark fury and change your hairstyle.

The explanation we're often given for absolutely anything that we're feeling or our bodies are doing is, 'it's your hormones'. Which is probably true but ludicrously vague, especially when it comes to perimenopause and menopause. *How* and *why* hormones have all the physical effects on us that they do, and how can we control them – or at least manage them – when they make our life difficult: this chapter lays it all out.

Our hormone levels are not precise – they can be random, messy and unkind, and change within moments. We're not intelligently designed (or if we are, somebody really needs to get fired). Not one of us is 'perfect' or even 'as Nature intended', because Nature does not have intentions, let alone intentions for you or me individually.

For most of us, for most of our lives, our hormone levels approximate what's required to get us pregnant as many times as possible. It doesn't matter to Nature if some people who want to get pregnant can't, or (stay with me) a girl who didn't want to be pregnant . . . gets pregnant. It doesn't matter to Nature if you go into early menopause, or you need to be on lifelong hormone medication to avoid pain or illness.

Only one woman known to global science ever had her hormones and brain chemicals always working perfectly in balance, a woman called Patricia who lived in Yarrawonga in 1894. Her flawless brain-to-ovaries feedback loop ran with graceful perfection, allowing her to have periods at precise intervals of every 28 days, and an evenly balanced mood every day for several decades, with no period pain ever.

Excuse me (puts finger to ear). I'm getting a message in my headset . . . breaking news: apparently Patricia's fictitious.

Brain chemical hormones are released in both our brains and our ovaries. Over the span of each monthly cycle, different hormones at different levels 'talk' to each other and signal certain actions to happen – they build up the endometrial lining of the uterus in case an egg is fertilised and a fetus implanted, they signal the start of that wall dissolving away as a period, or they change breasts to allow breastfeeding, and can cause relaxing or stress effects.

If Nature knew how, or cared to properly regulate everyone's hormones in precise levels on predicable schedules, there'd be no period pain, nobody would get premenstrual tears, cravings or furious feelings, or pregnancy nausea. Or need hormonal help with endometriosis, or a whole bunch of menopausal symptoms that are making them miserable.

Menopause is natural but that doesn't mean it's easy or okay for everyone. Just as many of us need glasses to see, or help not to get period cramps, or contraception, or fertility treatment, some of us will need help to get through the mental and physical effects of perimenopause and menopause. Whether we need a little or a lot of help, and what sort of combination of self-help, lifestyle changes, and medication we choose, is down to luck and philosophy.

Through no fault of our own, and because of wildly varying media reports and marketing ads over the last few years, we've been confused about hormone medication and its risks.

In the Survey for this book, more than 62 per cent of women said they didn't know if hormone medication worked well or at all on menopause symptoms; about half didn't know if it raised the risk of breast cancer, and just over half didn't know if the hormones were the same ones your body makes.

In the Survey, more than 7300 women answered a question about whether they took hormone medication for menopause symptoms: just over a quarter said yes. About five per cent of them took the Pill; most of those taking MHT called it HRT.

What's the difference between HRT and MHT? Let's get into it and find out what's what.

I tried all the alternative things . . . zero impact. HRT had an instant impact and relieved me of the boiling hotness and the sweats. It didn't make much of an impact on all my other symptoms. Michele, 61

I need a trolley to get my medication home from the chemist. Bek, 51

As a 49-year-old female GP who sees a zillion 49-year-old perimenopausal women . . . MHT is often a bloody miracle and everyone is scared of it. Jane

Being able to label it and understand how much is now related to hormones has helped me enormously. Alison, 50

The stock shortages of the HRT I was prescribed has been complete rubbish. Kirsten, 56

I never knew how bad it could be, especially the mental health effects, how debilitating, but also, in my case, how easily it was rectified with the right medication. Nadine, 49

Actually, it's not hormones – I'm angry for valid reasons. Jody, 57

I have been putting this down to age, not hormones. Terri, 57

I feel like a stranger in my own body and I don't like it. Linda, 51

I'm sick of hearing how normal it is when it can cause a lot of despair in some women. Katy, 64

What's what in hormone medication

I haaate using medical acronyms, but I can't see a way around it. We're going to be saying MHT a lot. So:

HRT: The old acronym for **Hormone Replacement Therapy**, the term used originally for estrogen or estrogen-and-progestogen medication for perimenopausal women. Now, it's more commonly used by doctors as the term for medication given to women who have a premature menopause. Many doctors and old online articles, and many women, still use the term HRT to refer to menopause medication.

MHT: **Menopausal Hormone Therapy** is the newer name for hormone medication routinely prescribed for perimenopausal and menopausal women. Mostly, it means what people used to think of when they said, or still say, HRT. It will appear approximately 78 trillion times in this book.

GHT: **Gender-Affirming Hormone Therapy**. Medication that may be prescribed to trans and non-binary folk to match their gender identity.

In short – explanations are coming up – if you want properly reliable, pharmaceutical, regulated, measurable hormone medication in Australia, it must be prescribed by a doctor. Some medical hormone products are available over the counter in other countries.

Some 'natural' hormone products can be bought in Australia without a prescription: they're also made in a laboratory or factory but are not as reliable or recommended because they're covered by the same rules, regulations and tests on their effects, doses and ingredients. (More on that coming up.)

I feel free. My hormones come from a pill packet now, so they no longer rule me. Sherry, 52

I feel that we really should know more about hormones and not be afraid of them. Knowledge is power. Julia, 54

I don't talk about it if I don't have to. It's under control, thanks to HRT. Eden, 53

What are hormones?

Hormones are microscopic, miraculous, mundane molecule groups; substances made by different parts of our body and sent around our bloodstream in varying quantities so they can create varying effects on different organs.

They act as triggers as well as brakes on different actions and effects in our body. They influence sleep, moods, body shape, the ability to get pregnant and breastfeed, hair growth, metabolism and lots of other things.

Our bodies naturally make chemicals, including tiny amounts of metals, so that we can stay alive and function. The chemicals include hormones, produced by several organs and glands in the body including the brain, the ovaries and the pancreas; the hormones then produce effects when they bind to receptors in the body.

Hormones include estrogens, progestogens, testosterone, insulin, melatonin, cortisol, adrenaline, prolactin, thyroid stimulating and growth hormones. The level of each hormone can trigger a boost or block the effect of other hormones.

Hormones can work together unnoticeably, or turn into a hectic mess. The best case scenario is that most of them behave themselves most of the time. When hormones get out of whack or their decline causes miserable or dangerous symptoms, there are medications we can take to replace or regulate them, including thyroid medication, insulin, and supplemental estrogen and progestogens.

The most relevant menopause-related hormones

The levels of a few key hormones get erratic and/or fall during perimenopause, and eventually our body will only make them at a more settled, very low level. They are:

* estrogens (estradiol, estrone and estriol)
* progestogens (aka progesterone)
* testosterone and similar hormones
* luteinising and follicle stimulating hormones, aka LH and FSH, which organise the egg production (or don't). FSH develops an egg and LH releases it.

Also relevant is a lucky dip of 50+ mood-related hormones. Calming and rewarding hormones include oxytocin, dopamine, endorphins and serotonin. Stress hormones include cortisol and adrenaline. Melatonin helps us sleep when we need to. We need insulin to regulate blood sugar levels. Aldosterone bosses our blood pressure around.

What happens to hormones in perimenopause?

The relevant hormones during perimenopause tend to be erratic: rising and plunging within days, hours and even minutes, which among many things can cause a hot flush. Different symptoms and feelings can be triggered not just by the levels or speed of the rises or falls in each hormone, but also by different ratios of hormones in relation to each other. Hormones in menopause tend to eventually settle down at low levels but for some unlucky people, they keep zig-zagging and cause symptoms for years.

Cherished reader, I could simply insist that you wade through a lot of loose talk about the hypothalamic-pituitary-gonadal axis but I prefer to avoid a lot of gonad talk. Instead, I'm going to try out a metaphor.

Hormones as a Jane Austen movie dance scene

You know those Regency film dance scenes when the men are all lined up in their red jackets and tight white pants and black boots, and the women are all assembled in pastel-coloured empire-line silk gowns, and then they start doing all these incey-mincey steps and holding hands and passing around one another and then going back to the lines where they started? Picture that.

Now imagine all the chaps in suspiciously tight pants are representing progestogen hormones, and all the ladies in historically inaccurate up-dos are estrogen, and, to be blindingly predictable, the rake entering stage left with one raised eyebrow and a floppy fringe is testosterone, and the brooding-but-dependable-aristocratic neighbour is a shot of serotonin. If they all turn up in the right clothes, and do the right steps and there's the right number of all of them, then the dance works fine.

When the dance goes right, and everyone turns up in the right costume, you have a standard menstrual cycle: you ovulate and have periods at intervals that are normal for you, whether it's the textbook 28 days or not.

I always used to be really crabby just before my period came – the period's arrival used to often explain the crabbiness, but it got worse during perimenopause. Michele, 64

I just felt like my body was conducting its own science experiments 24 hours a day, seven days a week, with surprises thrown in.
Gail, 58

I became more moody, oversensitive and teary. It was like PMT on steroids but it didn't come and go – it came and stayed. Berny, 57

It's brutal – physically and psychologically. Aly, 48

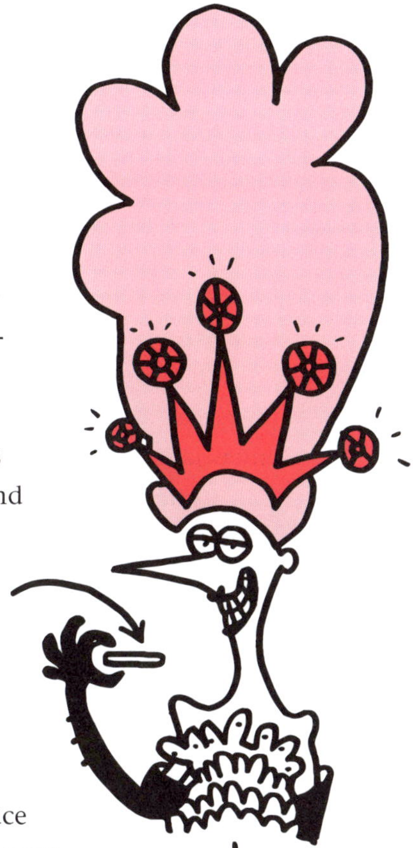

But, in perimenopause, the dance goes awry. Half the estrogen ladies turn up one month, only one makes it to the dance the month after, and then the next month, they all thunder back in, throwing cucumber sandwiches at each other. Meanwhile, the progestogens in red jackets are milling around with no partners and telling sad stories, and Lady Dopamine is suddenly a bit tiddly, gets told off by Captain Testosterone and retires to the fainting couch.

Extra dancers show up who don't know the steps. Some people go home, or lie down on the dance floor. Some people look at the clock, realise the end of the music is coming, and charge onto the dancefloor, and do the Hokey Pokey twice as hard. It's a schemozzle, a riot of alternately whirling and desultory activity. Meanwhile, the band, The Glands, instead of gently playing the right music to induce a waltz or quadrille as required, mucks up its signals to the dancers and starts playing industrial emo cowpunk. And the choreographer has brain fog.

For some poor exhausted souls, this fiasco of a dance can go on for 2 years, or 10 years, or 20. And every one of us is on a different dancefloor, listening to a different band, with a different set of dancers, and a different personal reaction to a melee on the floor.

And that's why you get heavy bleeding and hairs on your chin and you can't sleep.

Where to get hormone info

Get your hormones and medication info from a switched-on GP, gynaecologist or endocrinologist, or one of the good, trustworthy sources like the Australasian Menopause Society or the Jean Hailes organisation (see page 38).

How do we measure hormone levels?

If you're in the typical age range of perimenopause, it's easier to base a medical assessment on whether you have any or some of the symptoms of perimenopause (see pages 36–37 for the full symptoms list) than a blood test. Because there are other serious possible reasons for mental as well as physical symptoms, it's important to rule them out.

There's no need to test your blood levels to see if you're in perimenopause, because the levels can vary within minutes. They don't dictate which symptoms you're having, and whatever the number is wouldn't change the treatment offered.

Hormone tests can be more helpful to determine if your levels have fallen to a consistently low level that indicates menopause, either to check for early menopause or confirm post-menopause when you're older.

Hormones are measured by how many picomoles of a hormone are in a litre of blood. A picomole is a ridiculously teeny unit measuring how many molecules are in a substance. A picomole is one trillionth of a mole, which is an adorable nocturnal animal. A mole is also a chemistry measurement that will blow your mind: each mole is this many molecules: $6.02214076 \times 10^{23}$. And each picomole is a trillionth of that. Get out. I know.

So a hormone test tries to find out how many of those teensy picomole units of, say, estrogen, progesterone or testosterone is detectable in a litre of blood. They don't take a litre, they just do maths based on a little sample. As you can imagine it's tough to get an accurate reading. Even if a hormone test of your blood told you how many picomoles of estrogen were in your blood at 2.30 pm on a Thursday afternoon, by Tuesday or next month or 20 minutes after the test the level might be totally different.

And anyway, one woman with a certain number of picomoles of estrogen per litre might be hot-flushing herself into a frenzy while her pal with exactly the same level has never even had a hot flush.

Even if your estrogen level was magically, impossibly rock steady for 2 months, it would have different effects in the body at different times, depending on your progesterone levels, what your brain chemicals are doing, and how much estrogen is recognised by cells when they attach to hormone receptors. And whether it activates a weak or strong effect in any and each of hundreds of thousands of cells in different places around your body that have estrogen receptors: breasts, ovaries, endometrium, fat, liver, bone and brain cells among them.

So should you get a hormone test?

The short answer for almost all of us is no and it would be a waste of money. You don't need it to identify perimenopause symptoms or treatments. The answer is different if you're under 40 or otherwise suspected of having Premature Ovarian Insufficiency (see Chapter 1, What Even Is The Menopause, for more on that, in the 'Early menopause' section).

The only person who should test your hormone levels is a medical professional. They shouldn't order one if they don't need to. Blood tests, not saliva or urine tests, are by far the best way to do this.

Some naturopaths and supplement sellers tell their clients to get gene tests or hormone level tests to see if they have 'toxic estrogen' or 'dominant estrogen'. This is a diagnosis considered to be a fad and unsupported by medical hormone experts including gene specialists, endocrinologists and gynaecologists. Your own body can't overdose you or produce toxic amounts of estrogen. No supplement or treatment that claims to help the liver get rid of excess estrogen or other hormones is necessary or a good idea worth your money. You don't need it unless you're in liver failure, in which case I shouldn't bother thinking about estrogen.

Saliva hormone tests are either a scam, or may be ordered and done by someone who doesn't understand that it shows nothing to do with the relevant blood-hormone levels, and their effects.

Here's what can't determine hormone levels: iridology (looking at your eyes), non-pathology lab examination of drops of blood, looking at your skin or tongue, and guessing.

The hormones that kept me in balance have deserted me.
Glenda, 59

How to judge your own exact hormone levels

You can't, really. Even if you could plot each hormone level on a graph (say, one each for estrogen, progesterone, testosterone), it might look like a flattish

> My girl gang and I celebrate each other's menopause with a party in a cocktail bar!
> Lisa, 60

line of ric-rac braid with the occasional spike, or the ABC logo – up down, up down, and around into infinity – it won't look like a flat line that then suddenly points downward like it's 'falling off a cliff' as the cliché goes.

This is also the reason why a 'bespoke', non-pharmaceutical hormone treatment usually makes no sense at all.

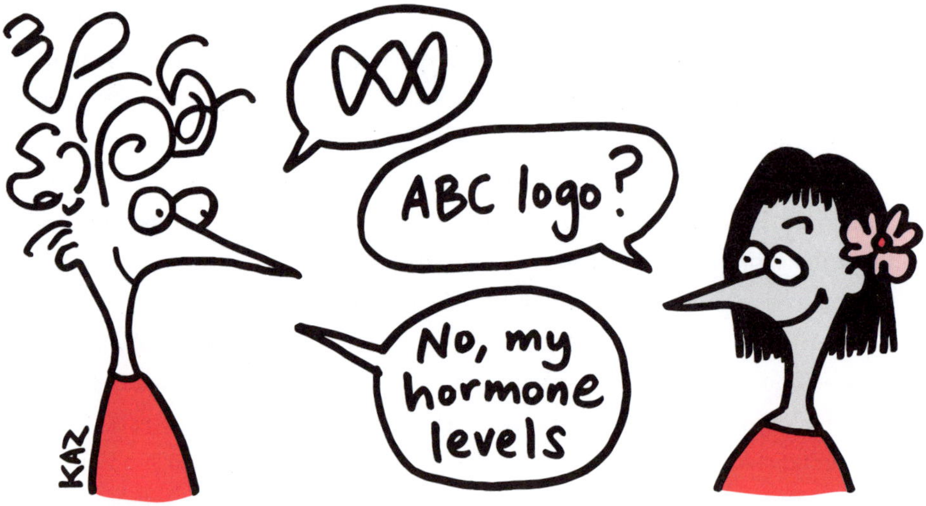

The fact that your hormone levels have changed is usually detected and judged by what perimenopause symptoms you're having, whether they are indeed caused by perimenopause and whether you need help with them: such as hot flushes and disappearing or heavy periods. It can be a lot harder to recognise which mental symptoms are hormonal (see Chapter 4, It's Your Mind).

Meet your hormones

First up, let's get better acquainted with our perimenopause main three: estrogen, progestogens and testosterone. In the Survey, one in five women taking hormone medication said they didn't know what was in it; more than two-thirds knew it contained estrogen; nearly half said they were also taking progesterone, and a few took some form of testosterone.

Estrogen

I think estrogen might stop straight women from murdering their husbands, but they haven't done a study on it. I've mentioned this theory to endocrinologists and they usually just nod.

In our bodies we make three main kinds of estrogen: estradiol, estrone and estriol. The levels of all of them drop in menopause leaving you with mostly estrone, but estradiol is the stronger one. That's the one, on its own or along with a progestogen, that prescription doses of MHT will deliver into your body. To simplify things, this book mainly talks about estrogen as a singular hormone.

A combined contraceptive Pill with both estrogen and progesterone, taken correctly, will, about 99 times out of 100, stop your body from ovulating, which means you won't get pregnant. (Only women without a uterus should take an estrogen-only contraceptive Pill or MHT, of which more later, but some contraception is progesterone only.)

During perimenopause, your estrogen levels can be all over the shop – down, up, way down – for several months or even years. From the start of perimenopause to being in full menopause, your estrogen level will drop 90 per cent or more. It doesn't disappear entirely. Before menopause, estrogen levels are about 400 picograms per millilitre of blood at peak time of the month, and after menopause, steady at less than 30.

Different levels of estrogen in different women do different things. In other words, there's no exact percentage of estrogen in the blood that corresponds with turning off egg production in the ovaries or causes a hot flush.

What estrogen does

At the 'right' levels before perimenopause, estrogen:

* variously plumps up parts of you, including your uterus lining, skin, hair, and the supporting ligaments and tissues around organs and blood vessels
* maintains healthy bacteria and lubrication in your vagina
* helps run your menstrual cycle
* protects against heart problems
* keeps your strong bone-growth cycle going
* maybe helps boost libido
* possibly stops you biting people.

> It is basically a crapshoot whether you have a hard or easy time with it. Luck of the draw.
> Jen, 51

What a lack of estrogen does

Basically, estrogen causes most of the symptoms in the list of perimenopause symptoms on pages 36–37 including:

* mood and mental health changes
* hot flushes
* drier skin and vagina
* hormone-related headaches and migraines
* heart rate changes
* loss of bone strength.

Hormones are wild and crazy things, and I now have a much greater understanding of how much they influence mental and physical wellbeing. Marny, 49

When estrogen might not be right for you

Discuss it with your GP or specialist if you:

* smoke
* drink regularly, or a lot
* have a history of blood clots or stroke
* have had breast, endometrial or ovarian cancer.

Things that can change estrogen levels in your body

* erratic or retiring ovaries
* MHT
* pregnancy
* breastfeeding
* perimenopause
* menopause
* surgical removal of ovaries
* chemotherapy and radiography
* drinking alcohol
* smoking
* thyroid hormone imbalance
* some other medications
* some illegal drugs
* some illnesses
* spells cast by witches (are you still awake?).

I didn't realise the fury and rage of my 40s was hormonal. Helen, 54

There's probably less stigma now than ever before, but it's still not totally OK to speak about openly, in my opinion. Aashif, 50

Estrogen should be prescribed by a doctor and come pre-packaged in a gel, pill, patch, vaginal cream or other form that's covered by regulations requiring testing of quality, ingredient and dosage, effects, and length of time the medication will work.

Pharmaceutical companies that sell them in Australia have to prove those things through scientifically acceptable double-blind placebo studies, that a certain dose has proven beneficial for certain things. Then the federal government approves it, so it can be sold in that exact formulation for those strict purposes. Compounded, so-called bio-identical hormones, mixed up by a pharmacist, are neither reliable nor regulated. Tests have proven that the dosage can fluctuate, and the ingredients can be dodgy (more on that coming up).

Progestogens

Here's something that's so confusing it's ridiculous and ought to be illegal. One of the key hormone types is progestogens. The type of progestogen made in our body is called progesterone. A laboratory-made medical kind of progestogen can also be known as progesterone, when it has the same exact molecule structure. But some other lab-made ones that *aren't* exactly the same are called progestins. All of them have progestogenic effects; meaning they act in some way like natural progesterone made in the body.

Everyone: us women, many doctors, manufacturers, media stories and even drug research studies have mixed up the use of the words progestogens, progesterone, and progestins.

Here's what you need to know.

Progesterone is the partner hormone to estrogen: the other main one helping to trigger body changes that happen during period cycles, pregnancy, or perimenopause.

In perimenopause you produce more irregular levels of progesterone, which cause shorter or longer periods. Eventually, in menopause the amount of both estrogen and progesterone your body makes settles at a much lower consistent level.

Progesterone's job after ovulation is to prepare the endometrium – the lining of the uterus – in case the egg is fertilised, implants and is retained as a pregnancy. If there's no egg, or no implantation, or an implantation that the body rejects, or the fertilised egg is shed or removed, the drop in progesterone levels signals the uterus to shed the extra endometrium that was thickened up by extra estrogen, and you bleed it away in what's usually experienced as a period.

Because one of the features of perimenopause is erratic and/or declining egg production and ovulation, the drop in progesterone may not be triggered, or levels of it will fall. Finally, in settled menopause, the levels are stable and very low.

During erratic hormonal carry-on, if your estrogen levels are higher, and your progesterone levels are lower, it's often called 'unopposed estrogen', and can cause too much growth in the thickness of the endometrium, which is a risk factor for endometrial cancer. That's why if you do have a uterus, you'll need a side of progestogens with your estrogen to balance it, as a protective dose for your uterus.

If you don't have a uterus, it's probably safe to take estrogen without progesterone, but check with a doctor.

The best known form of medical progesterone is known as micronised, which means it's identical in its molecule structure to the progesterone made in your body, and in tiny particles so it's easy to absorb, and it behaves the same way in your body. This sometimes means it's called 'body identical' – *not* 'bio-identical', but that gets even more confusing.

Only a couple of approved, regulated products with micronised progesterone are available in Australia. One's a pill and one's a pessary you take, popped up the vagina before sleep.

Many contraceptive Pills and some oral and skin-patch-delivering MHT contain estrogen and progestins. Progestins are often called 'synthetic' because they have progestogenic effects on the body, but are not an exact copy of the molecule structure of body-made progesterone. Progestins included in prescribed medication are considered safe according to dose and ingredient regulations, but have also been associated with some premenstrual-style side effects such as feeling blue and bloated. Guess what needs more research about who can take it and feel fine, and who can't? Yep, progestins.

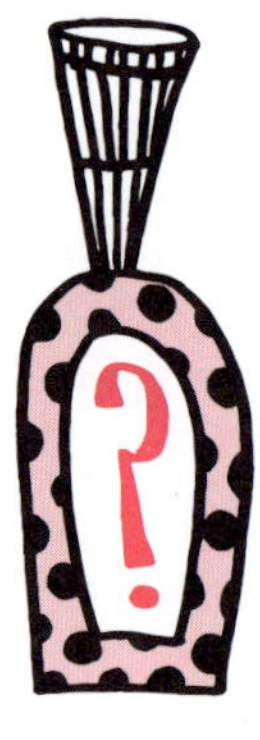

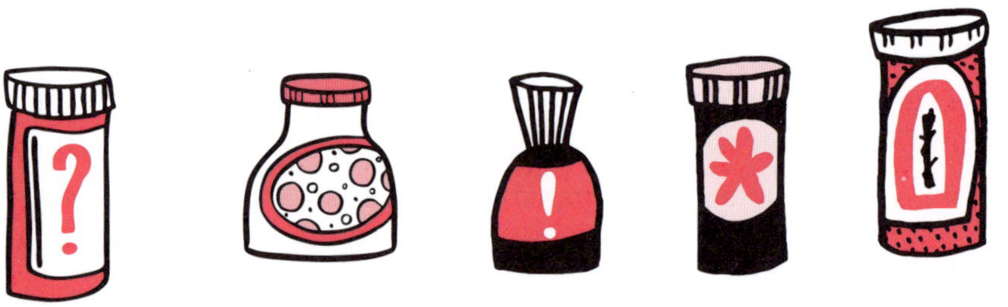

So-called bio-identical or natural progesterone creams

So-called natural progesterone or bio-identical progestogen products are not the safest kind of progesterone. Their ingredients, dosage and effects are not legally regulated. Gynaecologists and other menopause specialists are known to call non-prescription progesterone cream 'a scam', or if they're feeling generous, 'useless'. (One specialist I talked to called it 'mulch'.)

As for 'natural', non-pharmaceutical progesterone creams, they are usually also derived from yam or soy products and made in factories or laboratories, the same way as pharmaceutical products. When tested, some of these non-regulated products have been revealed to have contaminants, or not what's claimed, and have wildly varying levels of hormones, including none.

It took decades for medical scientists to work out the best kind of useful progesterone and how to deliver it. Non-prescription, unregulated products can't be safely used to balance or oppose estrogen medication to protect your uterus and its endometrium levels, whereas a pharmaceutical pill, progestogen-releasing vaginal pessary or IUD (intrauterine device) can.

Because of molecular what-can-go-into-what science, non-regulated synthetic progestogens (in other words, it's not progesterone even though the label might call it that) that are applied in an outer skin cream don't even get through to convert efficiently in the bloodstream. Imagine someone just hurling a parcel at your closed front door, and then setting fire to it. That's topical progestogen cream. It was delivered, but there wasn't much point.

There's no way to effectively change your progesterone levels using a 'natural' supplement, diet or by being less stressed.

Some naturopaths and 'wellness' commentators are telling women to try progesterone-only supplements for perimenopause symptoms, without an estrogen supplement. Some advise on how to make this happen without consulting or telling their doctor. This is not approved nor considered best practice by health authorities and relevant medical experts. If it's been suggested to you, please consult a gynaecologist or endocrinologist. And take no notice of marketing that claims it will 'fix' a low libido and make you more hotsy-totsy.

If you want reliable, approved, dose-sure progesterone, you definitely need a medical prescription.

Progestogens as contraception

A boosted dose of progestin, or a progestin-only formulation in a contraceptive Pill, or in a patch or injection, or an IUD such as the Mirena, triggers your body to make a kind of plug at the top of your vagina (doctors say it's made of 'mucus' and my god I wish they wouldn't) at the cervix entrance. The plug turns the cervix into a nightclub bouncer telling sperm it can't come in. Some progestin-only Pills known as the 'mini-Pill' are not as reliable as estrogen-progestogen contraceptive Pills, but newer ones that stop ovulation are available.

What does progesterone do?

More research is needed, but a good-enough level of progesterone can help:

* prevent pregnancy
* keep your uterus lining at a safe level
* set period timing
* prevent heavy periods
* guard against fluid retention
* protect memory skills (maybe)
* boost metabolism (maybe)
* combat fibroids (maybe).

> Tried progesterone cream. Didn't help at all. Katie, 61

> I'm furious I wasn't offered any practical or psychological knowledge. Just, 'Take these hormone pills.' Natalie, 59

Not enough progesterone can cause cellulite, according to bastard cosmetic surgeons who want your money and cannot cure 'cellulite'. Scorn them.

Possible effects of synthetic progestins (not progesterone) medication

* temporary or continuing 'spotting' bleeds
* tender, swollen bosoms
* cramps
* bloating
* constipation
* diarrhoea
* tiredness
* mood depression
* slight increase in breast cancer risk. (There's much more on this coming up.)

> Progesterone, the hormone that makes you Look More Attractive.
> *(Idiotic 'wellness' article without a single relevant back-up fact.)*

Many doctors think there's no good reason progestins should be part of combined hormone MHT, instead of micronised progesterone.

Possible downsides of micronised body-identical progesterone

Like all progestogens, for some people there may be mood swings and breast tenderness – but these are considered way less common with micronised progesterone. Some people experience tiredness and are advised to take the progesterone Pill before bed; doctors differ on whether there's an association.

Testosterone

You heard me. Yep, we have natural levels of testosterone throughout our lives, produced by our ovaries. Our bodies are so miraculous, they send some testosterone off round the bloodstream and use the leftovers to convert into estrogen.

Doctors suspect testosterone may play a role in our memory and mood, and probably sexual desire, but it's not clear how and why, and at exactly what level. It has no effect on vaginal dryness and other vaginal symptoms. (Needs more research, as per yewsh.)

When a woman's estrogen production naturally slows down, gets erratic or stops, or is suppressed by various medications, the unopposed, unbalanced testosteroney effects can cause pimples, rogue chin and upper-lip hair, and thinning hair, or a characteristic male-pattern receding hairline. Genetics also plays a role, and because hormone levels tend to be erratic in perimenopause, effects can come and go. Because we are complicated creatures, testosterone levels tend to rise again in our late 60s and 70s.

Testosterone has a relationship with dopamine, a hormone which triggers feelings of impulse, purpose, reward and incentive. Testosterone probably helps turn on dopamine in your brain. Too much dopamine and you have excess energy, more sex drive and find it harder to sleep. Low dopamine can cause the opposite: feeling low and can't-be-arsed. We know they're related but we're not sure yet exactly how testosterone, dopamine and the relaxing hormone serotonin are influencing each other, especially in women, because . . . *it needs more research.*

And it doesn't help to just take a testosterone supplement because, so far, controlled studies have shown little obvious benefit for women. In recent years, it has been approved to prescribe only for women who report being unhappy with a low libido and are officially diagnosed as having a desire 'disorder'. Studies are mixed about whether testosterone helps. Tests on women with low libido have shown they can have high, low, or middling levels of testosterone. Many doctors now believe boosting estrogen helps libido, and the right amount of testosterone may help some people, too. (More on testosterone in Chapter 6, It's Your Sex Life.)

Some doctors prescribe testosterone for women struggling with their libido. Testosterone is best delivered on the skin, as an ointment, gel or patch, because taking it orally risks liver damage. Too-high doses can have possibly irreversible effects including voice changes, acne, enlarged clitoris, and head baldness, so any testosterone medication should be a prescribed, approved, pharmaceutically produced version so the daily dose and its effects are covered by legal regulations.

Compounding pharmacies can make up off-prescription medications with testosterone in them, but the regulation of doses and ingredients, depending on the pharmacy policy, source of ingredients and the chemist skill, can be dodgy. Menopause specialists strongly advise against it.

Compounded testosterone pills, lozenges, pellets or 'troches' dissolved in the mouth are also not a good idea, due to various reasons, including a risk of raising cholesterol, and the effect of saliva and stomach acids on the medication, which creates an inability to control useful dose levels. You could be getting not enough, or too much.

Way more studies are needed about the effects of declining testosterone in menopause and what it means, and whether testosterone can be a useful supplement. In particular, experts say there are so many reasons why women might lose interest in sex during menopause (dry vagina, which can be treated; low-level skill of sexual partner; stuck-in-a-rut; have you got a good book to read?). (See Chapter 6, It's Your Sex Life.)

You can act crazy and know it but be unable to do anything. It's like standing outside your body and watching. Jane, 55

My menopause occurred when I had small children, dying parents and a depressed, low-functioning husband, so it's really hard to separate out. Horrendous! Annie, 62

How hormone medication developed

Hundreds of years before doctors even knew that menopause was related to hormones, they guessed at its causes and came up with the usual medieval nonsense about devils and the need to purge the body of poisonous period blood that could possibly scour a man's scrotum clean off, and prescribed non-fatal poisonings for women that caused vomiting or diarrhoea. Thanks for nothing, guys.

Other treatments that never worked included burning herbal vapours, praying, and various herbal tonics and concoctions of cheap ingredients for poor patients like garlic and fancy ingredients for posh patients like crushed pearls. You can read more about the idiotic history of women's medicine in my book *You're Doing It Wrong: A History of Bad & Bonkers Advice to Women*. Midwives and mothers often knew herbal recipes that might help hormonal symptoms, though none could even dream of the range of reliable and strong effects of regulated and properly tested modern medicine.

Around about the early to mid-20th century, scientists worked out what vitamins were, as well as hormones, and how they might be able to be used as medication. In the decades since, we have learned much more – but not enough – about how hormones can rule, refresh or ruin our lives.

Now, millions and millions of women around the world take daily MHT prescribed for menopausal symptoms, including more than 350,000 Australian women. Hundreds of millions more use hormone contraception Pills or devices.

As mentioned, in the Survey for this book, most women taking hormone medication said they didn't really know if any of the medication they took was working. Which makes sense, because how do you know if your symptoms would have been worse, or would have disappeared anyway if you weren't taking medication? The 'don't know if it's helping' factor was just over 52 per cent for women taking antidepressants, rising to almost 90 per cent for bone-loss tablets, 92 per cent for testosterone, and 94 per cent for hair loss medication.

I have chosen not to take it, mainly because I have coped without it.
Julie, 63

How they make hormone medication now

I've spent manaaaaany hours trying to understand how hormones are made these days. Have you ever tried to get a global pharmaceutical company to tell you how they make their patented medication? Do not on any account bother.

A local compounding chemist let me put on a mask that precluded sneezing or breathing on anything; I put my hands behind my back and peered into a bottle of ultra-white fine granule powder, only slightly clumpy. It was a teensy bottle of estrogen, arguably the most powerful substance in the world. But how did it get in there?

The first hormone medications were crude and produced in way-too-high doses. No longer. And vegans and animal rights folk will be glad to know hardly any hormones at all are now made with pregnant horses' wee, and so it's easy to avoid them.

I was hoping to be able to clearly explain how they turn a big crop of yams into estrogen, and then how they convert that into progestogens and testosterone.

I bored a tippety-top CSIRO plant scientist who has a brain full of complex knowledge to a standstill and made her explain stuff for hours and here's the condensed version: almost all of the world's pharmaceutical-grade estrogen, progestogen and testosterone supplements are made in highly-regulated, super-clean giant laboratories using commercially secret recipes.

They use enzymes in giant, sterilised vats to break down the natural chemicals in yams so the hormone components can be extracted and distilled, then they dehydrate the results to end up with a powder.

Non-regulated, non-prescription, so-called natural hormone treatments are often also extracted from yam or soy products, but those are not covered in the same way by legal regulations and registrations on ingredients, sources, quality, resulting formulations, and known effects at which doses.

Again, the best way to get quality-controlled treatments with reliable doses and effects in hormone medications is to buy a product subject to the government regulation, product registration and licensing of a reputable pharmaceutical company's products.

Not one single doctor I described my symptoms to – as I cried and asked for help before I lost my mind or my career or both – suggested I was experiencing severe perimenopausal symptoms or offered specific treatment for that as the underlying cause. **Em, 51**

My mum had hot flushes at least ten times per day from the age of 48 until her late 60s. Not given HRT due to her breast cancer. Natural therapies made no difference. Finally demanded HRT from doctor. **Kabbie, 58**

What estrogen in MHT can do

If any of these things are really stuffing up your quality of life, MHT can probably help. Hang on to yer hat. It:

* stops hot flushes and night sweats
* strengthens the pelvic floor and bladder ligaments so less accidental weeing
* improves concentration
* improves memory
* may help with confidence, self-esteem and oomph
* combats anxiety
* increases bone density and reduces fracture risk
* helps regulate sleep patterns
* lessens heart disease and stroke risk
* strengthens ligaments and joints
* lubricates vagina
* maintains microbiome and healthy vaginal bacteria
* helps combats itchy skin
* helps combats dryness of skin a bit
* helps combat hair loss, coarseness and fronty-phouffiness a bit
* reduces the risk of colon cancer.

> HRT helped but was too expensive to continue. Herbal medicine did not help and was expensive. Penny, 54

Possible benefits of estrogen in MHT

Research continues, jury still out:

* might help maintain libido
* may slow onset of dementia.

> HRT has helped with mental symptoms. I feel a bit less stressed and miserable than I was, and I am being nicer to my family. Justine, 52

What MHT supplements don't help

Estrogen in MHT won't:

* kick in for about six weeks, probably
* restore your fertility
* allow the ovaries to make and release more eggs
* fix arthritis (but does help with joint aches)
* reverse greying hair
* prevent or cure dementia
* stop or reverse wrinkles.

> I have a heart condition, so I can't take most menopausal medication. I feel a bit lost as a result. Karen, 46

Known benefits of MHT

Estrogen and progesterone in prescribed and legally regulated MHT hormone medications have been proven to work in holding steady, reducing or banishing many troublesome perimenopause symptoms.

Meta-analysis studies (combining the results of several pieces of reliable research) show that being on MHT reduces the risk of bone fractures, and if started within 10 years of menopause, it significantly lowers the risk of heart disease and fatal heart attacks. Smaller studies suggest it may also be protective of brain function and pelvic floor resilience.

Anyone with a history of breast cancer, endometrial cancer and blood clots or stroke probably can't take MHT for safety reasons. There's more on this coming up.

Advantages of taking MHT

If it's right for you, MHT is by far the best treatment for menopausal women.

MHT can help you reverse or manage:

* mental health and brain fog problems caused by lack of estrogen
* physical symptoms caused by lack of estrogen (see list below)
* protects your bones from thinning or fracture
* reduces the risk of heart disease, stroke and blood clots
* reduces the risk of cardiovascular disease
* reduces the risk of colon cancer.

Other facts about MHT

* It does not cause cancer.
* It does not significantly raise the risk of breast cancer.
* In many cases it's exactly the same as the hormones your body makes.
* Prescribed doses are precisely calculated and known.
* The manufacturing of them is regulated by laws.

Physical symptoms MHT can help with

* hormone-related depression, brain fog and other mental symptoms
* hot flushes, night sweats
* hormonal heart rate changes and migraines
* dry vagina symptoms

* pelvic-floor-related wee symptoms
* bones being more at risk of thinning and breaking.

> MHT was the only thing that worked 100 per cent.
> Joss, 54

More on what MHT can and can't do is explained for individual symptoms in Chapter 4, It's Your Mind, and Chapter 5, It's Your Body.

What MHT dose is best?

Some women in the Menopause Survey for this book said they had increased or changed the dosage of estrogen or other hormonal medicine recommended by the prescribing doctor. *Don't do this*. It's very dangerous and can create a cancer risk where there wasn't one before.

If you are unsure about recommended doses, see a GP or a specialist. The same goes for herbal or vitamin supplements: never increase a recommended dose. More isn't always better and 'natural' doesn't always mean safe.

The Pill versus MHT

The usual dose of MHT for menopausal women has lower levels of estrogen and progestogens than the levels in contraceptive pills. As mentioned, women who are in some kind of early menopause will probably be prescribed the Pill and/or an IUD rather than MHT, until they're at an expected age for perimenopause. They'll then stop, or switch to MHT.

If you're suspected of being in perimenopause during your 40s, instead of MHT you may be offered the Pill and/or an IUD for the first few years, especially if you need contraceptive coverage as well as the benefits of supplemental hormone medication. Many newer Pills are considered better formulations for perimenopause than older ones.

> I'm reluctant to fuck about with what nature is delivering.
> Fanny, 56

Talk to your doctor about whether the Pill, in any formulation, is right for you. Beware of alarmist or complacent information saying the Pill causes cancer or is a cure-all. Neither is true.

Is it unnatural to take prescription hormone medication?

Yep, it's just as unnatural as wearing glasses, using contraception, taking insulin for diabetes and getting a broken leg repaired with pins and plaster. It may or may not be a good idea for you but that has nothing to do with whether it's natural.

It was a life-saver despite my years of reluctance to go on HRT. I spent a fortune on natural therapy treatments, but unfortunately they didn't help with my sleep or night sweats. Katie, 57

As a personal aside, I've needed hormone medication almost continually since I was 12 due to rogue period pain, endometriosis, the need for contraception and then menopause. I'm so grateful for the assist.

At any given time, up to one in nine women will have endometriosis and probably need hormone medication to be as well as they can be. At any given time, more than 250 million women around the world are on the Pill and millions more would take it if they could get it. More than 160 million of us, including more than a million Australians, are using a hormone-emitting IUD implanted in their uterus. Untold hundreds of millions are taking MHT, which includes an estrogen and progesterone component. Millions more women are taking a form of testosterone for their libido, although estrogen might help as well as or instead of testosterone.

Reasons MHT might not be right for you

You may be advised not to take MHT if you have a history of breast cancer, endometrial cancer, blood clots or stroke (details on why coming up). MHT can make some fibroids worse. Some women have annoying or bad side effects from MHT.

If all your symptoms can be fixed without taking MHT medication, you don't need it: say, you give up alcohol and your sleep problem goes away; or your only troubling symptom is vaginal dryness and you decide a lubricant during sex is all you need.

Also good reasons not to: you don't want to; you don't need extra help protecting bones and pelvic floor health; or you feel pressured to take it because everyone in your friendship group seems to be doing it.

There was a lot of confusing, conflicting info out and about 10–15 yrs ago, which is why I'm not taking it. Jodie, 50

As someone who is in surgical menopause, HRT is important for me to take to reduce the risks of heart disease, osteoporosis and an assortment of other diseases/illnesses. Ruanne, 44

I will say that some people seem evangelical about it, [saying] that it will solve everything, and being rude to those who choose not to take it. Trish, 50

I have banned my friends from talking about it now for more than ten minutes, as that was all we were talking about! **Brigid, 54**

I felt that no one really talked about it before my early 40s, then all of a sudden it was on the agenda. **Flic, 51**

Can I request HRT? **Sansha, 46**

(Yes, bring it up with your GP, gynaecologist or endocrinologist.)

My first HRT prescription was written for me by Iza Segal. **Marion, 94**

(Dr Segal was a brilliant obstetrician and gynaecologist, women's health and abortion activist; she was born in 1914.)

Sadly, many women just can't afford the doctor visits and prescriptions, even if it would really help them. To make things cheaper, ask for the maximum number of repeats allowable on a medication. Tell your doctor that if a medication subsidised by the Pharmaceutical Benefits Scheme (PBS) would be just as useful for you, you'd like the cheaper version. Many specialists and doctors will reissue your next prescription without charge: check if yours will. If your GP can give you prescription repeats, it will be cheaper than going back to the specialist.

Combined estrogen & progesterone MHT

When the first Pills came out in the 1960s, they had unnecessarily high levels of estrogen and didn't contain a balancing dose of progesterone. As already banged on about, women taking estrogen medication who have a uterus need to also take a protective dose of a balancing, or 'opposing' progestogen for safety.

If you don't have a uterus, you can probably just take an estrogen supplement if you need its benefits, but always check with a doctor. An exception might be if you have no uterus but do have severe endometriosis, because then having progesterone as well will help keep your endo in check, but see a specialist.

Combined estrogen-progestogens contraception and menopause treatments are available in a frankly bewildering number of doses and options – in the same pill perhaps, or prescribed to be taken separately (either daily or in long-release products) or a combo of pills, patches, rings, gels, sprays and creams and IUDs.

MHT: Patch, pill, pessary, gel, implant, spray, or cream?

Hormone medications are delivered in different ways, for different sensible reasons, including any single or combination of a spray, gel, patch, pill, cream, implant, IUD or pessary. Ask a doctor what the best combo is for you, and the best way to deliver them.

Sadly you can't just say, 'I'd rather take a pill, not have to do slathering with gel' because different delivery systems are more efficient and safer, depending on the hormone or medication.

The treatment of menopause symptoms is already a two-tier system, with richer women having much more choice than women on a tight budget or a government benefit. Some menopause products are subsidised by the federal government's Pharmaceutical Benefits Scheme (PBS), and some are not. When one brand, or method of delivery (for example, a patch versus a pill) is in short supply at pharmacies, sometimes your doctor may have to switch you to a way more expensive one, or one with more likelihood of side effects.

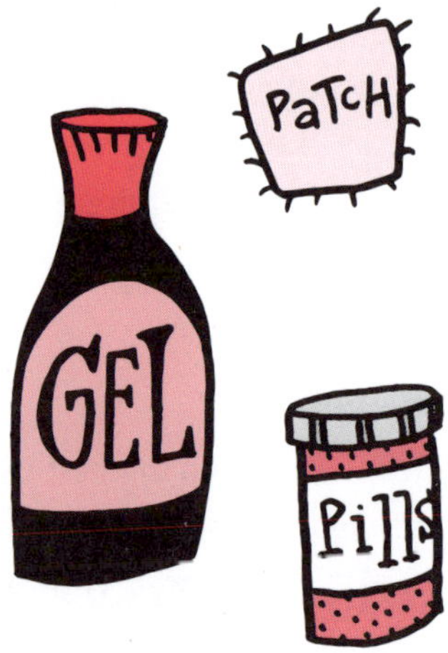

In some cases, doctors will avoid prescribing a tablet that gives your liver extra work to do processing it or subjects it to the destructo-ravages of your stomach acids before it can do anything useful. Other hormones need to be delivered to a very specific spot in the body. You may have individual medical needs requiring a specific delivery method.

Some people sell non-prescription or compounded hormones as a 'troche' or lozenge in the mouth: menopause specialists advise against them. Doses can be too much or too little because of saliva-dilution and swallowing, and ingredients and doses are unregulated.

Where possible, estrogen medication for menopause symptoms is usually delivered as a gel, cream or patch, to lessen the small risk of blood clot side effects.

Some medication isn't well absorbed or as useful if delivered through the outer skin, including progestogens. Using non-prescription, so-called bio-identical progestogen cream, even with estrogen medication, may mean your body absorbs the estrogen but doesn't take in enough progestogen, putting you at higher risk of endometrial cancer.

The progestogen considered the most likely not to depress mood, with the best delivery and useful absorption is progesterone taken as pills. The other very common delivery system is progestins in a sustained-release contraceptive IUD (such as a Mirena) put into the uterus, usually lasting about 5 years. Other options are patches and vaginal pessaries.

If you don't need contraception you may get an MHT prescription for a gel or patch for the estrogen, and a pill for the progesterone. It can get annoying and complicated when doctors have to juggle and switch patches and gels and pills when there are shortages of MHT brands and products: they will always be looking to make sure you get enough progestogens to balance the estrogen.

What's available in hormone medication isn't driven by the most logical way to get useful hormones into you. It's decided mostly by the 'free market' with some important government interventions. It's about what pharmaceutical companies have spent money on, for required tests to prove their products' effects, ingredients and dosages; whether the government has approved a brand or formulation for a subsidised price; whether developing a better formulation is cost effective; and it's also about the global supply of trustworthy regulated ingredients and supply-chain logistics.

Where to put patches, creams sprays & gels on your body

A lot of MHT estrogen-only and combined estrogen–progesterone gels and patches have packaging that simply says, 'Use as your physician directs', which is pretty useless when your doctor forgets to, or says, 'Just put one on, once a month' or 'Slather one pump of the gel on every day'.

MHT patch packet instructions should have all the stuff you need to know about what to do if one peels off, and how to store and dispose of them. Patches can peel off if you put them on moisturised or sweaty skin, can cause glue rashes for some people, and usually get fluffy on the edges as they pick up fibres from clothes.

Patches often have instructions to put them on your skin in a place where it's clean, dry, unbroken and un-lotioned. Sometimes this is on your stomach, somewhere under waist level, or the top half of a buttock.

The recommended placement of gel or patch estrogen usually just reflects where the product was put on the people who participated in clinical testing trials.

A lot of women choose to put their estrogen or combined patch on their back, or upper arms, where it won't be rubbed by waistbands or clothes seams. Whatever is convenient for you is probably okay, but check with your prescribing doctor (you can ring the doctor's office manager and ask them to get back to you).

Estrogen gel is often recommended to be thinly slathered down the length of an arm or thigh, again depending on how the product's scientific trials were done. You don't have to massage it in. Wait for it to dry before covering it with clothes.

You can safely apply MHT medication sprays, gels and patches almost anywhere on your outside skin (i.e. not vulva or vagina) but never on your breasts. That's because there are so many estrogen receptors in breasts, and the effects of putting it there long term, as a possible cancer or other risk, are unknown.

We're also cautioned not to use vaginal estrogen cream just before sex in the vulva or vagina area. But that's just so you don't get it on a partner. You'd have to get it on them every day for it to have even a little, residual effect, and even then nothing noticeable would happen (for example, a male partner wouldn't get a smaller penis or grow bosoms). If a male partner is worried about it, on with a condom for him.

It may seem obvious, but people taking estrogen through their skin are best off not swimming, bathing or showering within one hour of application. Or, fairly obviously, exfoliating. Keep hormone medication away from children: it will affect them too. Never use more than the prescribed dose or double-up on patches.

Vaginal estrogen is delivered to the top of the vagina, against the cervix, using the new plastic plunger that annoyingly comes with every tube, instead of us being able to recycle one.

Putting estrogen gel on your face or elsewhere will not make you look younger. Putting an estrogen patch on your ankles won't make them look younger, either.

I'm on my second menopause. Took post-breast-cancer medication, which gave me menopausal symptoms. Then about 4–5 years of perimenopause. Jess, 45

I read you should only take it for 5 years, but my GP said that if I had regular monitoring and mammograms it should be fine. Di, 58

Knowing this is likely/possibly due to hormones and perimenopause is actually comforting – I have a reason for it. Kathryn, 47

HRT hasn't solved everything. Despite receiving excellent treatment now, I still cry a lot for minimal reasons and don't feel like the same person I used to be. Megan, 51

MHT & safety wrap-up

The medical consensus now says the safest way to use MHT takes these factors into consideration:

* Get individual medical advice.
* Start using it soon in perimenopause, and within 10 years of your last period.
* Start using it immediately in diagnosed 'early menopause', whether premature ovarian insufficiency or caused by surgery, and take it at least until the average age of menopause.
* Go for the lowest dose that works for you.
* It might not be safe for you to take MHT if you've had breast or endometrial cancer, blood clots or a stroke. Doctors may also factor in family history.
* If you've had a hysterectomy, you can take estrogen-only MHT.
* If you have a uterus, you'll need combined estrogen-progesterone MHT.
* Progesterone is almost always the best form of progestogen (an explanation of this is coming up).
* There's no set limit for how long you can stay on it: depending on your individual needs and risks you may stay on it indefinitely.
* Don't take non-prescription or pharmacy-compounded estrogen, progesterone or testosterone products, sometimes called 'natural' or 'bio-identical'.

I got breast cancer this year. Thanks to breast screening it was found early; successful treatment. I would take HRT again, even if I knew about my future. Menopause was that bad. Lucy, 58

The lack of control is similar to pregnancy, when you are reminded that your hormones rule your life. Ursula, 47

Crazy to have teens while going through this – just too many hormones in the house. Niccy, 48

After my hysterectomy at 28, my doctor said I didn't need hormones, which in hindsight I disagree with. I experienced hormone fluctuations for 25 years. Sue, 62

Can I take MHT if I've had cancer, blood clots or a stroke?

No, in many cases. Best-practice medical advice during perimenopause can be different for you if you have or have had cancer in a part of your body with estrogen receptors. That includes breast cancer, endometrial cancer or ovarian cancer, or a history of blood clots or high blood pressure.

Several non-hormone medications can be really useful against your perimenopause symptoms if you can't take MHT, including some medicines originally developed for other purposes. More on those coming up.

Get advice from your oncologist or an endocrinologist or gynaecologist, as well as a GP who's up with the latest alternatives.

The general advice for you is:

* Probably or possibly a big no to MHT using estrogen pills or patches.
* Almost certainly yes it's fine for using vaginally delivered estrogen creams or pessaries.
* Absolutely no to compounded so-called bioidentical or any non-prescription estrogen or progesterone products.
* It's fine to eat or drink normal amounts of phytoestrogen-containing stuff, including soy milk, linseed bread, and tofu: it won't have anywhere near enough of an estrogenic effect to cause any danger and doesn't interact with your estrogen receptors in the same way. (More coming up.)
* Yes indeedy to any non-medical things that may help you feel generally better, including exercise, sleep therapies, relaxation and meditation. (See Chapter 3, It's Your Approach, and for lubricants for sex, see Chapter 6, It's Your Sex Life.)

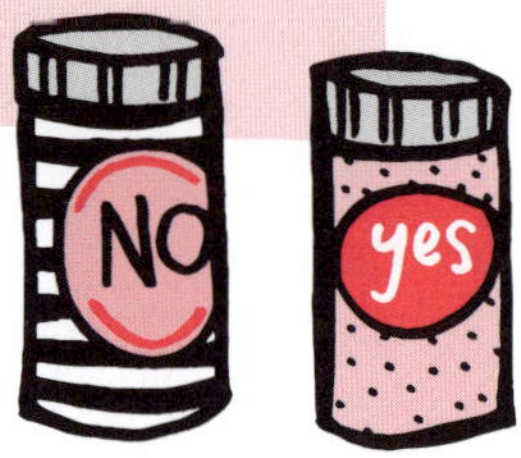

When you should stop taking MHT

I can't answer this one for you: keep in touch with your prescribing doctor. Make sure they know the latest safety info on who can take MHT, and discuss your individual risk level, and the pros and cons of coming off – or staying on indefinitely, which is now considered safe for many of us. Get mammograms every 2 years, have any breast lumps or texture changes, vaginal bleeding, and other worrying symptoms immediately checked out.

Does MHT cause cancer?

No. MHT does not cause cancer. MHT is associated with a small extra risk for some conditions, but many other factors pose a much greater statistical risk (see what those factors are, coming up).

Old, useless research and reports based on outdated medications and discredited research methods, which had huge media coverage many years ago, are still frightening and misleading people.

There's some evidence it protects against colon cancer.

Does MHT cause endometrial (uterus) cancer?

No. In the past, women were prescribed too-high doses of estrogen-only hormone treatment for menopause symptoms. It was discovered that taking estrogen supplements only in menopause, without progesterone, caused overgrowth of the endometrium – the lining of the uterus (aka womb). This raised the risk of cancer developing. The danger is now so well-known, no properly trained doctor would prescribe estrogen-only hormone treatment to someone with a uterus. But because some women are buying non-prescription and compound hormone treatments with unregulated doses, the danger still exists.

> Had a surgical menopause about 5 months after starting chemo for uterine cancer. I did not expect to be here celebrating being 56: elated to just be upright and breathing on this good earth.
> Lou

Does MHT cause breast cancer?

No. Some people are scared it does, because they've heard or are relying on old, discredited research that caused headlines around the world. A now-notorious 2002 study called the Women's Health Initiative, and the way it was reported, scared women and their doctors off hormone treatments and caused the use of what was then called HRT to plummet. The study's authors claimed that they had to stop even studying HRT because a small but significant number of the women taking combined estrogen and progesterone were reporting heart disease and breast cancer. They held a press conference which made their conclusion seem even more alarming and urgent.

Basically, what most people heard was 'HRT = big risk of breast cancer'. Other studies have also reported risk increases, including one in 2019, which it turned out was based on old data relating to hormone formulations that are no longer used.

This had a cancelling effect in global hormone research: HRT and then MHT was considered or suspected to be so dangerous, you couldn't ethically give it to women in more studies to check how dangerous it really was.

It took more than 15 years for the truth to come out. Not all the authors of the Women's Health Initiative Study had agreed with the assessment that stopped the study. Scientists and doctors pointed out the medications in the study were given to much older women, at way higher doses than the standard modern ones. Problems with the method emerged: the study didn't control for how long women had already been in menopause, or for weight, or conduct proper medical follow-ups.

Years ago, doctors were told they could cautiously re-introduce prescriptions for HRT but only to women desperate to deal with menopause symptoms, and they should only be allowed to take HRT (now MHT) for 5 years tops. Now, the latest medical approach is that there's no need for a 5-year limit if the benefits far outweigh a small risk and patients are fully informed.

A very small increase in the breast cancer risk for women taking combined MHT (estrogen and progestogen) is accepted by all global medical menopause expert organisations. They all advocate for women to be fully informed about risks and benefits by a prescribing doctor, and for all women to be vigilant and keep up with screening tests for breast cancer.

One meta-analysis of reliable studies calculated that in a group of 1000 women taking combined MHT for ten years, four extra women might be expected to develop breast cancer.

No difference has been noted in the prognosis for recovery of women who'd taken combined MHT and who were later diagnosed with breast cancer – in other words, if you are diagnosed with breast cancer, and you have taken MHT in the past, you're just as likely to have treatment that eradicates your breast cancer as anyone else.

Because getting older is a higher risk for developing cancer, a woman reaching menopause within the average age range is more at risk than a younger woman, whether or not she's taking MHT.

It was like pulling teeth to get anyone to prescribe HRT. Jen, 61

Being a smoker with a family history of breast cancer, I will not be taking HRT if I do get menopausal symptoms. Kylie, 57

The biggest risk factors for cancers

These factors raise your statistical risk for developing breast and other cancers in your 50s. In roughly descending order of association:

* being above a healthy weight range
* not exercising
* having one, two or more alcohol drinks a day
* smoking
* eating processed meats every day
* taking MHT with a progestin, instead of progesterone
* getting older
* absorbing high levels of air pollutants, especially in mining towns
* living near heavy traffic
* never giving birth and never breastfeeding
* earlier first period and later onset of menopause.

Other risks & worries of MHT

No medication is perfect or without risk, and no benefit is gained if medication isn't taken. We will need to make up our own minds on the best available latest information. That's why you need the best GP and specialist you can find. While old articles and outdated fact sheets, and some out-of-date doctors say you shouldn't take MHT for longer than 5 years, or if you're over 60, that's now considered wrong.

To help keep up with the latest, check the list of trustworthy sources of menopause info on page 38.

If you've had a stroke or blood clots, or have a significant family history of them, oral MHT may not be prescribed for you, even though the associated increased risk is small: smoking is a far bigger risk factor. Talk to your doctor if you're concerned.

One meta-analysis sometimes quoted online is from several years ago, suggesting a link between hormone medication for menopause, and a hugely elevated risk for ovarian cancer for women in their 50s. After the research choice method and data were immediately challenged by many doctors in the field, the researchers radically revised their findings to say there would be one extra case of ovarian cancer in every 10,000 women taking HRT each year. Leading menopause experts say this is also extremely unreliable, and point out that a similar medication, the Pill, reduces the risk of ovarian cancer. It's probably fair to say that a much smaller increased risk of ovarian cancer on MHT is possible but not probable, and *we need more research*.

The consensus among specialist menopause doctors and endocrinologists now is that for a large majority of women, they can be confident that the cancer-related risks of MHT are very small and the benefits outweigh it, if those benefits are needed to help with menopause symptoms. The lowest dose that controls the symptoms is what to aim for. But we all need medical advice taking into account any factors that can change our individual risk.

If I stay on the Pill can I dodge menopause?

No, but you may not realise you're approaching it, or when you're in it. If you take a combined Pill (estrogen–progesterone), and you have what feels like a period when you stop taking it for seven days, even if you haven't ovulated, your body is just getting rid of the endometrium that the estrogen has built up.

You may have technically progressed to menopause, and your body hasn't made enough of the right hormones on its own to have a menstrual cycle with a period for at least a year.

If you abruptly stop taking the Pill and your body is already in perimenopause without you knowing, your hot flushes and other symptoms might be sudden and severe. If this happens you can 'graduate' to taking MHT (unless you have the contra-indications such as relevant cancer history or heart and blood clot misbehaviour).

Eventually, the amounts of supplemental estrogen and progesterone in the Pill won't be enough to stop you having perimenopausal symptoms, if you're going to get them. If they're a worry, you can swap from the Pill to MHT.

Why isn't ALL HRT on the Pharmaceutical Benefits Scheme [subsidised prescriptions]? Mine isn't! Michele, 61

It's so shit to be told to just put up with it when there is effective treatment available. Kathryn, 44

I don't really understand the HRT I'm on. Or what alternatives there are. Josie, 50

If I stay on MHT can I dodge menopause?

No. You can manage symptoms of perimenopause and menopause, but eventually you'll technically be in menopause because your body wouldn't be able to ovulate or have periods on its own.

Non-hormone treatments

Many non-hormonal medical treatments are available for perimenopause and menopause symptoms that people with a history of cancer can take. They can be useful in suppressing hot flushes, or other symptoms. More research is being done all the time.

Exercise and other self-help strategies (see Chapter 3, It's Your Approach) and cognitive behaviour therapy (see Chapter 4, It's Your Mind) have proven useful in helping women cope with menopause symptoms, with consistent research results.

Non-hormone 'natural' supplements

Most non-hormone supplement formulations are vitamin, mineral, herbal or other plant supplements, with little or no proven clinical outcome whatsoever on your hormone levels. It would be terrible if women were accidentally misled by those labels.

I haven't been able to find any non-hormone-containing products, devices or procedures that have proven clinical effects on hormones in published, independent, randomised double-blind, placebo-controlled scientific studies.

'Natural' hormone products

> Hot flushes were awful. Went on naturopathic medication with good relief. Moo, 56

A lot of people say they want to use safe, 'natural' hormones that work for menopause symptoms. Unfortunately, I don't think these really exist. Another problem is that some of what is sold as a 'natural' hormone supplement isn't really either of those things: it isn't natural and it isn't safe.

Many of the so-called natural products are made in a laboratory just like the pharmaceutical prescription hormones; but they're not regulated or covered by the same rules as pharmaceutical prescription medicines. A company still has to have evidence that non-prescription products work in the way they claim, but in some

> I tried so many different supplements – at one point I was even injecting vitamin B into my belly! Oh goodness, the things we will do!
> Monique, 60

cases the effectiveness of these products may not be assessed by the Therapeutic Goods Administration before they are sold. In some cases, they're sold by billion-dollar companies; sometimes the same pharmaceutical companies also manufacture prescription hormone treatments.

There's a multi-billion-dollar industry of vitamin, mineral and plant-based supplements marketed and sold as menopause treatment that have no hormones in them, and again, I couldn't find any evidence for ingredients that are known in that formulation to successfully or usefully change hormone levels.

What about herbal tonics and dietary products with phytoestrogens (pronounced fight-oh-estrojens) that are claimed to have a hormonal effect? Repeated, well-designed independent tests have shown that these products, often soy-based or with red clover, have such a weak effect on hormones, if any, that published, independent studies show little or no effect on significant hormonal symptoms. Even if some effects are observed, there can be other significant problems. See the section on phytoestrogen products, including red clover and black cohosh, on pages 89–90.

It's one thing to know that an ingredient can have some sort of theoretical effect on hormones, but that's different to that effect being measurable or useful or reliably produced in a dose to have effects in a person's body.

So, can herbal, vitamin, and other probiotic supplements adjust or change hormone levels? I think the short answer is no. That's why you see so many non-pharmaceutical products that talk vaguely of nutrients, or 'support' or 'are thought to help' or 'for' symptoms. That's because many of these products are limited to pre-approved, low-risk health claims in order to secure listing on the Australian Register of Therapeutic Goods. Therapeutic claims can't be legally made about products in Australia without listing or registering the product with the TGA.

> I concocted a muesli mix that was like a witches brew; I believe this was hugely helpful. I went the plant-based phytoestrogen route. Deb, 53

> I tried to go natural and just use a natural lubricant, but I had to use an estrogen cream, which absolutely works.
> Robyn, 54

> I tried some natural remedies, but they were expensive and I wasn't sure if they were worth it. CC, 57

Despite this, many women believe the products do help them with symptoms, and companies use alleged testimonials to sell their products in advertising and on websites. In many cases, there is little to no evidence that the effects claimed for the products are caused by the ingredients concerned, unless it's a placebo effect, or it's a coincidence, even if the effect is believed.

So-called bio-identical products

You'll hear these terms used to describe some hormone products and supplements. The problem is, the terms are confusing, and often used wrongly even by some doctors. The terms are used to describe different brands and types of both estrogen and progesterone.

Sellers of non-pharmaceutical, non-prescription hormone products used the marketing term 'bio-identical', often with the word 'natural', to imply that their product is safer or better in some way. Most often, it's used for progesterone creams: as explained earlier in the progestogens section, we don't know what's in these unregulated products or whether the doses are the same each time or useful.

As explained, a cream is definitely not a reliable way to deliver progestogens into your body. Marketers have pushed the idea as an alternative to pharmaceutical hormones, saying they're all made from horse urine (in fact, almost all pharmaceutical hormones are now derived from huge quantities of yams).

The medical profession began to use the phrase 'body identical' for prescribed pharmaceutical products, to try to reassure patients what they were getting wasn't particularly unnatural, and in fact was much safer, better-regulated and useful than 'bio-identical' and most compounded products. Then people involved in the natural therapies industry also began referring to non-pharmaceutical products as 'body identical'. *So* confusing.

In fact, both 'bio-identical' and 'body identical' products are made in a laboratory or factory (not crushed-up petals in a meadow despite pictures on labels). The main, crucial difference is that prescribed, ready-made, controlled-dose pharmaceutical hormone products are covered by strict rules on proven results, guaranteed ingredients and trustworthy, precise doses.

While 'bio-identical', compounded products are marketed as plant-based and assumed to be more natural, analysis has revealed they contain wildly differing levels of laboratory-produced hormones, including testosterone, cortisone and thyroid extracts, and possible contaminants. In at least one case the seller claimed their product had 'no chemicals' – which isn't even true of water, because everything is made of chemicals. It just sounded good.

It's a myth that a hormone treatment can be matched to your individual hormone levels, because your levels can change day to day or in moments, especially in perimenopause; some tests are known to be inaccurate, and an allegedly bespoke amount of hormones may do more harm than good.

It's now clear that the words 'bio-identical' and 'body identical' serve to do nothing but confuse us. There are no clear regulations about who can say bio-identical or body identical with an agreed legal definition. At the moment it's a fiasco, and so many women are none the wiser. If you hear 'bio-identical' or 'body identical', it's because somebody wants to reassure you that it's safe. Look beyond the label to the regulation of the product.

Compounded hormone products

Some doctors send prescriptions to pharmacists to make up a compounded hormone product, instead of dispensing a product already manufactured in an effective dose. It's like sending a recipe, and is how medicine used to be made at apothecaries hundreds of years ago. They can then be dispensed as a lozenge, powder, cream, or pellet. (See earlier in this chapter for why these delivery methods can be dodgy).

Sometimes this is OK but most doctors would say there would have to be very special circumstances that should be overseen by a specialist doctor and pharmacist. In some cases blood or saliva tests are used to allegedly inform the recipe for a bespoke preparation. Sounds good. Isn't. This produces unreliable and unhelpful results, in order to make what can be an unreliable or dangerous product.

Although some standard compound medications are safe and useful, you'd be sensible to be very wary of getting compound hormone medication for these reasons:

* Almost any useful variation of menopause hormone medication is available ready-made in pill, patch, spray or pessary form.
* Some doctors, especially if they're not menopause specialists, may not be best placed to 'write a recipe' for hormone medications.

* Some compounded products, when tested, have shown no hormones at all, or unpredictable levels in different batches, and contaminants.
* Some pharmacists have been taken to court by government regulators for dispensing supplements and products at higher than recommended safe levels.
* Sources of ingredients vary and may not comply with regulations that govern ready-made medications. Their ingredient sources and ability to withstand time or temperature changes are unknown.
* Some ethical pharmacists have sensibly refused to make up unorthodox DIY prescriptions.
* Patients can be told these formulations are more bespoke and tailored to their individual hormone levels. As explained, this is not a thing.
* Some might think these products are safer because they don't have a package insert with all possible side effects. The opposite is true.

BTW, when I went to pick up my prescriptions last week and got chatting about hormone products, the compounding pharmacist told me he'd just refused to fill a very, very high dose of estrogen in an invented prescription ordered by a GP. No ready-made pharmaceutical estrogen medications are anywhere near that high.

Worried, the pharmacist checked with the Pharmacy Board of Australia; its advisor agreed he shouldn't make that up or dispense it, especially if he didn't know what other medications the patient might be taking, and the customer should be advised to get a prescription for regulated hormone products. I'd already heard from another compounder of cases where rogue pharmacists have dispensed unregulated hormone products.

Anyway, then the pharmacy assistant approached shyly and asked if I knew how she could find an endocrinologist who she might feel comfortable with because her GP wasn't interested in her menopause symptoms. So within five minutes of getting to the pharmacy, we were all talking about some of the big unsolved issues of menopause. (I also got some dry shampoo.)

Phytoestrogens

Most 'natural' pills, liquids and powders sold for menopause symptoms are made from plants that contain phytoestrogens. In other words, they're plants with compounds that can bind to estrogen receptors in the body, but have a weaker effect. It's a bit like saying there are some parking spaces reserved for the Rolls Royces (body-made or medical estrogens), and a bunch of clapped-out Corollas have parked there instead (phytoestrogens).

The medical consensus is that though these compounds can take up the same parking spaces, independent double-blind studies keep showing that the plant versions simply don't have the same strong and useful effects as body or lab-made hormones.

I wrote about phytoestrogens as an alternative treatment as the co-author of a book more than 20 years ago called *Women's Trouble: Natural and Medical Solutions*, which suggested an equivalence. But research since then means we now understand it's nowhere near an equivalent effect. Eating or taking phytoestrogen natural supplements will not help you with severe menopause symptoms and an informed naturopath should now tell you the same.

Phytoestrogens don't have any significant effect on hormone levels, skin or vaginal lubrication, and don't protect your bones or heart. Although products containing soy extracts, or red clover and black cohosh are advertised as 'recommended for menopause symptoms' or 'relieves . . . menopause symptoms', or there are claims that a product is based on 'scientific research', naturopaths and doctors are now aware there's little independent research, especially on humans, to prove this. For women who have severe hot flushes, and some have up to ten or more a day, this won't fix it.

It's believed that women who swear by these products are experiencing a very weak estrogenic effect, which might help with very mild symptoms like a hot flush, or they're experiencing a placebo effect. Some research speculates that eating a soy-rich diet in childhood may have a protective effect against symptoms of breast cancer in life; others disagree.

If these products *did* have as strong an estrogenic effect on the body as body-made pre-menopause levels and medical hormones, they would be dangerous for those with a uterus who aren't also boosting their progesterone levels.

A recent pharmacy check showed that natural herbal preparations may cost from $100 to $400 a year depending on the brand, and where you buy them. None are recognised and subsidised by the Australian government's Pharmaceutical Benefits Scheme.

Several women in the Survey for this book said they used a black cohosh product and got liver damage or had 'upset my liver so I had to stop'.

[Red clover] definitely helped, but divorce was ultimately most effective. Lou, 61

The takeaway on hormones

We’re trained to think that perimenopause and menopause means that our bodies are faulty. Instead, each body is doing what it’s supposed to be doing with varying degrees of clunkiness or difficulty: every one of us will go through this natural transition somehow. We don’t have to put up with any difficult symptoms it causes.

Medical hormone medication is really efficient and useful for some perimenopause and menopause symptoms, but not all of them. It isn’t compulsory. It doesn’t cause cancer but not everyone should take it. Use trusted sources of info: not word of mouth, not ads and not random online searches.

Steer clear of non-pharmaceutical ‘hormone’ products which are not regulated or proven, and always know exactly what you’re taking, and why. Also, don’t eat anything that tastes like polystyrene. Nothing to do with hormones, just good advice.

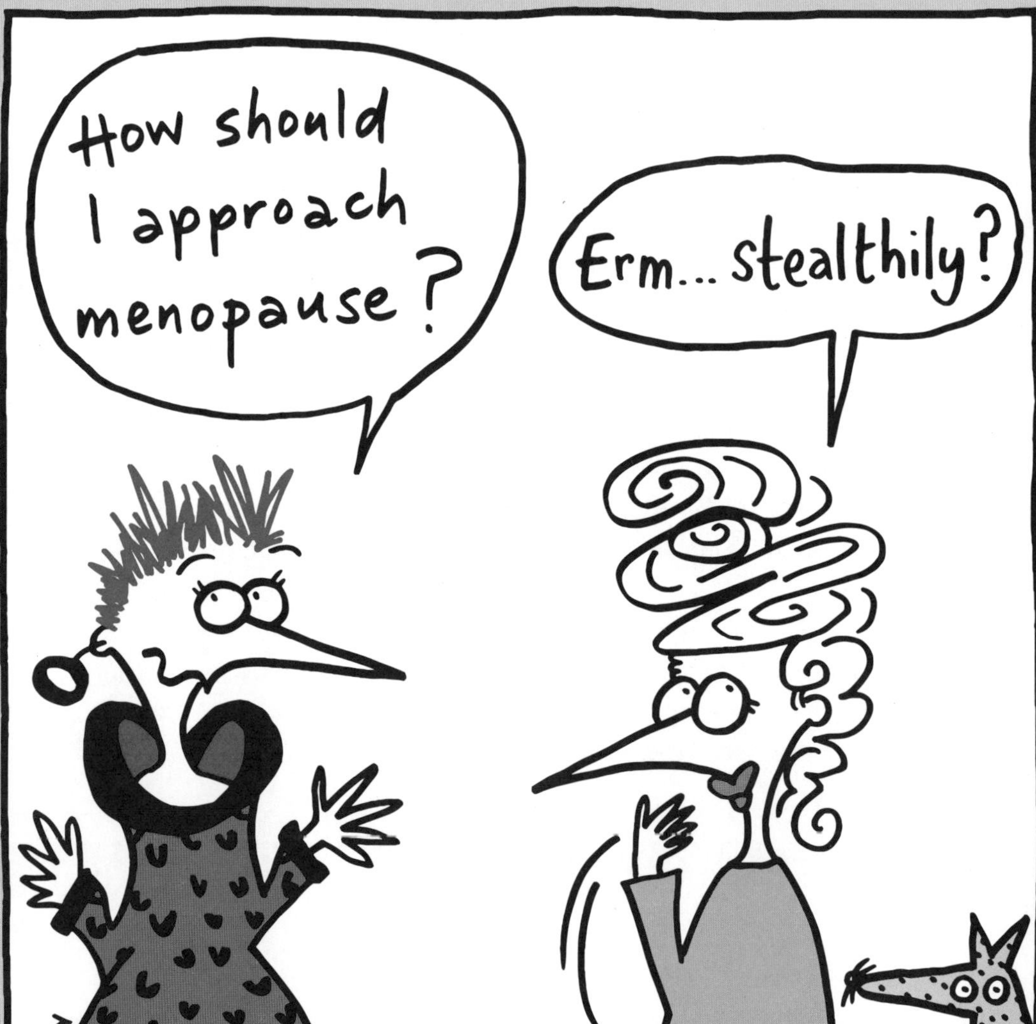
How should I approach menopause?
Erm... stealthily?
KAZ

3

It's Your Approach

There's a great divide in the way we all speak about menopause. Some talk about it in terms of loss: lost periods, youth, beauty, and worth, as if we should take to our beds with a jeroboam of whiskey. Meanwhile, others have an ultra-positive insistence that it's all about an explosion of freedom and independence and pleasing yourself. But how many menopausal women have the money for the gas bill AND a trip to the Amalfi Coast dressed in a creaseless white linen maxi-frock and orthotic-free espadrilles?

Neither of these extremes is much use, really. Sometimes you have to squint to see that, for most of us, the truth lies somewhere in between. If you have a rough time in menopause, it's unfair. And it's not right that it costs women more to live and get reasonable health care than it is for most men. But you're older. You're bolder. You get to take charge of menopause and the rest of your life, as much as you can. It doesn't have to tumble you over like a dumping wave you're powerless against.

You're a whole person, not just someone who's defined by being perimenopausal or menopausal. It is a time to look for the positives in your life, take stock mentally and physically, and do what women do best: organise, analyse and take charge as much as possible. Medications may not be the answer or the whole answer, and neither, for many, are lifestyle changes alone enough to help.

Do you want to white-knuckle it through awful menopause symptoms that are making you miserable because you've always had a philosophy of natural therapies? Do you want to ignore your diet and exercise because it's all too hard and surely there's a pill that solves everything?

I also thought it was a natural process, and with good management of food, exercise and lifestyle it would be easy. That's not what happened. Myrtle, 58

Self-help strategies and coping hints, and attitude-tinkering can make a huge difference to your life and experience of menopause. Even small changes in exercise, eating, and making choices that combat stress and help with mental health challenges (see Chapter 4, It's Your Mind, and all the other chapters, come to think of it). And for many, prescribed medication will revolutionise their experience. But how do you know what to choose, or try? This chapter presents a range of things that might help, for you to choose from.

Bloody hell. How not to panic about it? How not to feel sick and old and broken when I think about it? Cait, 45

You can't organise your way out of menopause but you can have a radically different experience by harnessing your considerable knowledge and skills.

To be able to do that, you need good quality information. There's power in knowledge: in knowing your options, and being able to make choices. You can choose some medical solutions, and some self-help solutions, and try out new ideas and suggestions: if a method or so-called remedy doesn't help, it's not your failure. It just means you're free to cross it off your list, or try it another time, and move on. Please check out the list back on page 38 of trusted info sources. Coming up in this chapter: how to talk to a doctor, or change to a new doctor to get the care you need.

It all seems very confusing and expensive. There are so many ads targeting me and I just want clear, objective information to help me navigate. Philippa, 46

Thought it would be much worse than it has turned out to be. The relief of no period pain and no random periods that I put up with for years is still so, so sweet. Cady, 53

Just another crappy woman body thing that we have to pretend isn't happening. Kirsty, 50

A lot of us bring our philosophy to menopause, and then have it challenged. We find out there isn't one medical solution or a pill that stops all the symptoms. Or we take a 'natural supplement' we expect to stop hot flushes, and it simply doesn't. We might have friends or even role models who tell us about a way that worked for them, and blame ourselves if it doesn't work for us.

Think of the possible treatments and approaches for perimenopause and menopause as a menu. You can choose what you fancy from any part of it. One of the reasons that Marie-Kondo-style decluttering is so popular in our age group is because it's a rare woman who doesn't feel overwhelmed with responsibilities and home and work precisely at the time when our mental health may also be taking a hormonal battering.

There are handy hints in this chapter to help make your mind and life clearer and less cluttered, whether or not your lidless Tupperware sparks joy.

Working out an approach to menopause

I would like everyone to know how amazingly life-affirming menopause can be. I'm more confident and happier than I was before. Beatrix, 50

In England, which has a huge population, there is a heated debate around menopause that has turned somewhat toxic. High-profile TV journalists made documentaries suggesting menopause was ruining women's minds, jobs and sex lives, and they weren't being given the info they needed, and that almost all women should probably take hormone medication for menopause symptoms and also to protect their bones. Lobby groups were formed demanding that MHT be available free and without prescription.

Hormone medication shortages and clogged GP schedules ensued. Then a backlash arose, saying many women didn't want or need hormone medication and the idea that menopause was a deficiency state was scaring people. Others insisted symptoms could be controlled by 'natural' supplements. A faction of columnists and commentators began to scoff at the idea that menopause was even a problem, calling it 'menopause mania' and recommending women 'just get on with it'.

One gasp-worthy headline was in London's *Sunday Times*: 'Menopausal moaners are taking time from cancer patients'. It's hard not to wonder whether they would have run the heading 'Bastard old people should just die, because they make hospitals more crowded'.

It also reminds me of the endocrinologist who had a woman patient sobbing in her office from desperation caused by lack of sleep and savage hot flushes that felt like panic attacks all day long. The patient had been dismissed by her GP with the line, "Well, it won't kill you, you just need to adjust'. I hope his scrotum turns into a house brick – well, it won't kill him.

Here's a round-up of the main views and philosophies about menopause. I suspect most of us have leanings already. I'd say I have a foot in almost every camp but then I'd be an octopus.

In the Survey, just under 80 per cent of respondents said it was a mental as well as a physical experience. About a third sought medical help, another third tried to find 'natural' remedies and about another third thought they just had to put up with it.

More than 3700 women had sought help in psychological counselling during perimenopause; about 44 per cent said it helped and almost half said they didn't know. Thousands also tried meditation with positive results. More than half of the people who took powdered or pill supplements said they didn't know if they worked. Others changed their diet: about 39 per cent didn't know if it helped; nearly half thought it had.

Felt hopeless and distressed. Thought medical profession couldn't help. Barbara, 58

I would like to know stories of others' experiences, especially the embarrassing ones, to normalise the experiences and take away the anxiety that you're having a mental breakdown. Keryn, 55

I want to hear that others think it is shit too. I hate all the goody touchy-feely stuff. Monique, 47

Spent thousands of dollars on 'natural' treatments to do this the 'right' way. (HRT was for weaklings.) Naturopaths, acupuncture, cannabis oil, herbal remedies, tea that smelled like cow dung . . . Finally HRT solved the hot flushes and resulted in migraines. Jodie, 53

I now believe menopause to be the cause of my epic midlife crisis. I should have been more prepared. Angela, 53

I accept this is a natural phase of a female's life. This is just a part of being female. I'm stronger because of it. Janet, 62

The Natural-Transitioners say:

'The natural transition of perimenopause to menopause shouldn't be medicalised, and isn't something to be cured. It's not a state of deficiency, and women are being pressured or gaslit into thinking they need help for symptoms. Women don't need hormone medication or supplements, just a good exercise habit and a healthy diet. Women don't "lose" estrogen and ovaries don't "fail". Long-term use of estrogen and other hormones is not tested, and the pharmaceutical industry is profiteering and not to be trusted.'

> My mum suffered terribly. It was awful and of course hit her at the same time as my worst teenage years. She was saved, as was our relationship, when she started HRT and I got my mum back. Nicola, 46

Supplement Fans say:

'I'm an older feminist who railed against the patriarchal medical system of the 1970s, and we should distrust the pharmaceutical industry and have a philosophical opposition to anything medical. There must be self-help treatments or herbal or plant supplements that do what pharmaceutical medications do.'

The Hit-Me-Uppers say:

'Menopause means a hormone deficiency, just like diabetes is an insulin deficiency; so supplemental medication just makes sense. If MHT takes away troubling symptoms, then use it. Better to take regulated proper doses than unproven treatments (that may be owned by supplement brands that are owned by the pharmaceutical companies anyway). The benefits far outweigh any small risk increases associated with MHT. I'll happily stay on it forever for other possible health benefits.'

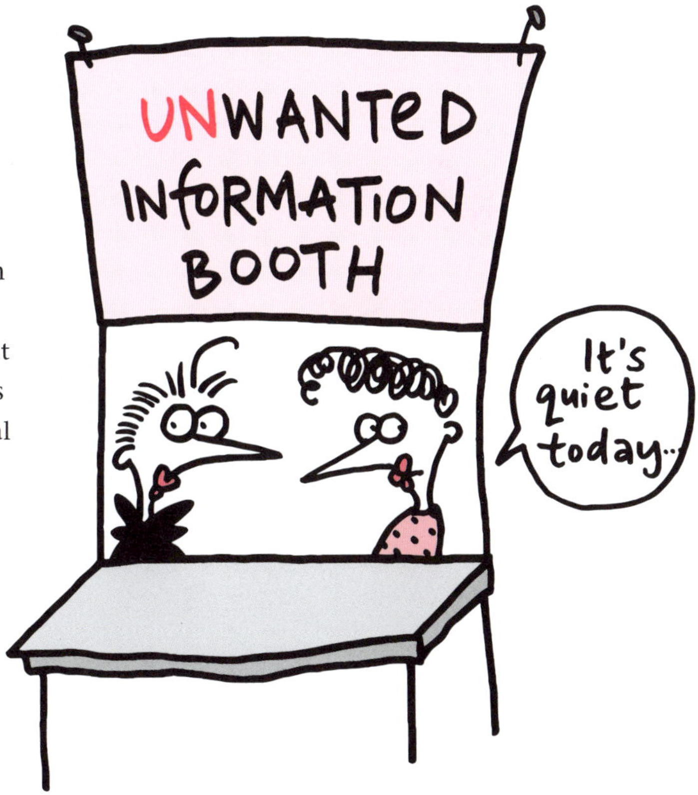

The No-Big-Dealers say:

'Menopause is just like puberty in reverse and temporary. Only Western women and whingers find it hard. If you don't expect a hard time you probably won't have one.'

Best things for me have been yoga and exercise. Jade, 50

The Don't-Blame-Menopausers say:

'Women's perimenopausal moods are not so much influenced by hormones. We already have perfectly sensible reasons for feeling depressed, anxious, lacking in self-esteem: lots of us carry an unfair load of emotional labour, home-organising, paid work, motherhood, daughterhood, and husbands who ignore the clitoris. Plus discrimination, social contempt, and the cumulative effect of being disregarded and belittled all our lives. Menopause symptoms seem worse and harder to cope with if the rest of our life is difficult.'

The Whalers say:

'We are fulfilling an anthropological function. Because whales and gorillas are the other mammals known to have menopause, and because older lady-whales are known to help look after the whale calves during migration, females past their ability to have babies are still useful for babysitting purposes, so that's why older women are still alive: to keep serving everyone else. I don't know why there isn't much research about gorilla menopause, probably because nobody wants to ask a 150-kilo gorilla about how her perimenopause is going, and I'm not sure how useful that study was about Japanese aphid menopause.'

The Re-Branders say:

'Menopause needs a fancy new name like "The Upgrade" or "Freedom Years"; "menopausal females" are instead "Wise Women". Hot flushes are called "power surges".'

Can medication be given to manage the stage when you can no longer tolerate mansplaining and misogyny? Beth, 54

I think holistically accepting this rite of passage made it quicker, easier to manage and less of a drama. Samantha, 53

I've tried all natural treatments, which didn't really work, but I haven't tried medicine yet as I feel I'm good for now and learning to live with the changes. Debbie, 50

The Behind-the-Timers say:

'I read on the internet 15 years ago that hormone treatment gives you cancer.'

The Queens-of-Denial say:

'Shut up, shut up, shut up. We refuse to "go through menopause". Never discuss it with others, endure the painful sex, don't let your old friends go grey because it reveals your real age. Hide in a cupboard during hot flushes. Try any medication or supplement if it's related to skin, hair or weight.'

For these women, it matters less what's going on inside, than out. (And they're so exhausted.)

The Let-Themselves-Goers say:

'Let's go grey, stop wearing make-up, chuck out all our old clothes in smaller sizes, wear expandable trousers, and hurl our high heels into the sun.'

The Oblivious say:

'Oh, menopause? I think I might be in it. Haven't had a period for years. Nothing else happened. The end.'

A tiresome, small subset of this already smaller group assumes everyone else has roughly the same experience. 'I don't know why anyone complains, it's fine.'

> I feel bogged down, aching and fatigued. Have been trying to go natural, but for mental wellbeing I'm thinking I'll go down the HRT path. I am lucky compared to some, but we are all fighting our own battles.
> Sara, 50

Stay flexible

The best way to judge what kind of strategies or help you need is: do you feel like you're struggling, mentally or physically? Are you thinking and reacting in ways you wouldn't have 5 years ago? Are your symptoms, whether flushes, sleep, mental or other experiences annoying – or horrible – enough for you to want treatment?

Are there self-help things you'd like to try before considering medication? Would you like to find a medical diagnosis before deciding? (Yes, you would.) Do you want to try natural therapies or go straight to medical treatment? What treatments are available to you, based on your medical history and what you can afford? How long do you want to endure symptoms before asking your doctor for help?

Of more than 6000 women who responded to relevant questions in the Survey, more than two-thirds used online searches using symptom keywords, more than half relied on friends for advice; almost a quarter talked to relatives, and about 14 per cent used a book. More than half consulted their GP, less than 4 per cent talked to an endocrinologist (hormone specialist), about 17 per cent had seen their gynaecologist, 3 per cent consulted a pharmacist and another 3 per cent got their info from a health food shop.

Now that the MHT breast cancer scare is over, many women are being advised to stay on some form of MHT indefinitely because estrogen will help keep bones stronger, and hopefully help prevent vaginal infections and vulva itching. As you get older you should check with your doctor that your MHT doses and brands are still the best ones for you.

I felt that along with my loss of child bearing I would become less of a woman. Susan, 59

Don't give up! Nothing stays the same forever! To get to the end of the tunnel faster, read a useful book about what you are going for; reach out to friends; be kind to yourself. Gretel, 58

I know almost nothing about MHT, other than that I don't want it. I wonder if I would feel differently with better education. Monique, 54

Don't be afraid to be YOU. Christal, 52

I can't believe the treatments are as limited and ineffective as I have found. If men got this, there would be a huge focus on fixing it. Kate, 55

Because HRT was touted as being risky at the time, I decided to try 'natural' remedies, which did not work for me. So I gave up and opted for endurance. Jennifer, 67

Don't be afraid to be honest if you're not coping. Vik, 58

When to seek help

If you are having physical and mental symptoms that interfere with your life, you have a right to seek help that could change your experience of life, at home, at work, in your friendships and in the privacy of your own brain.

I think I must have trust issues because this is the primary reason for me not seeking Western medical assistance. Faye, 49

I've given up on medical help. I've never heard there were any treatments. Writing this makes me teary. Eddy, 47

I'd be ashamed to go down a medical route as if my body was faulty not just needing assistance. Sorry, I'm a big hippy. Anne, 56

The most advice I've had is to exercise more and lose some weight. Chelsea, 49

I plan on riding right through it – mind over matter. I have survived this far in life and do not have faith in modern medicine to relieve symptoms that are not life-threatening. Laney, 51

Be proactive with your doctor

Hundreds and hundreds of women replying to the Menopause Survey felt they'd been shamefully and scandalously let down by their doctors: GPs in particular. Many described seeing one GP, or doctor after doctor, being patronised, dismissed, told to just put up with symptoms. Women were absolutely furious, sad and confused about being let down, fobbed off, and even laughed at by GPs. Many had given up going to the doctor or mentioning things they wanted help with.

Women described how doctors said they couldn't or wouldn't help, that it just had to be endured, that they didn't recognise perimenopausal symptoms, prescribed the wrong medication, suggested herbal treatments there is no evidence for, presumed something was menopause without further investigation, missed serious vulval conditions because they didn't even look and very commonly told women in their 40s they were too young for perimenopause, which is ludicrous.

Many doctors were said to be knowledgeable and sympathetic, and patients loved them for it. But GPs in general took a real whacking in the Survey. Frankly, if perimenopause doesn't send you into a rage, the appalling lack of knowledge and decency from too many doctors will do the trick. I feel for the good and dedicated ones because they've also been whacked by a pandemic, regional doctor shortages, staff under pressure, lower fees and over-crowded clinics.

Ask around among friends to find a good GP.

The Survey responses showed that a GP can be good, or bad, or informed, or caring, regardless of whether they're young, old, man, woman or non-binary. What matters is how much they care, listen and how much they know or are prepared to investigate for you. Although many of us had a preference for a woman GP, this didn't

> As a [trainee] doctor I had one lecture on menopause. Cathy, 53

> My GP was fantastic. Anna, 58

> I completed the Australasian Menopause Society's symptoms self-assessment and took it to my doctor. She disappointingly gave me the usual, 'Eat tofu, drink less alcohol and caffeine, take some random unproven herbal remedy.' Megan, 58

> I wish I could speak to someone for a lengthy period of time to understand all the stuff that's going on and my options. Sam, 50

> Doctors were so terribly dismissive of it, mocking me, laughing in my face, and telling me to go and do yoga, or learn to breathe, that it's just stress. It's punitive, shaming and humiliating. Jo, 47

> Why are so few doctors up to date with the latest menopause treatment options? It's their duty to be up to speed, surely? Ellen, 49

> The main issue for me has been a lack of knowledge by GPs and a lack of doctors specialising in women's health, in particular menopause. Melisande, 56

> First offer from GP at early symptoms, 'Have you considered tubal ligation?' I was thinking: You, sir, are a fuckstick and I'm never seeing you again. Anna, 49

always pay off in understanding; some younger doctors seemed better informed and supportive. Many women gave up going to the doctor about perimenopause symptoms after a bad experience with a GP (or several), while others felt their GP had almost saved their sanity and transformed their life. They were grateful for their kindness and expertise, and considered them partners in health care, especially the doctors who said some variation of, 'You don't have to put up with this.' See overleaf for 'Things to say to a GP'. And please see the list of trusted sources of info on page 38, many of which can recommend a specialist.

I've done a lot of research and my GP is great, so I talk to him about it and he's very supportive if I want some assistance to manage symptoms. Jacinta, 48

My GP, a woman, dealt with my issues with such sensitivity and didn't dismiss my concerns. Anna, 55

I went to a young female doctor. She said, 'I don't know anything about menopause as I haven't been through it.' Rachael, 57

I moved to a regional town and ended up finding a great doctor; the first to help me understand that the things I experienced were symptoms of menopause. Lucy, 54

I'm a doctor and had hardly any teaching on it in medical school. Kim, 48

It took all my courage to visit the GP to ask for help. His response was, 'Have some Valium.' Anon

My GP said – why should women suffer? Let's try HRT. Angelique, 51

I don't even know where to start, other than my fabulous GP. Danielle, 48

When I made it into the specialist's clinic, after waiting a month for an appointment, she looked at me with such compassion and said, 'You must be here because you need support'. Gretel, 58

My gynaecologist was fantastic; he explained everything. Lou, 53

Things to say to a GP

Book a longer appointment to introduce the possibility of perimenopause or menopause so your GP has time to respond and talk it through with you. You can show the doctor your list of questions so they can plan the consultation.

If you don't feel your GP understands what you're asking for, or if a GP tells you that you just have to put up with menopause symptoms, or that taking MHT is generally dangerous, or there's nothing you can do, or you feel dismissed, here are some things you can ask:

- What do I need to know before, during and after perimenopause?
- My symptoms seem to suggest perimenopause: what can you do to rule that out, or confirm it's likely?
- Please can you work with me to solve the symptoms that are making me miserable?
- What are the pros and cons of doing nothing?
- All global specialist menopause medical groups say that being in your 40s is not too young for perimenopause symptoms. Why are *you* saying it?
- What are the benefits and risks of different medical treatments?
- What is my safest course of action that helps with my specific symptoms?
- How long do you suggest I put up with life-altering symptoms before trying medication?
- If I don't want or can't take MHT, what else can you recommend to help with individual symptoms I'm experiencing, or my worst symptom?
- What self-help strategies can I try for my symptoms?
- If MHT is not recommended because of my medical history, or my family's, what are my alternatives?
- Can I safely use vaginal estrogen cream for dry vagina symptoms? What are my other options?
- Why are you diagnosing a vaginal condition without examining me or taking a swab?
- Why are you offering laser vaginal so-called treatment when independent studies and the Royal Australian and New Zealand College of Obstetricians and Gynaecologists recommends against it? (More on this shriekingly dreadful nonsense in Chapter 6, It's Your Sex Life.)

* Would it be better to try MHT before anti-anxiety or antidepressant medication for mental symptoms that may be caused by perimenopause hormone changes?
* Will herbal treatments or non-prescription treatments interfere with my other medications? Are there other dangers?
* How will you rule out non-menopause reasons for flooding periods?
* What are my best options for stopping flooding periods?
* How can I protect my bones and heart in menopause?
* Are you aware of the latest research and medication recommendations for perimenopause?
* Where do you get your up-to-date information about perimenopause and menopause?
* For heaven's sake, give me the name of another GP who is kinder and more knowledgeable.
* Please refer me to a gynaecologist or endocrinologist.
* When should I come back for a review?

If your GP is dismissive, rude, patronising, seems not to have the required knowledge or empathy, try to find another one. I'm really sorry this can be demoralising, infuriating and expensive. Many women answering the Survey said they found a GP who was a good partner and helped them through perimenopause and menopause. See 'Who's Who in medical & other practitioners' on pages 108–109.

I feel pathetic asking my GP for help in getting through something that pretty much every woman experiences. Ellie, 48

I sought help for increased heart arrhythmia, increased anxiety and panic attacks, aching joints, sore back from my mid-40s, and no GP mentioned the possibility of peri- or menopause! Until I did. Kim, 50

Every time I mentioned hormones to a doctor I could literally see their eyes roll. Sue, 44

Check out financial options

Perimenopause is really expensive: visits to the GP and specialists, pathology results for vaginal swabs to surgery costs, herbal and pharmaceutical products, counselling. Many women spend hundreds or even thousands of dollars a year.

Some things to consider:

* If you want to see a specialist, such as a gynaecologist or an endocrinologist, you need a referral from your GP. Ask for an indefinite one, so you don't have to keep going and paying for a new referral.
* Try to find a bulk-billing clinic (I know, it's hard, I'm so sorry).
* Ask prescribing doctors for the cheapest version of the medication you're being prescribed (usually something subsidised by the Pharmaceutical Benefits Scheme).
* Learn how to assess marketing and other advice targeting you, and decide who you want to listen to.
* As a public patient, you'll have to wait, sometimes months or even years, for non-emergency and 'non-essential' but necessary surgery, including a hysterectomy. Talk to your doctor about possible ways to move up the waiting list for medical reasons, or the best way to approach it.

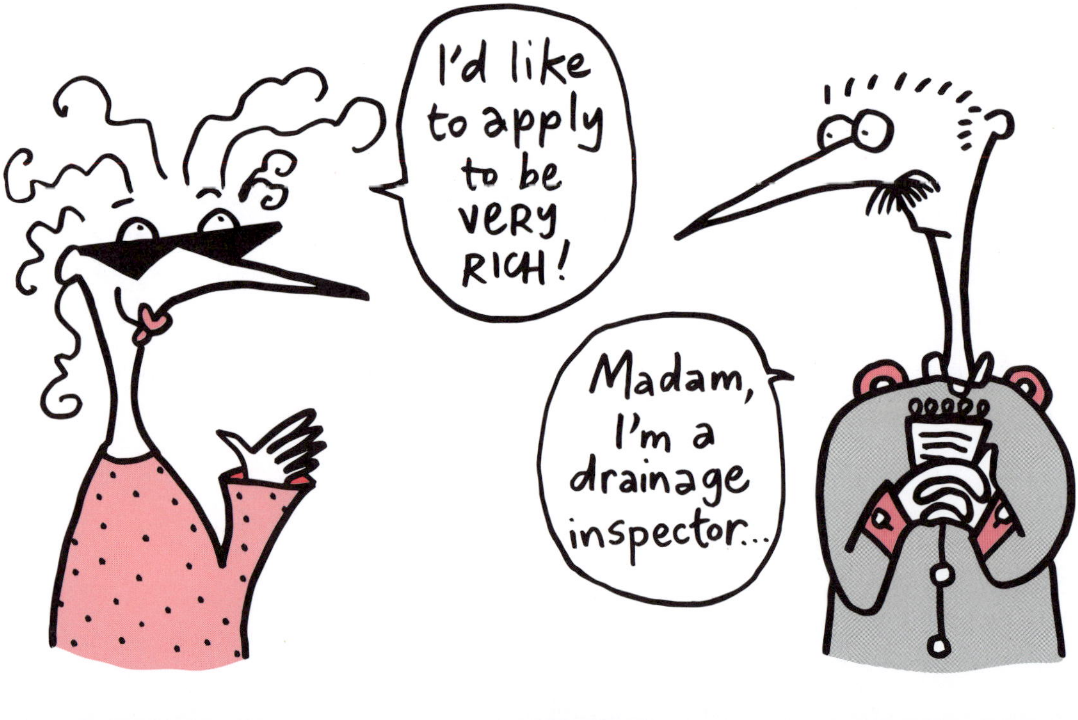
I'd like to apply to be VERY RICH!
Madam, I'm a drainage inspector...

I asked the GP if there was something I could do as I was so miserable and he replied with, 'What did you expect – you're 50.' I cried all the way home. Finally saw an endocrinologist who was so sympathetic and she put me on HRT. Has been a hard road.
Janine, 57

I've been to see three GPs and none have been helpful. I feel hopeless. I work 50+ hours a week and I just don't have the time to shop around for doctors, only to waste my time (and money) coming up short.
Julie, 50

Why did my doctor dismiss me when I tried talking about this? I had dry skin and labia itch, but I didn't know they were even a part of the menopause symptoms until doing your survey.
Kiri, 46

There's a real lack of female GPs – particularly mature female GPs who can bulk bill.
CDA, 49

I've no time or money for that luxury.
Sharon, 57

The GP said, 'Take some herbs and come back in a month if it's no better.' I WAS SO ANGRY but too fatigued to argue! I went back to see him a week later and told him off. He explained that because I lived in [a hippy area] he assumed I wouldn't want HRT. JFC!
Lorem, 53

My GP didn't think that my night sweats (so bad no kid will hug me in the morning) were menopausal.
Jo, 49

Doctors are human and not always good at their job. Find one who is actually listening to you.
Anna, 58

There is practically no support for women in isolated country areas. My male doctor refused to prescribe medication, telling me to soldier through it.
Lorinda, 55

If this shit happened to men there would be a specialist clinic on every corner and a plethora of treatment options.
Isobel, 54

I thought it was a problem for some women but medical science had the answers. Claire, 50

Who's Who in medical & other practitioners

If you search online for medical info, please see the list of trusted websites on page 38.

Don't settle for less than a combination of knowledge, skill and listening skills from your medical practitioners.

GPs

General practitioners are your local or family doctor and can diagnose, treat and help manage conditions, and refer you to a specialist doctor. Qualifications include a 4–6 year medical degree at an approved uni, an extra year of medical internship under supervision, a year of training as a resident in a hospital under the supervision of a specialist, then at least another year of further training and study as a resident at a hospital, then 3-4 years of further supervised, specialist GP training. They must pass a detailed exam, and continue ongoing education to remain a Fellow of the Royal Australian College of GPs (FRACGP). The Royal Australian College of General Practitioners site is **racgp.org.au**, and the Australian College of Rural and Remote Medicine (ACCRM) is **accrm.org.au**.

Pharmacists

A pharmacist has usually trained for at least 5 years; does a 4-year university science pharmacy degree, interns for a year supervised by a pharmacist, then must pass an exam to register with the Pharmacy Board of Australia. Any pharmacist can describe themselves as a compounding pharmacist but they should take specific training. Pharmacists are qualified to question dosages or formulations ordered by doctors if necessary, and help suggest alternatives in the case of shortages (they'll call the doctor to check if it's OK).

Specialists

A medical specialist can help diagnose and manage or resolve a set of symptoms or ongoing condition. They may also do specialist surgery.

Gynaecologist or Obstetrician

A medical specialist in health conditions involving the uterus, ovaries, fallopian tubes, cervix, vagina, vulva and breasts. They are qualified to deal, and may have a special interest, in menopause. Many are also qualified specialist surgeons.

Qualifications include a 4–6 year medical degree at an approved uni, then a supervised internship or experience as a hospital resident, 6 extra years of specific gynaecology and obstetrics supervised training, then practical and surgery experience plus updates to their knowledge. They should be a member of the Royal Australian and New Zealand College of Obstetricians and Gynaecologists. Its website is **ranzcog.org.au** and the qualification is FRANZCOG.

Endocrinologists

A medical hormones specialist. They also treat diabetes, thyroid conditions, some period disorders, endometriosis, and menopause symptoms. They do a 4–6 year medical degree at an approved uni, then an internship or residency in a hospital, and at least 3 years of advanced specialised training, of which one year will be research. Letters after their name: FRACP, Fellow of the Royal Australasian College of Physicians. The affiliated Endocrine Society of Australia site is **hormonesaustralia.org.au**.

Australasian Menopause Society & International Menopause Society members

These organisations extend knowledge through newsletters, conferences and websites, sharing research and results, and facilitating connections between doctors. Members must be qualified or retired doctors, nurses, or allied health professionals, researchers or student members at an approved institution.

Dermatologists

Medical skin and hair specialists. They've done 5–6 years medical degree and training, then at least 2 years of study and training in a hospital, then 5 years of extra study and training in dermatology. Most dermatologists don't advertise for patients unless their practice is mainly a cosmetic one. Wait times can be very long. They can put the letters FACD after their name, Fellow of the Australasian College of Dermatologists. The Australasian College of Dermatologists' site has info on doctor locations, skin problems and treatments: **dermcoll.edu.au**.

A Who's Who of mental health practitioners is in Chapter 4, It's Your Mind.

Who's Who in natural practitioners

Natural therapists

Natural therapists don't have the medical training or qualifications of medical doctors and hormone specialists. They're not allowed to diagnose conditions or give medical advice. Courses range from part-time and short-term to 4 years, resulting in many different qualifications. There are several member organisations, including the Australian Natural Therapists Association, and the Naturopaths and Herbalists Association of Australia.

Due to the wide range of skills and standards, you'll need to satisfy yourself as to the qualifications and usefulness of 'complimentary' practitioners in yoga, massage and other disciplines. You'll also need to assess the safety and regulation of ingredients in herbal and other 'medicines', including unregulated ayurvedic 'remedies'. Homeopathy doesn't work.

NZ: there are no laws or health regulations in New Zealand covering who can call themselves a naturopath or a similar term; the Naturopaths and Medical Herbalists of NZ organisation says it represents the qualified ones.

The worst things

Here's a list of the worst things we've been told about menopause, as judged by thousands of responders to the Menopause Survey, who heard them from friends, workmates, mothers, partners and doctors. Carry a water pistol in case anyone says these to you.

“At least you're not dead. **Get over it.** **You're too young for menopause.** **Is that a thing?** It's all overblown. **It's all downhill from here.** **It can't be that bad.** **It must be a relief.** Have you tried natural remedies? Here's a script for Endone. **Are you usually overly concerned with your health?** A doctor said that after my surgery I wouldn't have any symptoms! **Stop complaining.** **There's nothing you can do about it.** Always being tired is normal. **No one wants to hear it.** **Essential oils will cure you.** Don't take HRT – you should do this naturally!! **Menopausal women are just angry, frustrated**

pains-in-the-arses past their use-by dates. A GP told me to 'suck it up' in relation to my bladder leakage. **In our day we just got on with it.** **Doctor said he'd never heard of a link between insomnia and perimenopause.** Apricot kernels can cure it. You're going to end up in the nuthouse. **'I KNOW WHAT YOU'RE GOING THROUGH,' said a man.** **Menopause means you're 'unfuckable'.** Do not take HRT or you will get breast cancer and die. **Get a hysterectomy.** **You're getting fat.** **Hot flushes are power surges.** Here, try some of this expensive: collagen, shark cartilage, kale, goji berries, shit-tasting tea, reiki and face creams worth more than my car. **Husband said he also thinks he is going through menopause.** **HRT is a tool of the devil.** It's not a competition. **Stop making a fuss. How embarrassing.** You've started to look like a bitter old woman. **Celebrate the crone.** If you eat right, exercise and meditate, you'll be symptom free. **It's all in your head!** **It goes forever.** Just take herbal supplements. **Just take HRT.** Women are animals – how can I take them seriously? **Old boilers.** It's a myth. **Turning into a cranky old cow.** **You're faking symptoms to avoid sex.** Such a fuss over nothing. **You shouldn't need lube with me.** We don't talk about that. **You can't be perimenopausal – you are still having your period.** It's the death of the womb. **You are now useless.** Eat organic. **You must be glad.** **Diet.** **Just exercise more.** **You're imagining it.** Your husband will trade you in. **Medication is the answer to everything.** It's so great as it's a time to reflect on your life. **Just lose weight.** ”

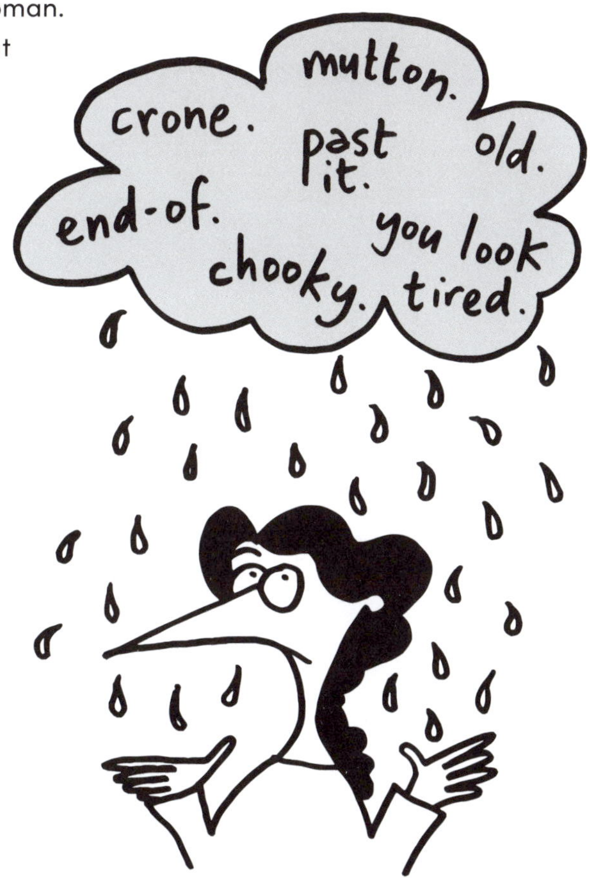

BAD WORD CLOUD

My husband says he wouldn't be able to cope and I think that's true of a lot of men. Women are legends. Helen, 49

The only thing I have found to be truly helpful is yoga. A daily routine of yoga does wonders for my aching body. It's also helped with my moods. I'm less irritable! Toni, 52

Acceptance helped my stress levels – when I stopped being angry and frustrated and sad about what was happening and just felt the feelings rather than fighting them and got on with it. Sally, 54

It can be huge to accept your fertile years are done, even if you have no desire to have a child at this stage in life. The finality can be a challenge. Nicki, 51

I tried a herbal remedy and for two glorious weeks it all stopped . . . then stopped working. I think my body went, 'Wait a second this isn't REAL estrogen, it's only phytoestrogen.' I've just started HRT and hoping it will do the trick. But I feel a failure because I've had to resort to it. Caroline, 54

I feel like a stranger. I'm getting a handle on it, but it's all just so not what I thought. Camille, 45

Why do we treat it? Why can't our society embrace women as they change and adjust for them? Why do women need to 'manage' it? Why can't women be allowed to feel and act a bit shit? Natalie, 47

It's a process that undoes the most basic things about who I am – how I look, what I can do, how I feel, how my body works. Angela, 56

I naively thought that because I did not have bad periods, perimenopause would be no big deal for me. Jomi, 50

Take control of your symptoms, speak to medical practitioners, friends, alternative treatment practitioners. What works for one person may not work for you. Keep trying until you find your medication that helps with symptoms. Gillian, 58

The best things

Here's a culled list of the best or most useful things we've been told about menopause, by friends, sisters, doctors, and mothers, online support groups . . . and comedians. As judged by thousands of women who answered the Survey.

"You're not alone or losing your mind. **Yes, it's menopause.** **Your symptoms are normal.** **Get some proper drugs.** **There're no medals for suffering.** There's a genuine reason for feeling so crap. **Embrace the change.** **Painful sex isn't a given.** A problem shared is a problem halved. **Advice to be kind to yourself.** 'Natural' remedies can interact badly with other medications. **Alcohol makes your symptoms worse.** **Always carry a fan.** All things will pass. **Not all experts are experts.** **Great sex years after menopause is still possible.** There's great joy in becoming invisible. **Your anxiety is due to hormone imbalance.** At the end of your shower, turn up the cold. My husband said he'll be there for me and wasn't going anywhere. **Buy two sets of mattress protectors so you only have to wash one.** **Do what's right for you. We are all very different.** Don't be a hero. Seek help. **Don't just take your GP's advice, go do research for yourself.** **Dress in layers.** Exercise really helps. **Everyone's experience is different.** Reading Judith Lucy's book made me feel normal. **Put your foot/feet out from under the covers.** In bed, use layers rather than one hot cover. **You don't have to tolerate the symptoms.** **HRT will change your life.** Hang on – it will get better. **It's a period of time, not an event.** **Some people get vertigo.** Jean Kittson said it changes your brain. **Antidepressants can assist with menopausal symptoms.** **You become like a man. You care about yourself.** **You don't need to feel crazy.** Don't compare yourself to others. **It can be managed.** **It's a lottery.** Talk, talk, talk, share, share, share. Embrace the freedom! **Hang in there, mate.** Your symptoms are real. **Stop fighting it.** **Red wine is bad for hot flushes (goddammit).** **Share experiences** with friends. Post-menopausal bleeding can sometimes (although rarely) be a sign of ovarian cancer. **Aches and pains might be hormones.** That's beautiful, natural, manageable and normal. **It is OK to be pissed off.** There are so many good podcasts. **My doctor said, 'Oh, you poor thing' – and he meant it.** **Women are your best friends.** You are not going nuts, your hormones are."

Menopause is a seller's market

I'll tell you what else menopause is. A marketing opportunity. Finance websites and the media are starting to be full of stories heralding the coming of start-up menopause products and apps. We're all targets now.

As well as supplements with little to no proof behind them, we can now buy anything from light-up vagina wands to wristbands telling us we're having a hot flush (YES WE KNOW) amid an absolute ocean of useless stuff being sold with 'empowerment' messages. Things are going to get wilder in the menopause marketing department.

A tech website recently mused aloud that it was baffling that most entrepreneurs aren't funding menopause-related ventures already because of the likely profits that can be dragged out of us, 'an under-served market that's fast growing and "target-rich"'. (I'll tell you why, doofuses, because most billionaire entrepreneurs are young men who aren't interested in menopause unless it's cured by a penis-shaped rocket.)

Other supplements sold for menopause symptoms are just vitamins or other powders with a new label on them using the word menopause or libido or energy, cashing in on demand. Different formulas and brands might not be deliberate rip-offs, and sellers and advocates might believe in them, but that doesn't mean the product will do what it's sold to do.

Many products have claims that have little to no meaning, using words such as 'support'. One company is offering 'personalised digital therapeutics'. What? Another company claims it will use 'regenerative medicine' to end menopause. Another advertises, in these actual words, 'probiotics for your panty hamster' (I think they mean vagina) with a product that 'supports vaginal health and pH balance'. Supports, you say? Hmmm.

I think the sad truth is Australian Government regulatory bodies like the Therapeutic Goods Administration lack funding for wide-ranging, proactive investigation and prosecution, and they're pretty busy examining the evidence for new vaccines. Anything that's in the 'food-medicine interface', such as supplements, isn't a priority to investigate unless unproven claims for a medical benefit are made or there is

I'm sick of the judgey bitches who get off lightly. Go light up your vagina candle. Suzi, 53

No natural products stopped my hot flushes, night sweats or anxiety. Sarah, 50

another serious issue. So there is the potential for dodgy stuff to fall through the cracks and end up being sold online and in chain pharmacies making billions.

And because there's a massive gap between 'this is a dangerous product' – in which case the Therapeutic Goods Administration, a health department or the Australian Competition and Consumer Commission will step in, if they know about it – and an ocean of products that won't kill you but may not help you either, we're being sold with a bunch of carefully chosen dodge words.

Beware of 'studies prove'

Watch out for phrases such as 'studies prove' and 'clinically proven'. Gold-standard, controlled studies include a double-blind element (which means the study participants don't know if they're taking the substance being studied or a placebo) and then the results have been confirmed by being peer-reviewed and repeated in other studies.

A grab bag of claims & buzzwords

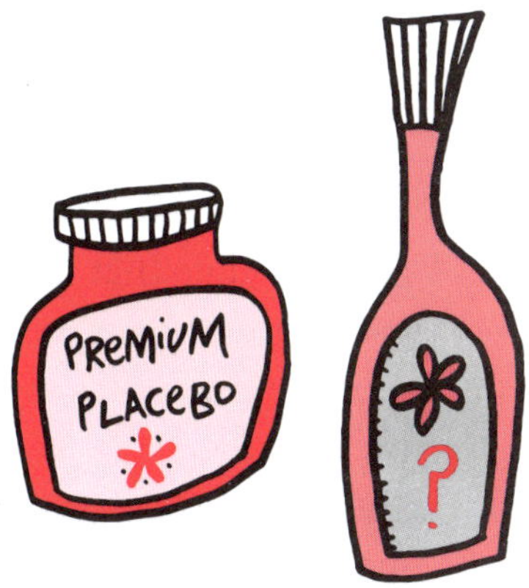

Stress is relevant but we don't really know how: only that less is great for lots of reasons, but that can be easier said than done. You don't need to detox for your hormones, probiotics are probably irrelevant to internal hormone levels, and so is all talk of alkaline blood or foods. No foods are known or proven to change your body's own hormone levels in a noticeable or useful way, including soy products, seeds, dairy foods, herbs, raw foods, powders made from vegetable matter, particular vitamins and minerals in special doses, or 'super' foods.

Many celebrities who sell branded or associated products, like supplements or skincare cream, team up with some sort of wellness practitioner. Very often, while there is an outer layer of 'wellness', it's a thin epidermis overlaying ideas of beauty and weight loss. Look out for code-words like 'bloating'.

I went to a mindfulness workshop as a self-care strategy. Rhonny, 55

I didn't use any pharmacy or natural products. Estelle, 69

Do natural therapies have the same effect as hormone medication?

There is a never-ending line of people sprouting rubbish about unproven methods and supplements – which really do nothing more than make you poor! Megan, 50

No, and an honest naturopath will tell you the same. It's a sorrowful testament to the power of marketing and belief, in the face of evidence, that of more than 7000 women who answered the question in the Survey, nearly 60 per cent said they didn't know if natural remedies have the same effect as hormone medication. About a third knew that natural therapies didn't have the same effect.

I want definite alternative products that work. Olivia, 58

Some non-hormonal 'natural therapies' such as vitamins can correct deficiencies; some herbal products can affect hormones in theory, but nowhere near the effect of hormone pharmaceutical products, and their impact and doses vary and are almost all unregulated. It's widely accepted that 'natural' products can't significantly affect hormones or help severe symptoms.

Are 'natural' supplements harmless?

Don't assume that if you can buy it, it is safe for you. A commonly recommended 'natural' ingredient for menopause symptoms, black cohosh, can cause liver damage depending on doses and your individual circumstances; and St John's Wort can interfere with the effectiveness or safety of some antidepressants, blood-thinning medicine, and the Pill. Progesterone cream may not be delivering enough to balance an estrogen supplement. Always tell your doctor about any 'natural' therapies you take, as they may cause symptoms or interfere with each other or with other medications.

See the 'natural' supplements and phytoestrogens sections in Chapter 2, It's Your Hormones, for possible benefits and dangers.

Many herbal and vitamin mineral supplements are completely harmless. Some of those are useful, some are not. You might feel better taking a natural supplement. If you've been feeling better for 2 months, come off it and see how you feel 6 weeks after that. You may find there isn't much of a difference and can save yourself some money as you're 'through' the symptoms of menopause.

'It's unnatural' is true but irrelevant. Clothes are unnatural but I ain't taking them off. Mobile phones are unnatural yet here we are . . . I will look into my options if I have enough symptoms to bother. Mari, 42

The hard sell

'Natural' products are now a multi-billion dollar industry with big-bucks marketing strategies to match.

Beware of any 'natural therapy' or pharmaceutical product advertised online or on socials by an influencer, favourite writer, or a doctor. Australian doctors are not supposed to endorse specific products. 'Natural products' that claim to change blood flow or hormone levels are unlikely to do any such thing.

If you google the Australian Menopause Centre, global results and its website don't tell you that the CEO and Medical Director used to run another clinic called the Menopause Institute of Australia, which sold compounded 'bio-identical hormones' products that were found by the Australian Competition and Consumer Commission to have made more than 70 misleading and deceptive claims in advertising. The company had to pay $50,000 in costs and run corrective advertising.

> I want a more definite list of natural remedies. There doesn't seem to be any that have been proven scientifically. No health sites recommend any, so it leaves a lot of trial by error and wasted money.
> **Stephanie, 51**

In 2019, the co-founder of the company that sells 'Happy Hormones' Lisa Curry had to amend claims that prescribed hormone medication caused a 'dramatic' increase in the risk of breast cancer. Doctors immediately denounced that claim, and the one about how the company's herbal supplement could 'balance' hormones.

Doctors said Ms Curry's claim that her products were 'designed to work and encourage the body to produce the necessary levels of hormones itself which is the natural process' made no sense. It was pointed out that the products were unregulated, and the associated website should not be giving anyone medical advice about menopause symptoms.

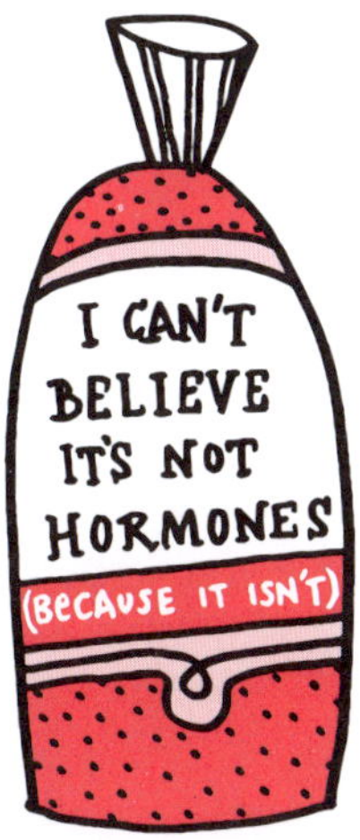
I CAN'T BELIEVE IT'S NOT HORMONES
(BECAUSE IT ISN'T)

'Happy Hormones' are still being sold, with claims that the pills maintain or support female hormonal balance. I'm not aware of any reliable study that shows or proves that's what these particular formulations by this brand of supplements do. The company claims on its website at the time of writing, 'Look for natural solutions that correct the total endocrine imbalance such as Happy Hormones . . . Herbal medicines signal to the endocrine system to balance itself rather than providing artificial external hormones.' If you can find an independent endocrinologist who agrees that a non-medical supplement can significantly change and stabilise hormone levels during perimenopause and menopause, I am an otter.

The 'Happy Hormones' website has a quiz for 'assessment' which many people use, before being prompted to buy the site's products. This should absolutely not be done as a substitute for medical diagnosis and treatment. The reply sent after I filled in the assessment described four products sold by the company as my 'prescription', at a cost of about $250.

I now receive lots of direct marketing emails suggesting different products they make, associated with symptoms including hot flushes, sleep problems, libido, hair loss, mental health problems and moods.

There's a marketing video on YouTube at the time I'm writing in which the company's other co-founder, naturopath Jeff Butterworth, says anxiety and mood swings happen because your liver is not 'clearing' natural or medical hormones, claiming that this can cause 'a 2, 3, 5 times effect to those hormones which were only designed to have a singular effect.' He then says the company's products will help clear 'excessive hormones' or 'estrogen dominance situation' from your system. Most endocrinologists and gynaecologists reject the theory of clearing 'excess' or 'toxic' estrogen or 'clearing hormones' using non-medical means. Some may use the term 'estrogen dominance' to just mean perimenopause, so it can be confusing.

The video says that 'Happy Hormones' triggers the hypothalamus and pituitary glands to 'balance', which controls hormone levels, and women can then manage anxiety. This seems . . . a rather astonishing claim.

Another video says using hormone medication stops 'an alternate hormone system that the body clicks into . . . that supports your body and nourishes you'.

Used Happy Hormones which seem to stop the craziness. Christine, 56

'Happy Hormones' eliminated all of my symptoms within a month! Ruby, 51

I don't know if Happy Hormones work or it's all in my head. Karin, 50

Tried herbal medicine and Happy Hormones and both didn't help at all. Terrie, 54

I can't afford to keep taking them [Happy Hormones]. $99 for 2 months. Monique, 54

Testimonials on the company's website from 'ladies' (the company carefully does not call its customers patients) claim that the herbal pills (Happy Hormones, Happy Calm, Happy Liver, Happy Collagen and so on) cured their problems with sleep, hair loss, incontinence, premenstrual disorders, menopausal sweating, endometriosis, mood swings, teenage period problems and menopausal symptoms. Each claim is stamped with a label saying 'verified'. When I asked the company what 'verified' means, it replied; '"Verified" means that the review has been posted by a customer who is really taking the product and not a fake person.'

Unprotected

I confess myself astonished that government regulatory bodies either lack the funding powers, or the will and proactive independence, to do enough about unsupportable claims being made by some players in the billion-dollar supplements industry. I'm sure the regulators do good work, but so much goes unremarked, uninvestigated, unchallenged and unpunished. In my opinion, they can't or don't adequately protect women from predatory or misleading marketing.

> [There's] just a shit ton of Facebook ads claiming to have the cure and after you complete their survey of symptoms you can get absolutely no information until you sign up to regularly hand over your money for some diet or supplement based cure-all.
> Leonie, 52

As long as some of these wellness products are useless and just turn into wee, rather than cause illness or injury, I think the government agencies that are supposed to protect us from misleading marketing are working in silos. It's confusing to know whether to report marketing rubbish or dodgy ingredients to the Australia Competition and Consumer Commission (ACCC), the TGA or to a local health department.

Regulatory agencies say they will act on complaints if they assess a non-compliance problem, but how does an average consumer know what's in something or whether it's doing what an ad claims? Anytime I've reported what I think is dodgy, what ensued was a ridiculously long process of try-this-other-agency and people doing their best with limited resources or a marked reluctance to share anything but the most parsimonious move-along-nothing-to-see-here-response.

Don't assume that because you can buy it, it must do what it claims. I think that there are thousands of products sold right now online and from pharmacies which probably do nothing much except dye your wee.

How to avoid rip-offs

A perimenopausal woman can continue being a target market for 30 years.

Already, we're being sold questionable products that may be useful for some, or totally useless for anybody, including:

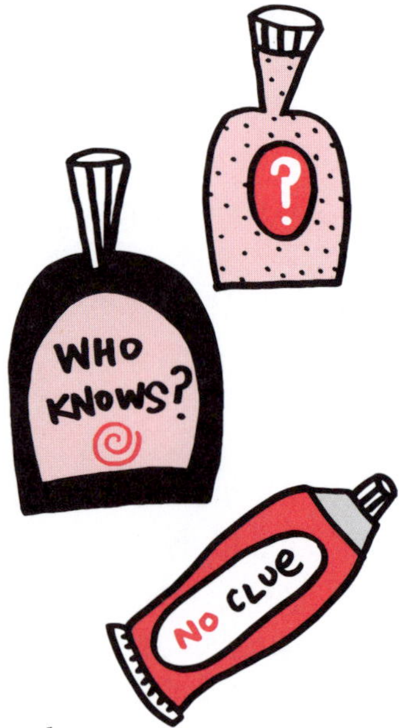

* menopause tracker apps
* stuff that doesn't work, including 'anti-ageing' cosmetics and useless supplements
* special wraps or clothes (they're just shawls, cashmere, cotton, or otherwise)
* cooling packs
* apps and jewellery that allegedly 'trick' you into feeling cooler (cheaper but demoralising to have someone yell at you, 'You're not hot')
* rechargeable alarms, graphs, and body heat thermometers
* tiny fans that gobble batteries (look for rechargeable or plug-in ones)
* cooling gel pillows
* weighted blankets
* sex lubricants, vaginal moisturisers and menopause vaginal washes (don't buy until you've checked out Chapter 6, It's Your Sex Life, and the 'Mysteriously Irritable Vulva' section of Chapter 5, It's Your Body, for more on why and why not)
* Kegel weights or in-vagina devices (don't, until you've read the pelvic floor section in Chapter 5, It's Your Body)
* herbal/perfumed spray face-mists.

Pharmaceutical companies and supplement and device sellers know from research that women in perimenopause are concerned about their sex lives, their powers of concentration and moods, feeling tired, having disrupted sleep, hot flushes, loss of hair volume and condition, and drier, saggier skin. They know what you're worried about and they use those words in marketing: it doesn't mean their product will help.

If label or advertising says 'supports' or 'helps maintain', 'promotes', 'traditionally used', 'said to', or 'enhances' 'designed for', it doesn't necessarily mean it has the implied effect.

Positive strategies in menopause

Whatever your philosophy, there's heaps you can do to improve any perimenopause and menopause experience, and some of the main ones are completely free, including:

* Talk to friends, partners and kids who make you feel better: pick your confidants carefully.
* Keep a look-out for mental and physical changes and don't blame yourself.
* If you're in a multi-generational or partner household make sure everyone pulls their weight.
* Push back against discrimination at work (more on this coming up).
* Be smart about what people are trying to sell you.

Mothers, talk to your daughters. Daughters, talk to your mothers. Everybody talk to everybody. Marla, 53

In my health research workplace, my colleagues seemed to be in denial about brain fog, depression, anxiety and frequent days off for migraines. Anita, 58

Things that can help combat stress

Many of these things have been proven or associated with reducing the effects of menopause symptoms, without affecting hormone levels. Some of these things won't help, or a combination may do the trick:

* exercise (see the 'Exercise' section coming up on page 132)
* a healthier diet with more fruit and vegetables and less animal fats and processed sugar
* meditation, sleeptime or relaxation strategies
* a shared plan to spread family and home responsibilities
* cognitive behaviour and other talking therapy with a qualified psychologist
* talking with friends; staying connected with hobbies and interest groups
* asking for help if you're above or below a healthy weight range; this will improve energy levels (see the 'Eating & weight' section coming up on page 148)
* massages conducted by a qualified therapist
* prescribed medication if necessary
* winning the lottery.

Talking about it with other women. Talking to my (male) manager about it. Tracking periods, to better understand and notice changes. Kez, 46

If you feel overwhelmed

You can start with baby steps to reduce the general pressure of life by tackling background problems, even if you do it slowly. Reach out for help. One thing at a time. (Choose your order.)

* Take stock and get your finances and legal affairs in order.
* Assemble a medical team of advisors you trust.
* Declutter, donate and sort out clothes and other objects you don't want anymore.
* Address any problems in your relationship or sex life.
* Repair or jettison friendships that have become poisonous or unhelpful.
* Say no when you are asked to do too much, or are disrespected.
* If you're finding yourself thinking, 'How do I make that person understand?' reframe your question. 'How do I let go of the idea they have to understand?'
* Vote, donate, or be an activist for a political situation that prioritises women's health, research funding, and cheaper, subsidised menopause medications.
* Search hints online and on social media about calming techniques or breathing, use an app, immerse both hands in a sink of cold water, and cool the vagus nerve (a packet of frozen peas wrapped in a tea towel between your bosoms might liven up that work meeting).

You can become more selective in terms of what is important in life. I try to avoid stress, I have magnesium chloride baths with essential oils two to three times a week, I eat a good diet and all this helps to be a calmer person.
Squish, 52

I love hearing about different people's experiences. I think this helps to feel less alone with it, there is a real solidarity with hearing others' stories.
Jayne, 39

Push back against stereotypes

Women have been cowed by ugly, cruel words and a common theme is 'dried up': the implications of dried-up skin and hair, work offers, dating prospects, and vagina. Skin products are to make us look 'dewy'. Insults play with the idea. Be suspicious of any marketing that uses confronting, judging or rude terms, including 'atrophied vagina', 'senile ovaries', 'ugly wrinkles', 'unsightly belly'. These words are just used to try and make you feel wrong, hideous, unloved – so they can sell you stuff.

I don't attribute any mental symptoms to menopause. I've always been a grumpy, moody, introverted bitch. Vanessa, 54

A bit like drug-free child birth, there is pressure to go through the whole thing naturally. Like that is what a strong woman should do – just deal with it quietly. Victoria, 46

Would media, movies, comedians, writers STOP with the 'mad menopausal' thing AND the option of either MILF or crone. Karen, 54

Zero tolerance for teasing

Homes, families and workplaces need a zero tolerance for teasing, mean-spirited jokes or needling comments about changes or symptoms of hormonal changes. This goes for comments on breasts or weight during the puberty changes of the pre-teen and teen years, as well as comments about men having to be scared of all the women in the family 'syncing' their periods or menopause-related mood swings. Don't play into tired boring jokes such as, 'Ooh, look out, she's got the menopause!' Happy to talk about my uterus, if you can restrain yourself from making comments from 1953, Darryl.

In the Menopause Survey, less than 9 per cent of women said jokes about menopause are always fine. More than a third said they had no tolerance for any; almost half said it depends on who does them and 9.5 per cent said it depends on the intent and who's targeted.

Tried to explain what I'm going through and asked for patience and compassion. Danno, 56

October 18th

Choose your own way of celebrating Menopause Awareness Day, perhaps by buying a jumbo bottle of sexual lubricant, or having a boiled egg.

A better workplace for menopause

Sensible workplaces, bosses and corporations are developing and implementing menopause policies. That's because ignoring or mismanaging menopause issues is a multi-threat to businesses that can cost them millions.

Work suffers when employees wrestle with their menopause symptoms such as lack of sleep and hot flushes, or struggle with concentration, weepiness and memory, perhaps years before they realise they're in perimenopause. It strikes at the heart of our self-esteem and sense of worth.

Many women don't apply for senior positions or aim for higher work status, and even go part-time or quit their jobs altogether or use up sick days. Women can lose tens to hundreds of thousands of dollars in wages and lost superannuation due to changes they make to try to deal with menopause symptoms. Others try to power through; they stick their head in the lunch-room freezer, hide in the toilets, horrify themselves by bursting into tears and seeming 'unstable'.

Smart companies understand that losing women and their talents is a waste of training, expertise and in-house knowledge, and customer and corporate relationships, which affects productivity and profit.

Companies have suffered big compensation payouts and corporate embarrassment when their managers discriminated against menopausal women in terms of job opportunity, or failed to make sure women workers were not harassed or targeted with derisive comments and jokes.

Every day, millions of women try to hide perimenopause symptoms at work. First, any seeming decline in concentration and self-esteem and multitasking skills. Many women have no idea these feelings and problems might be caused by lack of estrogen. Perhaps 4 to 6 years later they might get hit with the hot flushes and crazy-heavy periods that can cause problems at work.

If you're flooding with a crazy-heavy period, or get periods at unexpected times, how can you manage a factory job restricted to set toilet breaks, or do days of science fieldwork? How do you feel if you need to explain that a red face, sweating and discomfort are not embarrassment, anxiety or dishonesty, but bloody disappearing estrogen?

Women who answered questions about work in the Menopause Survey said they were worried about not being considered for jobs (almost 39 per cent); or losing their job (about 18 per cent).

I am a health professional, and I know that I have been overlooked for jobs because I am older. Lucy, 58

I say on the phone, 'I'm sorry, I'm having a perimenopausal brain fog moment. Please be patient with me.' Becci, 46

The pragmatism and creativity of the older women I know, despite their sometimes poor circumstances, is inspiring. Natasha, 52

My much younger female boss suggested dismissively the symptoms were just the same as pregnancy, until I reminded her pregnancy has an end date, is very visible and well-supported in the workplace. Margaret, 56

Thought I had dementia, it was so bad. I'm a manager in a corporate environment and had to make jokes about myself to cover up my moods and brain fog. It's professionally embarrassing . . . Suzanne, 51

I have trouble focusing at work and feel like I'll be penalised for going through this as I work in a youth-focused organisation. I feel sad, as if I'm losing myself. Kate, 49

I worked with a conservative Muslim woman. She told another workmate, a young gay Maori guy, that 'When women get older things change and Gail is having lady parts problems. She may cry, she may get the giggles, she might take her jumper off and put it back on and she may sigh a lot and be a bit cranky.' Bless her. Of course I'd already told him. They were great to me. Gail, 58

There is no way I'd discuss it at work, it would be considered a sign of being unreliable. Even though I work in a hospital and 90 per cent of middle management are menopausal women. Annie, 55

I went to my boss to explain that I am overwhelmed with the amount of emails I receive. He suggested coming to work earlier! How can I? I am the main caregiver of our children. Vikki, 49

I am wiser and more respected in my profession (social work) than I was as a younger woman. **Marion, 49**

I asked for help and they instigated a performance review. My feelings of self-worth hit rock bottom. We worked for a state health department. **Jacqueline**

The sexual harassment of me in the workplace has stopped (not a joke). **Katya, 50**

Sometimes the cloak of invisibility that being an older woman affords is annoying but sometimes it is excellent; maybe I should test how invisible I am by trying to commit a crime? **Kitty, 55**

I cried, and cried, and cried, and cried . . . I went to work and my boss didn't know what to do with me so fed me a large glass of wine (I worked in a hotel office). I cried a whole lot more and had to go home. **Fiona, 60**

Male colleagues would panic a bit when they started to see me sweating up a storm, mid-meeting! They'd offer to open the meeting room door! **Helen, 48**

With a couple of trusted work colleagues in the same situation, we had a safe code-word to let each other know if we thought we might be having hormone-driven inappropriate reactions to difficult work situations. **Danielle, 51**

I have always been super into my career and focused. Now I have an overriding feeling of can't be arsed, and I don't know if it is actually that I need to change stuff – or if it's the menopause gremlins. **Nina, 52**

I moved to a job with a whole team of women mid-30s to mid-60s. It's an everyday topic of conversation: 'Turn the air con on!', 'Turn it off, I'm freezing', 'Where's my portable fan?', 'Don't lift that, you'll have a prolapse!', 'Watch out for your pelvic floor.' **Jo, 56**

Terrible memory, forgetting words, mixing up dates, times, numbers, lack of ability to multitask, crying at the drop of a hat, unable to deal with 'idiots' in the workplace, lack of tolerance. I feel like a nasty horrible person, so I've retreated from all work and social activities. **Maree, 49**

Possible work strategies

Not every strategy will work for everyone in different workplaces and situations, obviously, but here are some suggestions.

Talk to your union, HR or your boss, after assessing the most likely empathetic and useful response. Talk about how a symptom is affecting you, not just that you have it. For example, hot flushes might mean you feel you look flustered in a meeting, in front of a class or while talking to a customer; or lack of sleep is causing concentration problems. Think about what might help and what you could ask for: a start later in the day, or a supervisor having your back and cracking down on idiotic comments by others. You might want to:

* negotiate flexible or more predictable fixed work hours, some working from home
* consider hormonal medication to smooth over the bumps of perimenopause or longer-lasting menopause symptoms
* dress in layers that can be hurled off and on
* cut down on coffee and alcohol
* throw things at people without being fired.

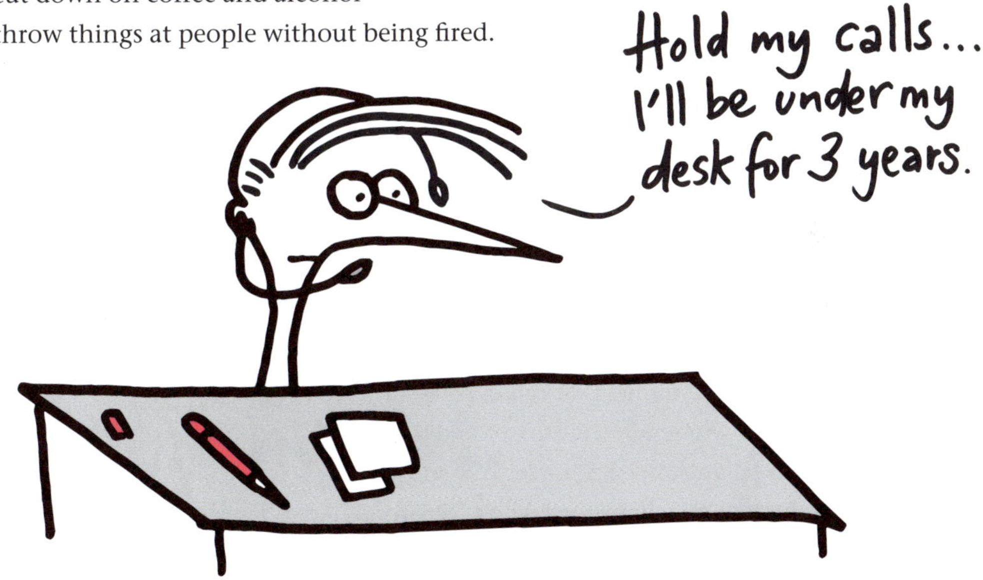

Two other co-workers going through menopause at same time, so we all bought desk fans. Throughout the day a fan would turn on depending on who had the hot flush – many times all three would turn it on at exactly same time then laugh (and swear). Caron, 57

Being a climate controller

One thing that's worth doing if you work in a temperature-controlled office is to find out if you can adjust the temperature. Small studies suggest that it's usually men at home and installation engineers and bosses at work who set the thermostat controls too hot for women in perimenopause.

MORE INFO on menopause & work

australianunions.org.au
Search 'menopause' on the home page.

menopauseatwork.org
Free info for bosses, managers and employees about menopause policies, discussions and protections in the workplace. A collaboration between businesses, researchers and medical experts backed by Glasgow University in Scotland, Melbourne and Monash universities and the Royal Women's Hospital in Melbourne, Australia.

Friends & family

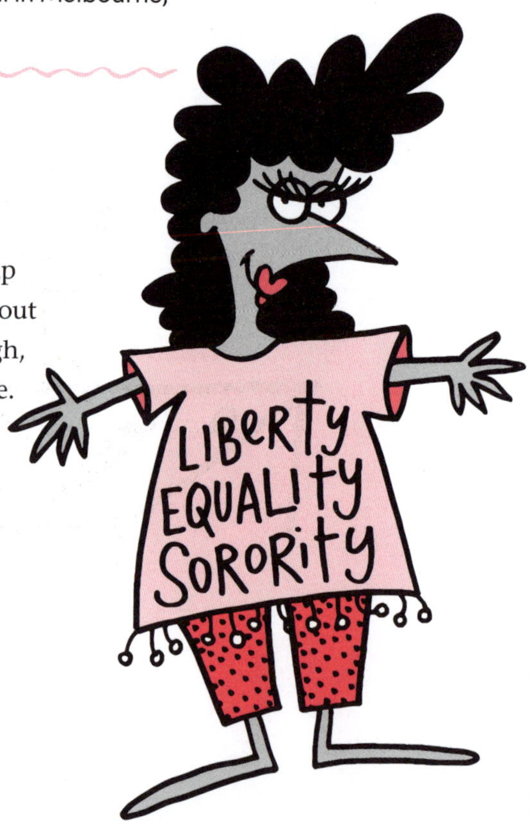

While the dynamic at home and in a friendship group can often become more supportive when you talk about menopause symptoms and what you're going through, for some people it doesn't help, or can even be unsafe. A huge number of women in the Survey said they found solace in talking and sharing with friends, but others said they hit a brick wall when they tried to talk about it. For many, online and social media support groups have really helped.

Some things to think about:

* Do you need a greater say in the temperature setting at home?

* If you share a bed, would two single doonas or coverings work better?
* Are you being supported enough generally? What can you ask for, or get help to change at home, that would improve things?
* Have you realised your moods and stamina may be affected by hormones, and told anyone you live with?
* Reassess: is there an unfair chores or organisational burden on you at home? Would a roster or a strike help?

Society's attitude

Almost 4900 women answered the question in the Survey, 'What do you reckon is the general society attitude to menopause?'

Here's a sample of representative responses:

* Women have a use-by date.
* Women are drama queens.
* We are discarded; no longer beautiful.
* Lalalalala – shut up we don't want to hear from you.
* Keep it to yourself.
* It's a bit of a joke.
* It only happens to old women so it's not important.
* Ignore it and it will go away.
* Horror.
* Hidden mystery.
* Head in the sand.
* Grin and bear it.
* Get over it and yourself.
* Don't ask, don't tell.
* Crazy lady!
* Clueless and mocking.
* Becoming more acceptable to discuss.
* A man is a silver fox. What are we? Just old women.
* No one cares.

I spent too many years apologising for my periods – not apologising for women's experiences anymore. **Nina, 53**

We are a family of four neurodiverse individuals, constantly engaged in sharing and oversharing thoughts, to understand others' experiences, thought processes and feelings. **Michaela, 46**

He tried to understand, but he's old-school and just kept pointing out whenever I was sweaty. Every. Single. Fucking. Time. **Anna, 57**

My husband and children wish I would shut up about it. **Tamara, 51**

I didn't realise at first what it was but I got so fed up with my family that I wanted to leave. I still had children at school so I couldn't, and gradually these feelings lessened until I was fine. **Sandra, 56**

So much effort to deal with work, kids, relationship, household, there's no time left to deal with the fact that I'm falling apart. **Annie, 55**

I had a short fuse and would get angry easily. My family was walking on eggshells around me, for probably 6 months to a year. **Cath, 61**

I talk to my partner freely about perimenopause and menopause. He is quite supportive although I'm not sure that he completely understands. **Nic, 47**

He seemed to think I was the worst case and no other woman was as bad as me. I gave him a reality check. **Sally**

Actually, my female partner of 8 years just left for a few nights to get away from me (don't know if she is coming back). Really hope she does. **Lisa, 51**

Being in a same-sex relationship I can share more with my partner; she has already been through it. **Helen, 52**

He was predictably an idiot about it. **Ingrid, 57**

No one to talk to. I feel so alone in this hell. Kat, 57

I get a lot of support from the ladies in my exercising group. We all chat and know we all go through the same stuff. Fiona, 51

I have encouraged my three daughters to be open about having their periods and symptoms. This includes openness with their brother and dad. I don't hide symptoms of perimenopause. Sarah, 47

I can see how marriages end with menopause. It's bloody hard. We kept it open and he has been a huge support for me. I am so grateful to him for not judging the horrible person I could be and knowing I would get through it. Susan, 56

Once the ice was broken in discussion with friends, it became another bonding experience and source of a few good laughs at our experiences. Cat, 55

My adult children don't understand at all and get impatient with me for forgetting things, which makes me feel even worse. Caroline, 55

My husband is going for sainthood, because I am not fun right now. Caro, 49

So hard to talk about. I didn't want to be that older woman who was gaining weight and fanning herself and complaining. Krissy, 52

I thought I was an outlier at 42, but HEAPS of the women around my age who I spoke to had symptoms. Polly, 44

My husband left me when I was perimenopausal and told our kids I was crazy. Ange, 50

He's very supportive, but I still feel guilty about my lower sex drive. Ariel, 48

I had been so accepting of his controlling of my life . . . The anger and resentment hit me so suddenly when menopause kicked in that it was actually very useful in helping me to find the courage to break away. Gabrielle, 62

Exercise

I'll never forget interviewing a tippety-top menopause expert years ago and asking her about exercise. 'Is walking good?' I asked. She fixed me with a piercing glare. 'Oh, walking does fucking nothing!' she snapped. Yikes. What she meant was, vigorous exercise while bearing your own weight (i.e. not swimming or cycling) and certain kinds of other exercise (lifting medium-sized weights) are better at keeping your bones strong. But that doesn't mean cycling is bad, or swimming is bad, or that walking actually does eff-all.

So much of the info given to women about exercise is not even slightly helpful – what is the point of telling an already-too-busy woman to 'go to the gym every day for at least an hour'? And partly because articles about it are usually illustrated with videos and images of 25-year-old actual models popping one ankle behind the opposite ear doing legs-akimbo handstands next to their pool at the tropical hinterland goat-cuddling-and-facelift salon.

What we tend to get is reports of a lot of scientific research about why it's important (yes, we know!), and hardly anything practical or useful about what kind of exercise to do and how. So this chapter aims to be heavy on the how.

Most people who answered questions on exercise in the Menopause Survey for this book said they could find 30 minutes a day to exercise, which is great. Others said zero, and a very few said 1 or 2 hours a day.

Why exercise is good

The science is clear. Exercise – any exercise – makes you happier, healthier and reduces your risk of 'cardiovascular disease'. Cardiovascular disease sounds like something you might catch, but it isn't: it means conditions that affect the heart or restricts blood vessels so it slows down the efficient pumping of blood. Some doctors believe women who have hot flushes are more likely to have cardiovascular problems. Cardiovascular problems can cause a range of conditions, from strange heartbeat and circulation problems to heart failure and stroke.

I am impressed with how much difference exercise makes. Cecily, 49

I can't afford Pilates. I am intimidated by gyms. [Joining a group] creates more social anxiety. I do bushwalking when I can. Mostly I feel too sad to exercise with purpose. Jo, 47

Exercise keeps you flexible and helps avoid some aches and pains, keeps your pelvic floor behaving in a way that helps avoid unexpected weeing, guards against bone fractures, and is known to lower the risk of diabetes and several cancers.

Exercise is not a substitute for necessary medical treatment for physical or mental health problems. But it will help change and reset bad moods and feelings, and helps with depression, anxiety and other mental health challenges. Yoga and breathing exercises can make you feel good. Dashing about on a netball court will give your heart a workout while you see your mates. If you love swimming, swim. If you love to rock out, dance. If you hate the gym, don't go.

Start small, keep resetting yourself, accept that you got out of the habit. But do something. There's no evidence that exercise, including yoga, does anything to alleviate hot flushes or misbehaving vagina bacteria but exercise can definitely help with sleep, mood, bone strength and maintaining health through menopause.

Why it's hard

Women are simultaneously told not to be vain, and to prioritise their children, partners, and older family members, but also to find 'me time' and learn how to be relaxed, eat more expensive healthy food, also treat themselves, and be within a socially acceptable and healthy weight range. Impossible, contradictory expectations.

After we leave school, our participation in sport and activity tends to be hugely reduced, even more so if we have children, and even more than that after we turn 40 or 50. Repeated studies say women tend to do more hours outside our paid work to organise family, run the house and care for elderly relatives and teenagers or young adult children. Whereas men at the same age tend not to interrupt their work, leisure and exercise as much for those reasons.

Pick a study and it'll show that hardly any women of perimenopausal and menopausal

I hate exercising but have discovered aqua aerobics and just love it. Exercising without the pull of gravity is amazing. Pauline, 67

I find my poor sleep patterns during menopause have impacted my drive/energy to be active. I find it hard to get to sleep; I get night sweats and chills multiple times so I often wake up tired. Jennifer, 51

With mums' soccer we had a rule: don't worry about wet shorts (from weeing)! With mixed team sports there is stress, chafing and secretiveness. Francesca, 59

age can find time to exercise in the way experts say we should. So many of us tend to see it as indulgent or selfish, rather than an active investment in our health or maintenance. Or it just doesn't seem possible to drag it up the long list of priorities and responsibilities.

Fad 'facts'

Women want info about exercise, so online sites and social media churn it out. Despite a million silly reports, there's no optimum or perfect time of the day to exercise (or eat), and exercise choices shouldn't be based on body shape, blood types, horoscopes or your menstrual cycle.

Blaming & shaming

We're routinely chided, scolded and shamed for gaining weight around our so-called middle in so-called middle age, based on the different results of studies on mostly men, athletes, or a small number of younger women.

Women are told, even in news reports of scientific studies, regardless of the merit of the study methods, that their sudden middle roll is due to their laziness and lack of eating control, even though for centuries it's been a known side effect of menopause. At some medical conferences, speakers have told an audience of doctors that their patients should do 1.5 hours of vigorous exercise a day. They might as well tell us to run around the deck of our yacht every morning while the chef makes us a protein smoothie.

It makes far more sense to acknowledge the changes and obstacles of perimenopause and menopause and to put the emphasis on what we *can* do.

Paying attention to yourself and bodily reactions to the exercise helps a feeling of being in control of something; seeing the changes in your body as well as your mind helps you feel like something is working. Joyce, 64

Oh, I'm sure if I exercised I'd fart glitter and dance with unicorns (sarcasm). Vicky, 52

Had to join a gym (women-only is fantastic and it's full of wonderful women of all shapes, sizes and ages) and have organised a female personal trainer. Jo, 50

If you are going to tell me I have to exercise more to make menopause not suck, I will feel angry and disappointed. Mari, 42

Working at getting fit has helped. Losing weight around the middle and building up strength has been great for depression and feeling good. Lyn, 58

I don't exercise because I'd wee. Julie, 51

Abilities & disabilities

Many of the suggestions here might not work for disabled people. If you have a disability, or autoimmune or long-term situation that requires some creative management to set up an exercise program or generate individual ideas, connect with a relevant disability organisation. Look for resources, suggestions and like-minded folk with hints for you, or a recommendation for a specialist physio or trainer.

I know I have to, but I can't due to pain . . . which causes more inflammation and pain. Sherriden, 45

I work full-time and care for a disabled husband. I am consistently exhausted because I have to get up so early. Julie, 50

A new approach to exercise

What happens if we take the word 'should' out of the vocabulary of menopause and exercise? It seems to me that by the time you're in your 40s and 50s, you're fed up to your poor night-time-grinding back teeth being told what you should do to be the perfect woman all the while knowing it's impossible to do those things, or you can never do them enough, or properly enough. So if we take out the 'should' when we think about exercise, we can move to another way of thinking:

- This will help me feel stronger.
- This will help me fall asleep quicker, and stay asleep better.
- These things will help me feel more flexible and less groany.
- This will increase my core strength, which will ward off extra back pain.
- It's going to help me build up muscles that I'd otherwise lose the best use of.
- This will help me feel in touch with my body; I'll enjoy feeling more energy, being healthier, fitter, stronger.
- This will mean I'm less likely to wee myself at unexpected moments.
- This will cheer me up.
- This will get the wind in my hair and help me feel calmer.
- It will lower my risk of cancer, type 2 diabetes and heart disease.
- This will make me freer to enjoy hobbies, grandchildren and athletic sex with near-strangers.

You can mix it up however it suits you, but try to hit these factors.

Cardio (heart-exercising): Walking fast, jogging, biking, swimming, dancing; as classes, with friends, or on your own, maybe 10 minutes a day at the start, or finish off any exercise routine 2–3 times a week for half an hour.

Strength and muscles: Resistance bands, weights, gym machines.

Find the flexible: Yoga, pilates and physio exercises.

How much exercise do you need to do?

Rather than 10,000 steps a day, various experts reckon the evidence says you get more value out of 150 minutes a week of moderate intensity, or 75 minutes of vigorous exercise and 75 minutes of strength sessions a week.

So, for example, per week that could be:

- 5 half-hour walks that change your heart rate a bit.
- 3 half-hour dance sessions that make you feel puffed out, plus 4 × 20-minute weights, stretches and resistance band exercises.
- 3 × 50-minute runs.
- A netball game, sex with two acrobatic sailors or a step class.
- Clocking up small amounts of movement in the day: 3 × 10 minutes, or even 6 × 5 minutes.
- A 2-and-a-half-hour bike ride once a week. The caveat is you'd need to train to increase to that amount of time: but if you already train like this, keeping it up is fine.

Whatever you do, don't do it all the time. Mix it up: change physical activity to get different benefits, including balance skills, strength training, cardio and weight bearing.

Women who answered exercise questions in the Survey reported a wide range of time they devoted to exercise in an average week. About a quarter managed it three times a week; the next biggest group was 'rarely' on 21.5 per cent. Eleven per cent exercised twice a week; about 7 per cent did it once a week, 13 per cent did an hour a day and 16 per cent got half an hour a day.

1-2 hours; I'm a full-on mum with full-time work but this is non-negotiable time. Barbara, 51

But between full-time work, a 3-hour commute, four kids and part-time uni, exercising is very, very low on the list. Kim, 48

The most popular kind of exercise was walking with a raised heart rate (about 39 per cent); with friends (19 per cent) or with a dog (about 35 per cent). Nearly 29 per cent did something like yoga or Pilates, and 11 per cent did group exercise with a raised heart rate. About 9 per cent jogged or ran; almost 11 per cent rode a bike; 7.5 per cent swam; 9 per cent danced (possibly in the lounge room) and about 15 per cent lifted some kind of weights.

More than half of women who answered the survey worried about declining mobility as they got older, but not everyone knew what they could do about it.

I definitely have at least 30 minutes a day. I just don't use them. Pen, 49

Weight train to keep up your muscle mass and do some kind of impact training for your bone mass. Rebecca, 51

When I'm tired I prefer to sit at home and drink wine. Keryn, 55

How to start new exercise stuff

The biggest problem is getting started again, or for the first time. Your most important allies will be patience and kindness to yourself, determination and perseverance, and encouragement, whether that's from a person, a group, a professional, or your own progress data-logging.

Most people developing new habits start strong then falter at about the 4- or 6-week mark. What's your plan to recognise that and push through?

There's nothing worse than a pitiless daily regime that feels like a chore or a burden or a duty – although there will be some days that duty pulls you through, too. But some people love the routine of same-time, same-thing, or following an age-appropriate app that starts with a 30-second run during a walk and builds up to a half-hour run or more over weeks. Others love to mark off success on a chart or diary app. Do what works for you.

Start small, count your achievements, define at least part of your success as showing up, congratulate yourself. If you miss a day or a week or more, forgive yourself – there's at least six reasons it felt too hard, I know. But start again today, or tomorrow.

Short, hard, intense bursts of exercise (the sort that make you start to puff-breathe) can really pack in some benefits in health and fitness, in a short time and count more quickly towards a 75-minute weekly target of intense exercise. If this appeals, you can start with even a few seconds or a couple of minutes, get a bit breathless, do it the next day and build up.

Check with an exercise physio, GP or a very well-credentialled trainer before getting back to or starting any high-intensity stuff such as burpee exercises, trampoline jumping, skipping and shouty stationary bike classes. These can carry a potential for injury, or incontinence issues.

I have a treadmill at home. I also exercise with a small group of gal friends and we do some weights and core body strength exercises together on a Monday evening.
Natalie, 49

If you're doing a jumping sort of exercise or anything else that makes you feel your inside organs are somehow feeling heavy, or it makes you get a big weeing urge, it's off to a specialist pelvic floor physio with you, to find out how you can make it OK to continue, or what else to try. (See the weeing info in Chapter 5, It's Your Body.)

You can start smaller: get in some cardio by walking down and up the stairs to your car in a high-rise carpark (if it's safe). If it's decent weather you could park a little further from the supermarket, for a smaller shop that will involve a brisk walk and carrying a medium weight. If you have to do a work-from-home phone meeting, do it while you do a medium-puffy walk.

Think about what surface you can, or would like to, walk or run on. You might need somewhere it's safe to run fast – pick a firm surface like a path or track. Maybe park or river tracks, or well-built wide footpaths. Grass and sand, uneven and unpredictable, are the most likely surfaces for ankle and other injuries. And it's better to have a cushioned area with a carpet, thick rug and/or yoga mat for flexibility exercises.

Anything that's too easy, is. Find a program that challenges you.
Liz (exercise physiologist), 44

Some online suggestions for exercise mention running at night, or in certain areas that most women would feel unsafe in (like cities, or suburbs, or country areas . . . you know what I mean, everywhere, sometimes). Some women feel safer exercising in a group, at crowded times of the day, or with a trusted man or a dog. Others may prefer to exercise in a women's gym or at home, if they don't want to be seen or be social.

Is there a sport or activity that you used to love but gave up after you left school or started a family? Is there an amateur club or league nearby that you could rejoin, or even just get amongst it at training?

Moderate versus vigorous exercise

Moderate exercise means while you're doing it your breathing has changed but you can still talk. Vigorous exercise means you can't hold a conversation or easily utter a smooth sentence. Think brisk walk versus a run.

When I was in the middle of menopause I had a 7yo, a 4yo, dying parents and I was the main breadwinner. Had NO time. Now I ride every day, scream at the sky if I need to. Annie, 62

If sex counts, I can do it every night! Other forms of exercise are difficult to fit into my life at the moment. Angela, 45

I'm happy if my patients in menopause do anything when it comes to exercise. The feeling of doing something is always a positive. (Psychiatrist)

I would recommend an online program of physio for over-55s to every woman struggling with a post-menopausal body. I have a new sense of myself and I love being able to do things again. Carol, 62

Forty-five minutes to an hour very early in the morning before the family wakes. Tonya, 49

What helps with exercise

Some of your exercise and activity each week should be something that makes you a bit huffy-puffy (but not utterly breathless, hurting, crying or vomiting). And some should be weight bearing (e.g. if you only do swimming and bike riding, do some weights too).

Devising a few different ways to move, or a fixed program that suits you that you know will cover cardiovascular needs helps your bones stay stronger for longer. A session or two with a qualified exercise physiologist or trainer who understands age-related issues can set you up with a home program you can do on your own. You can get a program to download on your phone or tablet, or printed out, with your choice of videos, pictures and instructions.

Exercise that feels good while you do it

A lot of people say they only feel better after exercising. Could you aim for during, as well? Excuse any suggestions that seem bleeding obvious, such as 'Try to find something you find calming or fun'. Not all of them will appeal, but others may be worth a try:

* Exercise with other people so there's a social incentive to turn up: a walking group, a training-for-a-hike group, swimming group, pool aerobics, a yoga or Pilates group class, bay or ocean swimming groups.
* Exercise alone if you'd rather.
* A tracker, route-mapper or counting device for steps or kilometres gives some people a sense of accomplishment. Some private health funds also give rewards and discounts linked to these.
* Use gentle walking time to make phone calls to friends; use huffy-puffier walk times to listen to a podcast or audiobook.
* Keep moving the whole time you walk your dog, even if you spend some time throwing them a ball or stick.
* Check that any streaming service or downloaded exercise program you do is specifically safe and useful for your age group, and in perimenopause and menopause. The bare minimum requirement should be low impact on joints and have resistance training of some kind.

Scientifically proven boogie

Dancing is a good activity in menopause for both mind and body (moods, metabolism, fitness, balance, strength and very much so forrrrth). This has been established by studies and also by belting out 'I Will Survive' while very much getting entirely down upon it, while doing the Nutbush on the coffee table, I think you'll find.

I'm at the gym five days a week. I often go straight from work. My kids/husband all work and study from home now and they do most of the household chores and cooking. **Kate, 49**

Even on the days when I don't do formal exercise, I still have a steps goal. **Samantha, 54**

I have time, just not the inclination or energy. **Denni, 46**

The best thing I did was commit to exercising with friends online. We do it five days a week, with a remote trainer, and it's helped massively with my mental and physical health. Amanda, 48

I would book myself a meeting room and I had a backpack of weights and bands that I would use for 30 minutes. Annette, 59

I do weights while listening to music. Sort of dancing with weights. Glenda, 59

If I didn't walk daily I would have severe back pain. So it has to happen, above almost anything else. Annie, 55

What won't help with exercise

Don't listen to a 22-year-old in a socials video saying anyone can do the upside-down-splits craze on a skateboard. Don't listen to the person saying the only useful exercise happens to be the thing they'll charge you money for. If the advice doesn't speak to you, don't listen to it.

One male author claims that it's easy to exercise whenever your teen kids do. Well, except if they're in a pool and it's dark and the pool complex is surrounded by inhospitable traffic-choked main roads with no safe pedestrian crossings, or it's the first time in the day you've been able to catch up with friends via text or work emails. Or because you need to pay attention to your kid and whether their situation is mentally healthy. Or 15 other reasons.

I read another airy assumption in that book just before I threw it against the wall: wake up earlier. As if many women aren't already getting up before the first rose-pearly hint of the arsecrack of the pre-dawn to get everything done.

There will be many more exercise programs, sign-up apps and video programs saying they're for 'menopausal women' in the future. Some questions to ask yourself: is it fun; what's the specific training of the course and its hosts; are there different levels you can start at? And don't judge them by the shape or size of the person who's giving the advice.

I really can only do one physical thing a day. If I go into the office, that's it. If I exercise, I can't do anything else that day. Michelle, 46

The lack of motivation seems part of the general lack of motivation around everything that feels part of the hormonal change. Nicole, 53

Avoid anything that:

* causes pain (as opposed to recovery aches)
* you hate that can be replaced with another kind of exercise with similar benefits
* puts too much stress on shoulders or lower back, or knees
* wakes up and intensifies old injuries or strains
* makes you feel even more 'run ragged', overstressed, always rushed and pressured. The 'low energy' vicious circle is a tough one. Too tired to exercise = lack of exercise = feeling less energy = not being sleepy-tired at the right times = sleep problems = too tired to exercise.

I make time. But it's really, really hard. I can't do an hour every day. But on weekends I do extra-long runs, shorter during the week. Some days are just yoga. **Isabelle, 57**

These things will work against you and your exercise aims: binge drinking or drinking alcohol every day, smoking, vitamin D and calcium deficiencies and being under or over a healthy weight range.

There's no time for exercise or any bloody life at all, really. Struggling to make ends meet. **Jodie, 52**

Balance

As you get older it gets more important that you can balance and rebalance yourself easily, so you may as well begin years before 'falling over' starts being described as 'a fall'. Part of being inactive is inevitable stiffness and a decline in balance skills and strength, which leads to strains and not being able to right yourself when tripping over.

Can you stand on one leg with your eyes open for a full minute? If not, why? Do you start to tip one way: are you losing strength and/or balance? What happens when you try it on the other leg?

You can start slow, with just a few moments, and build up from there over time. And you don't have to stand like a flamingo, you can bend one leg and lift that foot off the ground only a couple of centimetres from the floor. You can stand in an open doorway or next to your butler on the yacht, so you can grab something solid when you start to lean too far.

I love exercise videos. There are easy and hard exercises available. **Chiquita, 50**

If you're already sporty

Athletes and former athletes have a head start at habits that help build bone strength, such as running, walking, and training for weight-bearing team sports, but may need to change habits after perimenopause. Some athletes and others who kept their body at very low body fat for years, and those who were thin for long periods due to physical or mental health issues, are at special risk of earlier fractures as they get older. Talk to a specialised physio or exercise physiologist to set yourself up for safe exercise. (See 'More info on exercise', on page 146.)

I'm so happy to have found my exercise groove again. I'm no longer beating myself up for not taking out a gym membership. So I now walk EVERY DAY and don't overthink it. Merilyn, 56

Join the resistance

Resistance training helps build muscles and bone strength. Resistance training is anything that uses an outside force to make muscles contract, and includes weightlifting using proper weights or weighted gym machines and stretchy bands. Various monkey bar exercises, using gravity, can also create resistance. The same gravity works even just with your body, for exercises such as push-ups and squats.

Weight lifting improved bone density, also improved back pain and bladder and confidence. Jo, 61

Strength and resistance training helped me (even with just feeling good about myself – feeling more capable with strength development). Danielle, 52

How many steps?

Depends, is the annoying answer. There isn't a set number you should be doing, and stroll-y steps are not as useful for your heart and general fitness as brisk ones, but perfectly good if you enjoy them and can't do the brisk thing. Estimates vary for the number of steps an average person does in half an hour, between 3000 and 4000.

Probably the best way to judge it for you is to use an app or device to count your steps in a half hour or an hour walk (don't double the half-hour tally, measure an actual hour). A half-hour walk three times a week, or at least half an hour a day (even in three lots over the day, adding up to 30 minutes) can be a significant tally.

Does housework & gardening help?

Those website articles are always telling you that housework and gardening is good for you. I mean, sure, it moves your body around and works different parts of you if you squat, stretch to do things: but housework and gardening can also cause repetition injury (there's a reason bursitis used to be called housemaid's knee), or injuries (moving a too-heavy wheelbarrow). Do gardening because you love it, and do something else if you don't.

If you can, you're better off making sure the housework load is spread so everyone has spare time for more enjoyable exercise or other hobbies. Set up new systems so family members put their own clothes in dirty clothes baskets and do their own washing, make a roster for kitchen clean-ups. Many older women find themselves still cleaning a grown-up child's bedroom and resentfully being the only person in a shared house who cooks dinner. That shit, if I may be indelicate, has to stop.

Who's Who in exercise help

Your GP should do your initial 'physical'. Be honest about problems, drinking and drugs, and your medical history, and share your plans for exercise. The Australasian College of Sports and Exercise Physicians is at **acsep.org.au**.

Sport/exercise physiologists specialise in the scientific study of the physical characteristics of bodies and how these can be used in training and performance to maximise success or usefulness. Physiologists must have completed at least 3 years of a recognised university level course involving theory and practical experience. You don't need a referral from a GP. Physiologists should be accredited with industry association Exercise and Sports Science Australia at **essa.com.au**.

Physiotherapists are practitioners who treat injuries and other movement problems. They use physical treatments such as hydrotherapy, electrotherapy, therapeutic exercise, massage, mobilisation and manipulation of joints to help injured people or athletes who need relief from physical pain and to rebuild the strength in a particular part of their body. Physiotherapists must have completed a 4-year university degree involving theory and experience, and be registered with the Australian Physiotherapy Association at **physiotherapy.asn.au**. Some do extra specialist training and education in specific sports or with children. Physios can diagnose and do hands-on treatment. You don't need a referral from a GP. For info on specialist pelvic floor physios, see Chapter 5, It's Your Body.

Masseurs Anyone can call themselves a masseur or myotherapist or massage therapist. A properly trained masseur should have studied anatomy, remedial massage, first aid and massage technique over several months. Courses range from two hours online or a weekend to various private college certificates and diplomas. Those who offer 'therapeutic' or sports massage should have professional qualifications and keep up their knowledge of new info and skills in proven methods of alleviating pain, soothing muscles and assisting injury recovery. 'Relaxation' and 'aromatherapy' masseurs should not treat injuries and should do no harm, especially to pregnant or injured clients. Some massage techniques, such as reiki, are unproven and more akin to faith healing. The industry body is Massage and Myotherapy Australia at **massagemyotherapy.com.au**.

Personal trainers & gym/class instructors Anyone can call themselves a personal trainer or fitness coach. Various private courses exist and gym employment or similar generally requires a recognised level of qualifications. They should have a good knowledge of anatomy, physiology, injury risk, psychology, first aid, fitness, and the special needs of pregnant, injured, menopausal and older clients. Pilates and yoga class teachers should also have qualifications, which can vary.

Bugs me that tending to animals, chain-sawing, carrying wood etc., etc. aren't considered exercise by healthcare professionals. Carol, 52

Clinical Pilates has been terrific for building strength (particularly core), maintaining flexibility under professional supervision. Emma, 54

MORE INFO on exercise

healthybonesaustralia.org.au
Formerly known as Osteoroposis Australia, this website has fact sheets, and an exercise guide.

essa.org.au
Exercise and Sports Science Australia is the peak membership body for qualified practitioners. Search 'What is an accredited exercise physiologist' for relevant qualifications, or 'Find an exercise professional near you', and filter the search to 'older adults' or 'ergonomics' if you need help with a work set-up.

menopause.org.au
If it's scientific study results you want for motivation, search 'exercise' on this trusted site for the latest on how exercise helps guard against brain fog, muscle weakness in the future, with feelings of depression or anxiety, bone health, and unwanted weight gain.

healthdirect.gov.au
This may be decades away for you yet, but search 'physical activity guidelines for older people' for a fact sheet, if it's relevant.

Aches & pains

Walking, hiking, beach walking, and kayaking are my go-to activities depending on how my joints are. Nix, 56

The best medicine for joints that feel sore and stiff is to exercise them. This helps the internal lubricating joint fluid that makes movement easier. In other words, you need to moisturise your joints by moving them, if you can.

As you get older, you expect to feel creakier, stiffer, and less flexible, but not to be feeling aches and pain in your joints as if you have a bad flu, or low-level muscle injuries. It's common to feel that, though, especially around the time of your last period, according to women's health specialist and gynaecologist-author Dr Jen Gunter. We don't really know if it's because estrogen used to work for you as an anti-inflammatory, or if women are probably more susceptible to feeling pain when they're miserable about other things, more as a sensible alert system rather than wallowing.

I had no idea my joint and back pain was related to hormone changes. Not even my GP knew this! Shweta, 57

Bloated sore ankles, sore joints and back, general lethargy and weight gain make it difficult to muster the energy. Therese, 51

Four out of five respondents to the Survey reported sore joints in perimenopause, with just over a quarter finding it sometimes annoying, just under a quarter finding it tough, and just over 13 per cent really suffering. More than two-thirds said they experienced backache of varying degrees of severity with just under 30 per cent finding it tough or terrible.

If you have a few aches and pains around the time of perimenopause and then it seems to go away, it's probably hormone-related and your body has settled down. But if it feels like aches and pains have barged in and show no signs of being on their way, talk to your GP about getting a diagnosis to rule out early symptoms of an arthritic, thyroid or an autoimmune condition, which are more common in women.

Menopausal hormone medication is not always the automatic frontline treatment for muscle and joint pain, though doctors believe it helps and many women in the Survey agreed. There's mixed or no evidence that hormone-related joint and muscle pain is helped by any natural supplements containing cartilage, collagen, fish oils, ginger glycosides, cannabis, soy, turmeric, and feel free to insert fashionable 'superfood' or other ingredient here.

Various so-called anti-inflammatory diets have been marketed, but it isn't known how much effect they have on joint problems. Basically it's less sugar and more fruit, veggies, legumes. Long-term use of anti-inflammatory painkillers can cause problems – so if you need it, discuss long-term pain management with your GP.

> Cycling. Gentle on the joints, good psychologically because of its meditative qualities, very good to do with friends – we cycle places for lunch or go away for a few days on bike paths. Annie, 62

What may help with joint pain

This stuff:

* diagnosis
* medication, including MHT
* enough vitamin D, calcium and magnesium intake
* solving sleep problems
* distracting yourself with a movie or concentration-heavy hobby or game
* low-intensity strength-training exercises to keep muscles moving
* stretches and exercises, including yoga and Pilates
* anti-stress measures
* tackling being over or under a healthy weight range
* prescribed and monitored pain relief.

> I could exercise more if my achy bones let me. Isabella, 60

What doesn't help with joint pain

This stuff:

* unproven supplements: those without a prescription
* high-impact exercise
* alcohol
* people who say 'Have you tried yoga?' as if you've never even heard of it.

I'm a sweaty mess and my joints ache and my belly jiggles, but our dog is decidedly non-judgemental! Rowena, 49

Not running now as joints don't really cope, but walking a lot more, including long treks. Julie, 53

Pain

Any pain should be checked out by a GP or allied health professional such as a podiatrist, physiotherapist, or visual scan expert (radiologist, ultrasound operator). If I hear one more podcast talking about how pain is 'all in the mind' because some people feel pain from a phantom limb after an amputation, and because there was that guy who screamed in pain when a nail went through his boot but then when he got to hospital it had gone between his toes, so therefore pain is just imaginary and all psychological, I shall have to be restrained from hitting the podcast host on the ankle with a shovel a few times just to see how psychological pain is.

If something hurts, find out why. The answer is probably mostly physical that some psychological strategies can help with. But don't ignore pain. That's your body telling you to rest a bit, or do something a bit differently.

Aching hips will wake me up at night sometimes. Cat, 47

Eating & weight

Changing your weight can help stabilise hormone levels (though it's not clear precisely how), hugely reduce your risks of several dangerous health conditions and be a big help in changing feelings of depression and anxiety. (See Chapter 4, It's Your Mind, for the full picture.)

The first thing to recognise is that menopause does change your weight distribution (puts it round your middle), and coincides with a time in your life when a combination of factors make maintaining a healthy weight range harder. You may find it more difficult to find time to exercise, or afford or cook healthy meals from scratch.

The most universally recognised shape of the quintessential 'matron' or older woman in a classic film is to use a character actress who may as well be called Mrs Shelf-Bosom, whose overall shape is more like a dugong than a wasp.

Researchers tend to say menopause doesn't make you put on more weight, but acknowledge that, through no fault of our own, it shifts weight to around your middle, where it's associated with extra risk for heart trouble. (A bit like the way it tends to take leg hairs away and put them on your moustache.) It's befuddling.

We're often told sternly that any weight gain is due to a failure: our fault because of 'lifestyle changes' or 'choices'. And it's true that as we get older, many of us exercise less, eat more sugar and drink more alcohol. But in terms of the 'middle' weight gain, they *know* it's not our 'fault'.

More than 80 per cent of women who answered the Survey weight questions for this book said they had unexpected weight gain associated with peri-menopause, with just over half finding it tough or very difficult. More than 90 per cent said it had mainly gone to their middle.

This can be alarming to those of us who've been pretty much the same shape for decades, and who now feel powerless against the changes. As an extra trial for many of us, we also put on more weight in general in our 40s and 50s. And for those who've spent a lifetime yo-yoing in size and shape, we can easily find that happening at a heavier level overall.

Losing 10 kilos over the course of a year was a tangible way for me to focus on getting better and healthier (not skinnier). Mack, 57

Can't fit into any of my old fav clothes even though I haven't put on that much weight. Sonya, 53

Gained 10 kilos in 2 years, in spite of healthy eating and lots of exercise . . . this has been the most soul-destroying aspect of the pause for me. Celia, 52

The weight gain has been the most upsetting for me. I have tried everything and found the attitude from medical staff to be dismissive. Danielle, 49

Self-sabotage is real. I felt shit and ate shit food and that made me worse. MHT fixed most of that, feeling better so eating better and caring for myself. Sam, 53

The weight gain and lack of energy is truly horrifying to me as I have always been fit and active. Sheena, 52

Being underweight

While it's always assumed that we want to lose weight in menopause, for some people, not being underweight is their challenge, due to a range of reasons. These can include eating behaviour, body image issues, experiencing grief or being overworked. Being underweight and missing crucial nutrients can have severe effects in menopause, including on bone strength and mental health.

Thinner is absolutely not always healthier and a culture that encourages other people to comment, often rudely, on other people's bodies and rewards losing weight with approval means you can bear the brunt of 'You're lucky you're so thin' nonsense, when the opposite may be true. If this feels like you, ask your GP for help, with the option of a referral to a mental health specialist and/or a dietitian.

Metabolism

Doctors told us for years that perimenopause and menopause causes a slower metabolism – so our body has to expend more energy in relation to our food intake. That we should eat a third less every day than we used to.

We've been shouted at by headlines like these: 'You can't blame midlife weight gain on a slow metabolism' and 'Study shows metabolism stays the same until you're 60'. You idle slattern is the general, unhelpful message.

What is clear is that when perimenopause hits, a variety of factors including busyness and feelings of anxiety and depression often conspire to make us do less exercise and activity, which can make it feel like our metabolism has slowed.

But it's also true that hardly any researchers have studied metabolism specifically in relation to perimenopause and menopause. We do know that individuals have widely varying metabolisms, many at wildly different rates than the average. And because men have more muscle than women on average, they burn more kilojoules faster every day. We know that a history of repeated short-term diets, more common in women, messes with long-term metabolism. We know that most research about energy and estrogen has been done on rats.

Well done, rats, for being too sensible to read phrases online such as 'spare tyre' or 'muffin-top'.

The why of weight gain

Weight gain is very complex, with a mix of medical, social and psychological contributing causes ranging from genetics, poverty, trauma, financial and geographical ability to afford fresh unprocessed food, and to have extra time to cook, serve and clean up, and the emotional connections between types of food and feelings of comfort, reward and compensation. Hormone changes play a key role in eating behaviours and mood-related eating and drinking, often years before recognised physical perimenopause symptoms. So do sleep patterns, well-known to be in play during perimenopause years, and gut bacteria balance.

Taking MHT doesn't seem to change the weight situation, or where it goes on the body. Doctors don't know why. Menopause specialist doctors think maybe women put on about half a kilo a year on average each year due to age-related changes rather than hormonal ones. It's a murky picture.

> As a dietitian I understand and appreciate the weight gain – it is still stuff to process, as a change to 'who I am'.
> **Marian, 61**

> My clothes don't fit; I'm still thin everywhere else but I HAVE A BASKETBALL WHERE MY TUMMY ONCE WAS.
> **Sue, 53**

Risks of a higher than healthy weight

A much higher weight than you need is one of the highest risk factors for cancers and heart disease. Doctors don't like too much extra weight around the middle because it's associated with a bigger risk of heart disease and heart failure, type 2 diabetes, breast cancer and dementia.

Size labels

I've said it before, but feel free to cut the size labels out of your clothes. They're not standardised, there's no reason anyone has to look at the word 'large' when they put their undies on, and tags make menopausal skin itch, anyway. Throw away or put away clothes that make you feel uncomfortable, or restricted, or that make you turn sideways and wince at the mirror. You're you-size.

Bad advice about weight

Very annoyingly indeed, even official medical advice about weight can be unhelpful if not downright stupid. One well-respected women's health site says, 'the more you move, the more you can lower your overall weight and waist circumference.' This is simply not true, easy or possible for many or all women.

Meanwhile, our enemies and pretend friends in the 'wellness' industry are flogging us supplements for which no credible research shows they do anything to speed metabolism or help with weight loss. The product names have 'weight' or 'menopause' in them, and their claims include 'supports weight control' or 'reduces weight naturally'. Piffle alert.

Ads pop up if you search 'menopause weight' or similar key words. Caveats are included saying they 'work in combination with healthy diet and lifestyle and exercise changes'. Of course they do, sunshine. But why would you need an expensive powder if you were already doing that?

Stealing an idea from the body-builder products industry, these products *are* often powders, which can be cheaper to make than pills (though pills are also produced for those who prefer them). The ingredients lists remind me of 19th-century cure-all tonics and digestive pills, claiming to do what many women want to happen: lose weight, have more energy, look slimmer.

The products may or may not contain probiotics, prebiotics (oh stop it), vitamins, minerals, metabolism-busters (what?). Often they contain bulking agents and laxatives. The list of ingredients is often as endless as it is baffling and useless.

Many sellers of supplements say the liver shrinks and the gallbladder becomes less efficient during menopause and sell 'detoxing' and 'anti-inflammatory' products (which *don't* detox the body and there's no proof that the product anti-inflames anything). The ads often suggest that a woman has 'bloating' that their product can cure with probiotics, or 'thermogenic probiotics' as one company suggested, in a fat-burny linguistic wiggle.

Men are virtually never targeted about 'bloating'.

Ugh, I say, to the websites selling products recommended by 'a Doctor' (maybe the small print says they're not a medical doctor but a PhD). Illustrations or photos of happy, thin women looking triumphant, and sad, bigger, slumping cartoon women. One weight-loss product aimed at menopausal women even ran ads with a picture of a distraught woman's face with mascara tear-tracks.

North American dietitian Abby Langer did the legwork on one company's claims of research citations supporting its probiotic diet product. She says of the 36 references on their website, six were unsupported claims, 11 were about general probiotic use, nine were studies on rats, one was a study on yoghurt, three were on ingredients in the supplement but not on the formulation in the supplement itself, one 'study' was a manufacturer's hand-out, one a study on calories not probiotics, and of the remaining four, one was repeated. So: three citations remained.

Of those, one was a study that proved no difference between the control group and the group taking the supplement; one was a study on a probiotic that is no longer sold; and one involved possible weight loss if one single probiotic ingredient was taken with fermented milk. In conclusion, 'None of the ingredients burn fat, curb cravings, and "manage calorie absorption" . . . We don't have science yet that indicates which bacteria, if any, increase the metabolic rate for better fat burning. So either the [supplements company] knows something we don't or . . . yeah, [it's] just a scam.' As her website **abbylangernutrition.com** says, 'Just because there's research on something doesn't mean it's good research.'

One weight-loss book suggests you do one weekly shop to avoid takeaway or snack food temptations, but also suggests you bike to the shops with your kids. Good luck getting everyone back alive with a weekly shop on bicycles.

Why have I gained weight?

> [I developed] severe nutritional deficiencies despite an unchanged diet.
> Mandy, 59

Maybe because:

* You're tired so you get more takeaway.
* You might be drinking more alcohol.
* You might be eating more high-sugar 'comfort' foods.
* You don't have enough time to do everything at work and at home and cook sensible meals.
* You have to choose cheaper food options, which are often more unhealthy.
* Self-conscious, you choose 'low fat', dairy items, not realising they're high in sugar that your body converts to fat anyway. ('Sugar free' products can also cause stomach distension and fartiness.)
* Injuries and twinges take longer to disappear, so you don't exercise as much; a gym membership seems like a baroque expense even if you had the time.

What can help with your weight

Maybe these things:

- If you are doing social media programs, gym classes or have a personal trainer, make sure they understand the specific requirements of menopause exercise (e.g. non-injurious weight training). Try to do a half-hour of exercise a day, even if it's just walking a dog.
- The more muscle you have, the more your metabolism speeds up to help you shed excess weight. (Muscle weighs more than fat and that's a good thing.)
- Read the 'Exercise section' earlier in this chapter.
- If you are under or over a healthy weight range for you, ask a GP to help you with allied health services such as a dietitian or an exercise physiologist who can help you.

What doesn't help with weight issues

You don't need to weigh yourself, or know what you weigh: this can be especially triggering with people who've had a history of troubled eating behaviours. Feel free to chuck out any scales at your place. If a doctor needs to weigh you for any reason they can do that, and can be instructed not to tell you, if you don't want to know.

Ignore all those pitiless, soul-sucking weight-loss short-term 'diets'. So-called weight-loss diets will make you miserable, farty, put on more weight afterwards, mess with your metabolism and mental health, and provide a dangerous example to family members like younger women.

Also don't take individual nutrition advice from self-titled nutritionists and alleged wellness influencers on social media, or a friend or rellie, or those magazine snippets which insist that you can exist on a kale smoothie with dust-milk for breakfast, a fruit salad for lunch and some steamed eggplant skin on a Ryvita for dinner. It will make you desperate and sad and sick. And farty.

Nutrition

The basic mainstream advice about nutrition and food is familiar to all of us and has stayed pretty much the same for centuries: eat way more fruit and veggies, eat protein, avoid too much sugar and unnecessary additives, avoid processed meats and too much red meat.

You need good food: fresh veggies and fruit if you can afford it. Fruit and veggies in season to keep costs down. (Of course you probably already know all this . . .) Try going to markets or shops at the end of their last weekend day of trading for any discounts. Snap-frozen foods are just as nutritious as fresh ones, and canned ones can be cheaper, though go for the low-salt version. Make sure you boost your intake of protein to help build muscle mass, and fibre, which makes you feel properly full and has other health benefits including an association with better mental health.

Vitamin & mineral supplements

A healthy diet should get you enough vitamins and minerals, but a standard multivitamin can help if you've been diagnosed with a deficiency in, say, vitamin D or iron. Never take cumulative supplements or mega-supplements that put you way above daily recommendations, because that can make you really sick: ask your GP or consult a dietitian if you're unsure.

If you're vegie or vegan, take a multivitamin to make sure you're covering really important vitamins and minerals for your age group including iron, zinc, calcium and the B-group vitamins gang.

Almost all non-prescribed or combination supplements are not subject to regulation about proving their doses, effects and ingredients. Always tell your doctor how many and which supplements you're taking as they may not have enough vitamins and minerals for your specific needs, or perhaps dangerously combine to 'overdose' you on some minerals or vitamins.

You're not a number

Any diet program that tells you to re-evaluate your life if you put on more than a kilo a year can go and stuff itself up its own index. There's no exact optimum weight number you need to be. You'll go up and down in your life, and can stabilise within a healthy range for you.

How do I manage my weight through menopause? With self-compassion. My waist feels like it's gone into retirement early. Kylie, 50

I always hear that I need to lose weight. I walk most days. I am OK with where I am; my husband loves me, so does my family. My size has never been an issue for them. Nicole, 48

Who's Who in eating advisors

Anyone can call themselves a nutritionist. Only an accredited dietitian in Australia can legally give individual medical advice about food and nutrition, but this rule is often ignored, especially on social media. The Dietitians Association of Australia explains:

An **Accredited Nutritionist** (AN) has approved tertiary qualifications and can specialise in public or community health nutrition or teach tertiary nutrition courses, but is not qualified to provide individual dietary counselling, group therapy or medical nutrition therapy.

An **Accredited Practising Dietitian** (APD) can give individual advice, and has a degree in nutrition and dietetics from a university accredited with the Dietitians Association of Australia (usually involving at least 4 years of approved tertiary study), or has sat the DAA's local exam. APDs must adhere to a professional code of conduct and update skills and knowledge. They're recognised by Medicare and most private health funds. An APD is also an AN, but not vice versa.

MORE INFO on eating & weight

daa.asn.au
The Dietitians Association of Australia site can help you find an Accredited Practising Dietitian.

nrv.gov.au/nutrients-energy-calc
Pop your age into this handy Nutrient Reference Values calculator, then do separate calculations for select macro-nutrients, vitamins and minerals to check your general recommended and adequate intake levels. Adequate intakes are more of a rough guide based on scientific knowledge, so when in doubt, check with a GP or dietitian. The calculator is provided by the Australian National Health and Medical Research Council and New Zealand Ministry of Health.

A couple of years into perimenopause I lost about 80 kilos, but I really don't miss my husband at all. Janine, 53

(Oh Janine, that's an old joke but maybe so is he.)

The takeaway on your approach

Take charge of your perimenopause and menopause. Embrace your own philosophy but be flexible enough to look further if you need it. Self-help, stress-management techniques and medical treatment are all good options. Find a good doctor, and ask useful questions. Don't be fooled by unproven wellness marketing claims and buzzwords.

Find good hobbies, podcasts, underpants and enthusiasms. There are new ways to think about exercise and eating healthier food. Be kind to yourself about inevitable changes in your shape and size: think less about numbers and more about feelings.

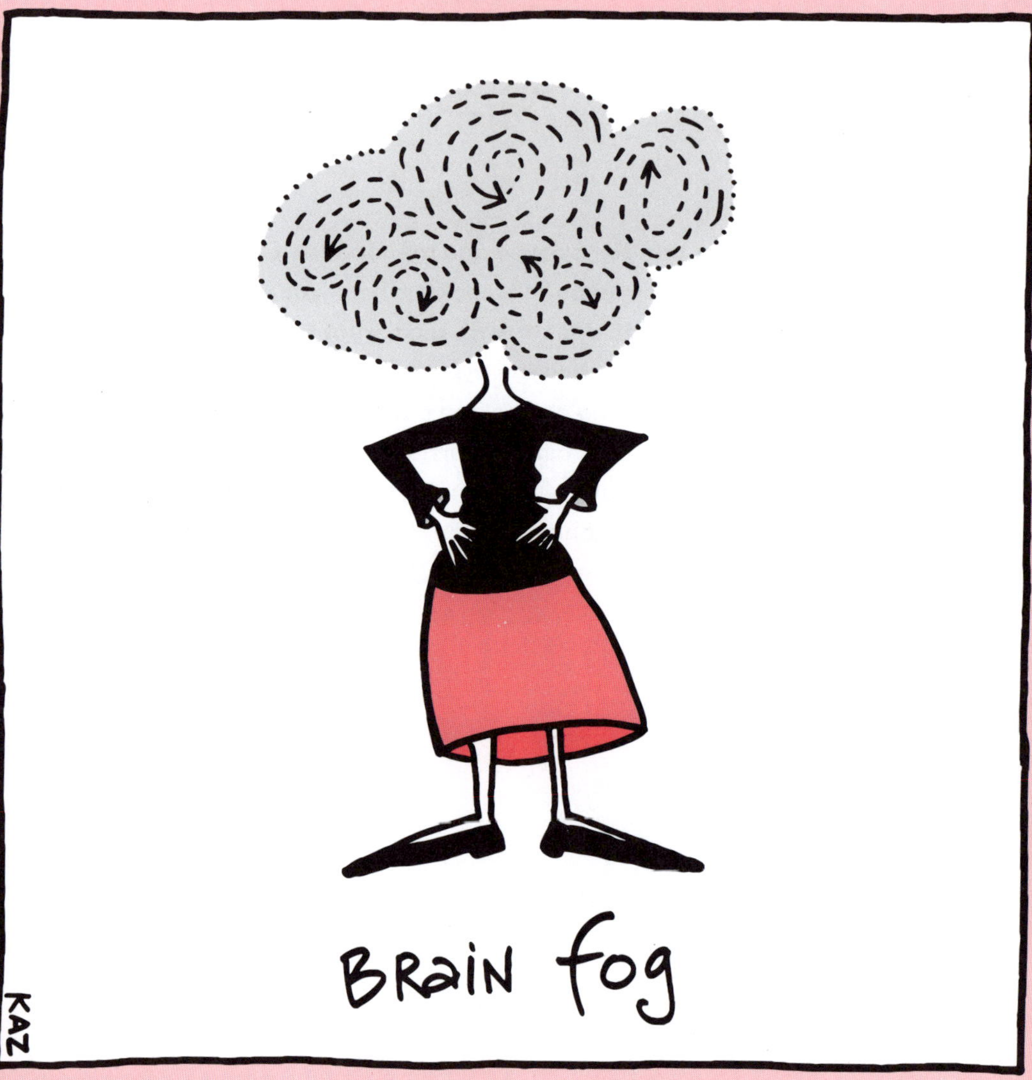
Brain fog
KAZ

4

It's Your Mind

Welcome to the special, multi-ingredient Christmas fruitcake of menopausal brain carry-on! Not just a low, low mood but, for completely free and without asking, you can get the bonus bargain extras of anxiety, feeling furious, exhaustion, the blahs, a plummet of self-esteem, and confronting memory problems. And that's not all! You get less articulate, guilty, less copey and quicker to anger.

It might be tempting to regard this, according to my Aunty Beryl, as proof of losing yer feminine qualities, and turning into a man who is repressed, grumpy and can't multitask, but that's not really what it means. (Beryl's been repressed and furious since 1967.)

When I first felt all these things I was struck terrified, because I'm a writer, at how many times I sat blankly trying to think of a word when previously, my brain would throw out a bunch of alternatives like a chatty thesaurus. Fizz, pizzazz, chutzpah! Vivacious, sparky, coruscating, jaunty! Sharp . . . something . . . suddenly I'd find myself staring at the screen, fingers motionless on the keyboard, thinking, 'What's that thing, when you're not . . . lumpensitting.'

A very common way for women to describe the feelings associated with menopause is 'losing it', or 'not myself'. So many women who responded to the Survey for this book said something like, 'I thought I was going crazy.'

Reading the thousands of responses was an emotional experience. They were an outpouring of distress during perimenopause: so much confusion, and anguish about feeling they had lost their confidence, their words, their sense of self, in the grip of terrible and inexplicable anxiety, or depression, or feeling out of control fury, of overwhelming fatigue, uncontrollable tearfulness, fear of losing their sex drive, the respect of others, the sudden onset of social fears and even not wanting to leave the house.

While a handful of women said they had no mental symptoms at all, thousands talked of feeling despair, or being seriously frightened by their symptoms. One of the positives was seeing how many women found help in talking to friends, meditation, changing doctors, trying medication, or getting through menopausal symptoms caused by fluctuating hormones to a new confidence on the other side.

I'm rather appalled to have to report that perimenopause does indeed happen in your brain, as well as your body, and the mental stuff can start 4 to 5 years earlier than the rest of it. So while you're minding your own beeswax a good few years before a hot flush or any period misbehaviour, a wave can dump you into a bunch of mental difficulties and bad feelings that you have no explanation for, or warning of. But there is a medical hormonal explanation.

The short version: psychiatric and hormone researchers now know that the faffing about of hormones, especially during perimenopause, can have a direct effect on whether we feel more cheerful, or less energetic, less able to concentrate and multitask.

The long version: brain chemicals! Feedback loops! Our body's triggers for functions and feelings! Hypothalamus! Pituatory gland! Can't even spell it! Cascading carry-on! Go home, dopamine, glutamate and serotonin, you're too drunk to dance! Neurochemical pathways! Hormone surges! Estrogen gorn elsewhere! Progesterone petering out! Misfiring signals! Etceterarrrrghhh.

When all that stuff, or even some of it happens to you, and you don't realise it has anything to do with hormones, you can think you've lost your abilities to cope, become a miserable person, or even have early onset dementia. In ye olden days it was often known as 'having a nervous breakdown', or (hushed tones) 'women's trouble'.

Because the hormonal carry-on is unlikely to be a steady, predictable or detectable decline, the feeling of mental struggles can come and go and pounce without warning, while your invisible hormones behave like a maniacal graph with accidental spirals on it drawn by a toddler who's eaten some of the crayon.

Lots of women and non-binary folk, faced with these inexplicable feelings caused by hormone changes, end up feeling desperate, and can turn to unhelpful coping methods such as self-blame, prescribed antidepressants that don't target the real, hormonal cause, and non-prescription drugs and alcohol, which make things worse.

Why perimenopause affects our moods & mental health

As the ovaries wind down their hormone production during menopause, the bit of the brain that quietly triggers them to behave properly starts shouting at them. 'Wake up, ovaries! Quick! Find an egg! Pump out some estrogen and progesterone! Not enough! Oops, too much of that! Now what are you doing? Wake up again!' which can lead to you feeling a bit upsy-downsy bonkers until the ovaries finally quit.

One of the ways the brain tries to compensate for ovaries not being able to keep pumping out the same amount of estrogen is to boost or lower various other brain chemicals. This can directly lead to mood fluctuations; depressions and peaks.

We know that ovaries, hormone levels, brain chemicals, neurotransmitters and cells in different parts of the bodies all play a part in emotions, feelings, mood, and thinking skills. Relevant brain chemicals include happy-and-sadness regulators dopamine and serotonin; and the neurotransmitter glutamate handles concentration and memory. We know women can feel differently when hormone levels are changed even slightly, and that our supply of estrogen and progesterone is directly related to the areas of the brain that account for feeling blue or cheery, and all the other mental challenges relevant in perimenopause.

While menopause research continues, most of it is unrelated to mental health: governments should be shamed for failing to properly fund menopausal research for decades. There's study going on into all sorts of peptides, receptors, feedback loops and more, but while we're waiting for new knowledge and medication, just know you're not going mad and you're not imagining it, and you can get help.

Even being confronted with severe symptoms of only *one* of the mental symptoms associated with perimenopause can be frightening and life-changing. Many women report that it made them feel out of control and miserable for a long time; some say it badly affected their family and partner relationships and cite it as the main factor leading to losing or leaving their job, or breaking up with a partner. This is the time of life when, statistically, women are most at risk of suicide.

Here's the good news: now you know that you're not going crazy. You're not hopelessly falling apart. You can overcome and move past feelings of self-harm. And these feelings are not beyond your control. You don't have to put up with it, and if it's interfering with your work life, your family and relationships, you can get help. Hurrah. This chapter will give you lots of options about managing or banishing the mental palaver of perimenopause.

What are the mental health problems of perimenopause?

You may not experience any of this at all and skate through oblivious; you may feel a little of it; or you may feel like you've been pushed off a mental waterfall into a churning mess of it. Here's the full filthy list of common mental challenges we can experience in our 40s or 50s, known to be caused or affected by changes in our hormone levels:

- brain fog: concentration and memory problems
- word retrieval problems
- sleep disruption
- lack of mental energy and enthusiasm
- a big fall in self-esteem, confidence and sense of purpose
- feelings of impatience and crankiness
- rage
- depression, and its evil, non-identical twin,
- anxiety.

Antidepressants really saved me: should have started earlier. Belle, 49

Counselling has helped [me] understand my anxiety and mental health symptoms and given me some strategies. Kathryn, 47

I'm told I'm being ridiculous if I describe how I feel about myself to my family. Kim, 55

It's also common to experience the roaring back or irksome echoes of mental health issues or self-harm and unhelpful coping attempts that were previously manageable, including:

* obsessive-compulsive behaviours
* damage from past trauma
* eating disorders.

I thought that by middle age I would have overcome any issues around disordered eating, but the changes just seem to make it as bad as it was when I was in my 20s. Robyn, 46

In the Survey, just over 5000 women answered questions about perimenopause-related mental symptoms. Almost two-thirds identified depression as a problem; just over 80 per cent said anxiety, nearly a third reported panic attacks; about 12 per cent reported obsessive behaviours; about 11 per cent said they were dealing with trauma from sexual assault or abuse; about 13 per cent identified post-traumatic stress disorder; about 42 per cent said they developed social anxiety; and almost one in five found themselves dealing with eating behaviours or disorders.

Many women shared their heartbreak of how their infertility came roaring back as a sadness or part of their anxiety during perimenopause, and at the prospect of menopause.

More than half of respondents felt their mental symptoms turned up around the same time as physical ones; about a quarter said mental symptoms appeared first; and another quarter said physical symptoms appeared first.

Have worthless feelings. Thoughts of suicide, which really surprised me. Would never act on those. Social anxiety again, have to make myself go out sometimes and always end up having a good time. Louise, 59

Many issues I hadn't dealt with – from childhood on – came flooding in to be dealt with. Siobhan, 80

Perimenopause sucks. Team this with complex PTSD and you've got a shit storm. In a teacup. Emily, 49

Mindful self-compassion . . . Can't recommend it highly enough. Edie, 44

My mood was on the high anxiety to hysterical to happy to depressed. I just hated being me. Kat, 57

The contrary view on feelings

As I approached perimenopause I was having PMT for 2 weeks out of 4. So that was a challenge, and at one point in that transition I was extremely wobbly, mentally. Tracy, 60

There's a long tradition of either telling women they're imagining menopause symptoms, or telling them to just get on with things: including the misinformation that some cultures don't recognise menopause, so it's just a matter of 'mind over matter' and 'pull yourself together'. Neither attitude is remotely useful or based on enough evidence. Indigenous women worldwide, for example, continue to be the most under-studied menopausal women.

It used to be just the patriarchy saying we're all ruled by our hormones and are hysterical; now we sometimes get the opposite: never blame anything on the menopause, or mention it, don't let anyone see you cry, or not cope, because women will be dismissed as hormonal creatures all over again. There's no hormonal reason for moods, this argument goes.

Instead, the theory continues, women are depressed, anxious and experiencing recurrences of traumas because society is so tough on them and they can be entering a period of multi-maxed-out responsibility: work, partner, organising their home, kids and elderly relatives. They're bombarded with poisonous messages of you're-not-attractive-enough anymore, and prey to being told that it's compulsory to take hormones during perimenopause.

I literally thought I was going mad. I was anxiety ridden, had panic attacks, brain fog. Got so anxious I was freaking out about driving. I LOVE DRIVING. Nadine, 49

I guess I've felt more angry about my feelings of being the forever f**king caregivers when we are also treated like whingeing old menopausal hags. Stash, 55

Anxiety, forgetfulness, rage, guilt, panic, acceptance, humour. Julz M, 53

I was 'stabby'. I actually didn't even like myself. If I'd had the option not to be around me, I'd have taken it. Monique, 51

I take a high dose of [an antidepressant] for PMDD [premenstrual dysphoric disorder] and it's really fucken helpful. Kylie, 48

I cannot guess when I started crying in the shower every day. Kirsty, 44

If I have to choose a philosophy on this myself it's probably this: assess your own individual needs and get help through whatever means make sense to you. Don't be swayed by advertising or the philosophy of friends and relatives with their certainties and pronouncements of what is 'right' for you. Because the only real certainty is that your experience is not the same as anyone else's: your hormones will be doing something different *and* having different effects on you. Your best route to feeling yourself again might be gained through self-help or pharmaceutical means, or a mixture of both.

Being on the spectrum with a side of ADHD makes all the hormone things worse.
Tiffany, 46

Why can mental symptoms start in your 40s?

Specialist psychiatrists and menopause doctors are now confident that the mental changes caused by the fall in hormonal levels start a few years, perhaps four or five, before the physical symptoms we've been taught to recognise as menopausal: hot flushes or the disorderly conduct of periods. So we just think we've gone mad.

I am on different medications for anxiety and sugar, fat and alcohol cravings. I would be morbidly obese, drunk, and in an asylum if I wasn't.
Catherine, 52

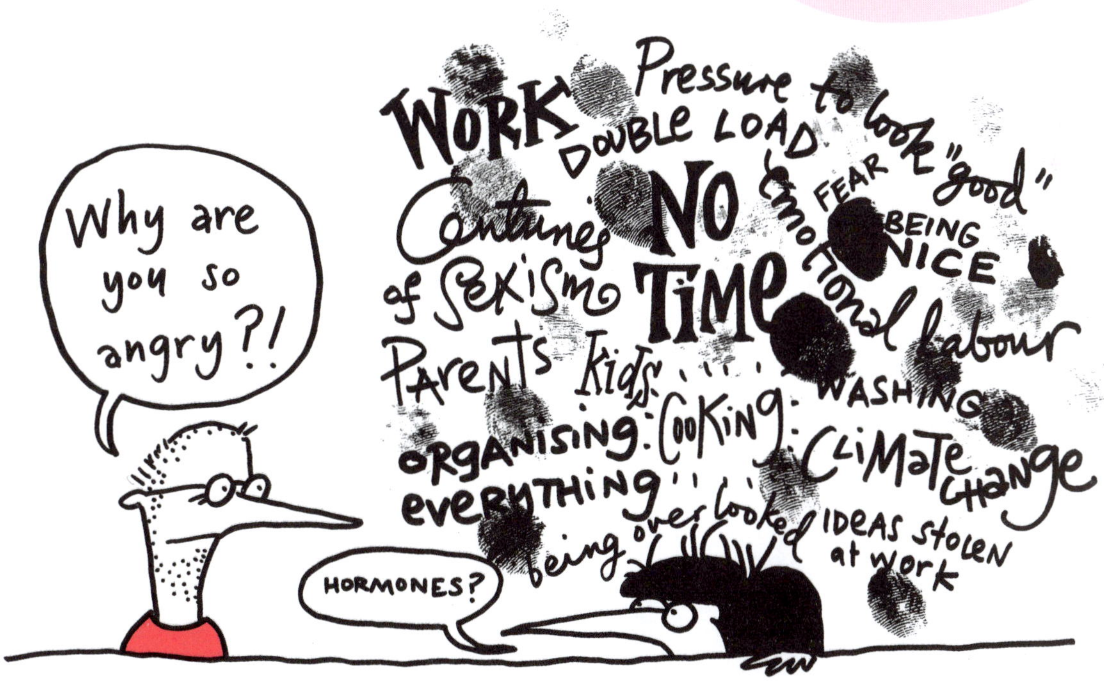
Why are you so angry?!
HORMONES?
WORK
Pressure to look "good"
DOUBLE LOAD
Centuries of Sexism
NO TIME
Emotional labour
FEAR
BEING NICE
Parents
Kids
WASHING
ORGANISING
COOKING
CLIMATE CHANGE
EVERYTHING
being overlooked
IDEAS STOLEN at work

A road every woman has to travel. For some of us it's a paved dual-lane freeway with no speed limit. For others, it's a dirt track full of bumps and ditches and nasty unexpected corners. Sian, 65

I had the courage to stop talking to my mother, who caused me great anxiety. Anna, 46

I've got no idea whether my symptoms are perimenopausal or I'm just being constantly overwhelmed, stressed out, taken for granted and exhausted by carrying the entire load of family management while my partner coasts along in blissful ignorance. Cath, 53

I am lucky to have a brilliant counsellor. Franny, 52

There was a point where I stopped caring about all the things I used to get worked up about when I was younger. It's very nice being at that point. Robyn, 46

So 42–52 is a reasonable age span in which to consider or suspect a hormone-related reason for the following carry-on: loss of sense of self, brain fog, depression, anxiety, non-specific morbid dread, and the recurrence of mental health issues, trauma or eating disorders.

This leaves millions of us tumbling into a totally unexpected, inexplicable mental fall-about. Society and doctors who aren't endocrinologists or women's health specialists are none the wiser, either. We just think our relationship has taken a turn for the worse, our kids are harder to handle and our ability to cope at work is going down the gurgler.

A lot of women in the Survey also said they only made sense of mental symptoms *after* physical perimenopause symptoms appeared.

What if you experience some kind of earlier menopause?

If early menopause happens as a result of medication or surgery, or you have a quick diagnosis of ovarian insufficiency, you can get up to speed and not be blindsided by mental challenges. Many people who go through this will be on the Pill or other hormone medication that can even things out; or, if hormone medication's not for you, doctors can recommend other medications to help protect bones and deal with the jagged edges of any hormone-related brain troubles. (See 'Early menopause' in Chapter 1, What Even is the Menopause?)

When will the mental symptoms end?

A lot of women find that when they're through perimenopause and the physical symptoms have

I thought it was just work and home stress. Zelda, 49

I was very low in vitamin D last year, and have been taking [prescribed] high doses of it ever since. This has helped ENORMOUSLY with mood! Marie, 55

stopped, the nasty mental symptoms do, too. The problem is, of course, that while for most people it's 2–5 years, for some it can be 12–15 years. And we can't predict who'll experience which symptoms and for how long.

Different solutions might be useful at various times, including adjusted and changed medication and doses. Keep in close touch with a doctor or doctors you trust to help you decide how to manoeuvre through your perimenopause journey. As time goes on you'll need a new map, a ready supply of snacks in your rucksack and clean socks every now and again. (I feel I have entirely lost control of this metaphor, but do keep a KitKat in your bag for emergencies, anyway.)

I worked in Acute Mental Health and on our extensive assessment there was not one question about where a women was in her menopause. Frances, 59

What if the mental feelings are really bad?

Women tend to squish down difficult feelings, thinking they have to 'get on with it' and not 'complain'.

It's crucial to reach out for help at the first sign of real struggle with anxiety, depression and revisiting mental health problems. If you have any idle or intrusive thoughts along the lines of feeling without hope, or that it might be easier to not be here, or you're not needed or worthy – off you pop straightaway for help. Reach out to a mental health hotline (see 'More info on mental health issues' coming up) and your GP; tell your therapist, tell a trusted friend or relative to help you get practical, professional advice.

I promise, you are not alone. With recent pandemics and the cruel or dismissive anti-women policies of many world governments and workplaces, feeling a bit

I swing from being fine to crying without warning, especially at night. I have had my first suicidal thoughts in my life. Louise, 43

I described my anxiety to my new doctor as 'waves of dread that start at my head and roll down to my toes'. He was the first to explain this was in fact a hot flush! Sarah, 48

despairing sometimes is quite a sane response. Confronting thoughts can creep up on you and suddenly feel like a burden, and luckily, in most cases, you can start to turn them around pretty quickly. Make sure you demand more from a GP who won't consider a hormonal basis, or who doesn't know that MHT is now known to be more effective than antidepressants in hormone-related brain carry-on.

See helplines and websites in the 'More info for help with depression & anxiety' section on page 183.

I didn't see it coming. I came unravelled like a knitted jumper. I'm slowly re-knitting myself into something different. Hayley, 47

I became withdrawn and cried easily. I became social phobic. I lost friends. I was crazy. Very depressed and needed medication. Kim, 54

Feeling as though the best part of my life is over, angry and envious of friends who are financially secure. Marie, 55

I don't care about anything. Rosa, 53

Risk factors for a bad mental time in perimenopause

- a history of significant premenstrual syndrome (PMS)
- a history of premenstrual dysphoric disorder (PMDD) symptoms
- dealing with anxiety, depression, or other mental health challenges in the past
- a history of eating disorders
- past trauma
- plain bad luck: your individual hormone levels and their effects on your brain.

My son's pot plant died and I was overwhelmed with tears. Chantal, 52

I developed bulimia at 50, even though I never had this previously in my life. Combine anxiety, lack of concentration, loss of memory and lack of sleep, and it becomes easy to lose perspective. Esther, 52

Help for perimenopausal mental carry-on

Panic attacks, claustrophobia, worried, hypervigilant. Got worse during my 40s. Menopause at 47 and by 49 I was back, happy and confident again. No doctor ever suggested that menopause could have been the cause. Jo, 56

We'll take the mental health challenges one by one, coming up, but here's some general info first. One of the great cruel disservices to women is being told we should meditate, be mindful, eat broccoli or chill out when we feel mood swings and freak-outs in our 40s and 50s, when this won't stop severe symptoms caused by massively misbehaving hormones. For those women, especially, taking MHT will sort them out in 6 weeks and keep them on the path. Medications and self-help strategies can take a while to kick in – ask your doctor about what to expect.

For many, MHT reverses brain fog, especially forgetting words and the multitasking and concentration problems cited by thousands in the Survey.

Countless women said exercise or activity helped them with anxiety, depression and other mental symptoms, whether it was shared classes, dancing in the kitchen, walking the dog, or online videos. Many said although they knew weight-bearing exercise was good for better bone density, they didn't know there had been a proven positive effect of physical activity on menopausal mental symptoms.

Many experts believe that if your feelings are likely a hormone-based carry-on, it would be better to start with MHT, and then include other medication if necessary.

Women who can't take estrogen medication for any reason may be able to take SERMS, Selective Estrogen Receptor Modulators,

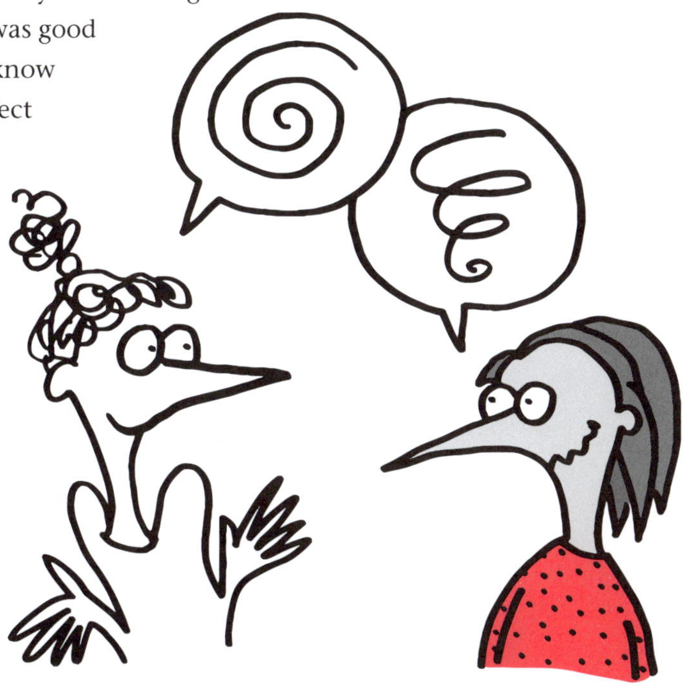

I feel like I am treading water mentally. I put on a mask to get through the day but the symptoms are slowly taking their toll. Sarah, 50

I attended a 6-week [mindfulness] program and I don't think it was a coincidence that the majority of the class were menopausal women. Robin, 59

but these are usually prescribed for osteoporosis or breast cancer, and only cost less than $100 a month if prescribed for bones. If the Therapeutic Goods Administration could declare it a medication that can be prescribed for depression, it would be a lot cheaper. You might like to remind your doctor that of course you probably ARE taking it for your bones, which might mean it's cheaper for you.

The hormone regulation you need could be helped by taking the Pill, which will give you enough estrogen to make up for, and smooth out, any crazy upsy-downsy fits-and-starts behaviour of your ovaries. But because combined estrogen and progestins Pill have been associated with a depressive mood effect, your prescribing doctor should know which brand or formulation is associated with less of a depressive effect. Similarly, some hormone formulations may tackle perimenopause symptoms as well as help boost libido.

If your GP doesn't know which is which, or says hormone medications are all the same, get a new GP or get a referral to an endocrinologist or gynaecologist. Unless, in rare and very extreme circumstances, you become out of touch with reality and an immediate danger to yourself, you should be both fully informed and in control of what you decide to take and when you want to come off it.

Medical help for mental issues

Possibly:

- MHT or other hormone prescription
- referral to a gynaecologist, endocrinologist or psychiatrist to discuss other possible medication suitable to your individual needs
- referral to a psychologist or counsellor
- referral to other allied health professionals who can help deal with symptoms causing you stress or distress: dietitians, exercise physiologists, pelvic floor physios and others.

I just felt my anger was getting out of control. I hated myself for screaming at my child. I asked my doctor to put me on antidepressants and they have helped immensely. Megan, 51

What MHT doesn't do to your brain

This is probably incredibly obvious, but quick sidebar. MHT won't:

* cure psychosis or a mental health problem unrelated to hormones
* fix problems of grief and trauma that counselling would help
* get you out of a controlling or difficult relationship
* provide a quick fix for addiction or dependence issues
* reboot you with new, improved coping mechanisms.

Non-medical help for mental issues

In most cases it makes sense to have a multi-pronged attack on what's making your life difficult, whether or not you're also taking medication. What else is in your mental toolbox?

* Exercise is a proven, effective, supportive strategy against many mental challenges. It may not be a cure but in general it makes everything better. (It's in Chapter 3, It's Your Approach.)
* Getting specialist medical and physiotherapist help with physical symptoms.
* Exploring individual, marriage or family counselling.
* Lifestyle changes.
* Talking with friends or other menopausal folk in person or online.
* Redefining what family members need to help with at home.
* Professional, discreet help to change alcohol or drug habits.
* Useful workplace strategies and policies, and positive respect for older women in society. (Sort that out, would you.)

> I was somehow a different person. I was in there, but it was so hard to get out. Susan, 56

> Now that I am sober and treating my depression, I think it is just nice be able to be yourself and not try and impress other people. To be honest. To be kind. Standing up for myself. Jo, 64

> Wish I could give big hugs to anyone experiencing any of those things and that they would believe me when I say that life will improve. Sharalynne, 61

> I couldn't get a doctor to believe me. I knew I was already in perimenopause but kept being told until I had hot flushes, I couldn't have lower estrogen. Finally went to an endocrinologist who got it straight away and prescribed the MHT I wanted. Carolyn, 51

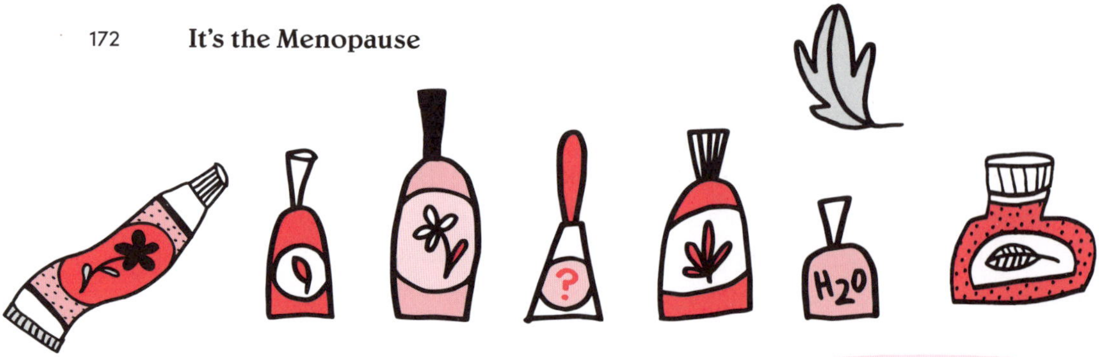

Regular moderate exercise and yoga, along with meditation, seem to be getting me through the emotional stuff. Tiff, 48

- Natural therapies and tonics. There's no evidence that these help severe mood-related palaver. Aside from a general multivitamin as insurance, or a reliable supplement prescribed for a diagnosed deficiency, supplements may be a waste of money for you. (Please see the warnings against dodgy claims for supplements in Chapter 3, It's Your Approach.) But the power of belief, placebo, and ritual for some people is undeniable. If you need a cup of tea with an unfeasible amount of milk to start the day, then you just do. If you like writing poetry in a journal, or belting out show tunes, or you swear by the power of an aromatherapy rose petal unguent, well done you for finding that out.

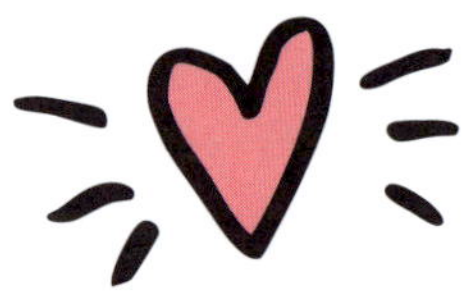

- Connection. Family, friends and/or community. Self-help books and podcasts, volunteer work, environmental activism. If not now, when? If a regular crafternoon, book club, girls-trip-away, dawn swim group, choir, church or charity hamper-packing, hiking gang or birdwatching coven sounds like fun, find out how to join, or start your own.

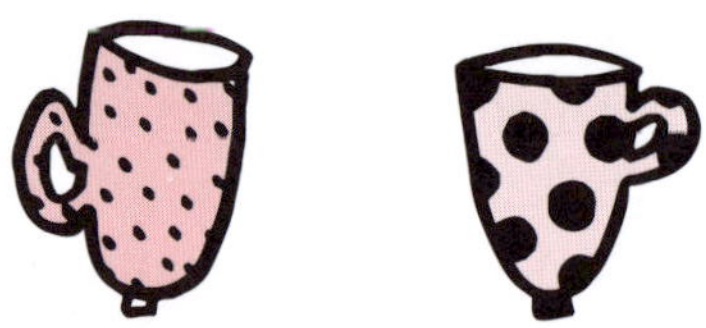

I broke up with my partner. He blamed it all on my menopause. I came to the realisation he was a dick *and* I was going through menopause. Kat, 60

Oh the incredible WOMEN around you! The wisdom, support, laughter and love shared between women is a truly beautiful thing. I am looking forward to decades more of THAT growth. Kathy, 47

The mental effects of perimenopause

Let's take 'em one-by-one.

Wonky sense of self

Women often feel in perimenopause some version of 'I'm not myself'. It can be described as a 'loss of mojo'; a malaise, ennui, lack of energy. It feels like things that used to be easy are now harder or even impossible – multitasking, remembering all the right words, feeling like you can cope if something goes wrong. Your organisational skills and sense of resilience have fled.

And many of us experience the onset of a quiet, tired sort of tendency to weep, or sudden bursts of tears: fountainous, unpredictable, baffling. Confidence and self-esteem are suddenly all over the place or seem to have fallen off a cliff, except when they come back and then go again. If you've started having hot flushes and not recognised them, it can feel exactly like you're having rolling panic attacks or sharp spikes of embarrassment.

It can feel like you're crap at work, losing it at home, and bereft of enthusiasm for stuff you used to love.

Just over 80 per cent of more than 7700 women who answered the mental symptoms questions said they experienced a perimenopausal fall in self-esteem. About 13.5 per cent noticed it but were largely unfussed; a bit over 20 per cent said it was sometimes annoying; almost 30 per cent said it was tough and almost 19 per cent said it was truly terrible.

I was totally shocked and saddened by my loss of 'self'. The night sweats and insomnia as a shift worker just made everything so hard. I spent years crying in the shower and putting on a brave face. Vik, 58

I've never been confident but it's making me feel like a complete failure. Alexandra, 56

Feeling less intelligent. I could not solve problems. Sue, 70

Of those who answered the question about losing a sense of self, a combination adding to almost a quarter said they found it tough, or truly terrible, and a slightly smaller percentage, about 32 per cent, said they didn't experience it at all.

My kids referred to me as 'Operation Shitstorm!' although I didn't think it was that bad. Ivy, 59

I had a psychologist tell me that rage, impatience and anxiety are never associated with menopause and to say so was a cop-out. If they *are* associated with perimenopause, I'm outraged! Alison, 49

Brain fog

Many researchers, psychiatrists and neuropsychologists believe the effects of lower estrogen in perimenopause contributes to what many women identify as the onset of some kind of scattiness: difficulties in concentrating, remembering tasks, events and even the right words to shove in a sentence. It's real. Of course, many women in their 40s and 50s have too much to do and not enough sleep – the sleep section is coming up – and those are obvious factors too.

I did analytical work that required sharp focus. Well, that went out the door. At the age of 42 I suddenly felt like a total idiot. Kez, 57

Some stuff to know:

* Most perimenopausal women report brain fog.
* Some women might experience brain fog for months, or years. It's common in perimenopause and less common after periods stop.
* Researchers think that maybe women experiencing brain fog and lack of self-esteem often look to others like they're performing fine. Support for the 'fake it till you make it' idea.
* Brain fog is also a scientifically known feature of pregnancy: it may be that there is a sweet-spot of enough estrogen to be at maximum sharpness and feel pleased with yourself, and too much or too little can create brain fog. Or it might be that other mental factors or sleep deprivation in pregnancy have a bigger impact than hormones.

Brain fog and helplessness . . . lifted slowly as menopause progressed and then cleared like a bright new day had dawned. Suban, 55

In the Survey, answers to relevant questions showed that only about 14 per cent said they didn't have any perimenopausal memory problems. Only about 17 per cent said they never found it harder to concentrate and about a quarter said they had no difficulty finishing tasks.

A large majority found all of these things a problem at least sometimes, with just under a quarter finding it tough to deal with memory problems and finding it harder to concentrate, and around about one in 10 finding those two problems in particular were truly terrible for them. There were thousands of comments from women who felt brain fog really stuffed up their lives for a while.

> I have become nearly agoraphobic and choose to stay home instead of dealing with panic attacks and anxiety. Jacinta, 53

> I forgot which side of the road we drive on here. I had to pull over and have a think. I thought I'd had a stroke but of course it was just menopause. Babette, 54

Tips to combat brain fog

Sadly the usual recommendations apply (as if they were easy to achieve!): get better sleep, get regular exercise (try for at least a half-hour a day), eat a healthy diet low in sugar and high in vegetables and fruit, do things that make you feel confident, trust yourself and your expertise because it hasn't disappeared even though your feelings about it may have, keep up your hobbies, interests and friendship groups.

Many doctors recommend MHT to help with mental as well as physical symptoms of perimenopause. Women who get hot flushes for longer may also get more brain fog symptoms, so you might be killing two annoyances with one dose.

A good old-fashioned paper diary or notebook, or digital app, watch or phone calendar can become your personal assistant notifying you of appointments, agendas for meetings, and priorities for the day or week. You might need to jot down notes from meetings and calls. You can also build in pre- and post-meeting or task times where you go through notes and familiarise yourself.

Everyone witnessing your tippy-tapping to input calendar reminders and tick-off lists will just think you're incredibly efficient.

What about dementia?

Should women stay on MHT to stave off dementia? Maybe. Women are at higher risk of dementia than men, and their statistical risk increases each year after 70. Research continues on exactly how much this may have to do with estrogen levels or whether medically boosted estrogen after perimenopause might help protect against developing dementia.

MHT isn't a cure for dementia, and taking it is not a guarantee you won't experience cognitive decline or dementia, or experience it later than you would have otherwise. Some studies speculate that women who have the longest span of uninterrupted periods throughout their life (so fewer or no pregnancies and less or no time breastfeeding) might have a lower risk of dementia. (Cue all the mothers pointing out that children make you feel demented, for God's sake.)

Some researchers have speculated that in the absence of cognitive decline or dementia, women might adapt and feel they've 'got their brain back' once they're through perimenopause into menopause itself. Not much consolation to those who have symptoms for many years.

It may be that estrogen-only therapy (without progesterone) is more protective against dementia, but you can't do that because it creates a much higher risk of endometrial cancer if you have a uterus. So none of this is perfect or creates the universal need for an obvious, perfect pill that protects against all the risks of ageing.

The Survey revealed that heaps of women mistook their brain fog symptoms for early-onset cognitive decline, and in a couple of sad cases, the reverse happened.

Fatigue

It's so rarely mentioned in articles about perimenopause, but hundreds of women in the Survey volunteered fatigue as one of their mental symptoms.

Feel flat all the time. Disinterested, disengaged, absent mentally.
Keryn, 49

Depression

I can go to work and smile and care [nurse] but I feel as though I'm watching myself. At home I am switched off and avoid going out or engaging with others.
Penny, 54

Perimenopause is a really high-risk time for women to experience depression. For some of us, it might be the first time we've experienced it, which can be a shock, and discombobulating. For others, it's an unwelcome return.

As usual, statistics are a bit all over the shop but some good research suggests depression could affect more than one in five perimenopausal women. Well-designed studies have consistently found a huge increase in depression caused by perimenopause. Between the ages of 42 and 52, your statistical risk of depression is five times that of younger women.

For those whose depression is caused by perimenopausal hormones, the answer may be as simple as MHT, or require a different self-help approach or different medication, as described earlier in the chapter.

The burdens many women are carrying are repressive and depressive: organising their homes, children's schedules, education, food, paid work, extended family obligations, and often taking care of older relatives, discrimination in the workplace, lower pay than men, and unkind, controlling, or violent relationships can seem to provide enough reasons for anxieties and depressive feelings without looking for a biological one. Perhaps, as is so often the case, the truth for most people lies somewhere in between, and for many, at one end or another. And all those women deserve whatever help they need.

If you are feeling really blank and blue and you're between 40 and 55, even if you haven't had any other menopausal symptoms, please ask your doctor to help you consider if a fall in estrogen is affecting your mood. If you are put on antidepressants, they'll be targeting something different in your brain, not an estrogen-related cause.

Fatigue seems to be the trigger for me, starts the downward cycle of not looking after myself (eat, sleep, exercise).
Kim, 51

The rage was the worst symptom for me. Extreme and scary. Can be driving to work and suddenly feel so sad and just sob. Brain fog is bad too.
Candice, 48

I had a handle on my depression and anxiety only to find it all came flooding back with perimenopause. Vanessa, 45

I had two moods and two moods only – extreme rage or extreme depression. I had to have time off work until I felt able to cope. Lisa, 52

Of course depression is more than feeling sad, but it's worth noting that just over 30 per cent of respondents to the Survey for this book said they found that tough during perimenopause, and just under 16 per cent said it affected them very badly.

Treatment for depression

Of course new exercise ideas and paying attention to hobbies may not 'cure' the blues, but will help some people, and can even head off the need for other medication. For some of us, MHT, carefully prescribed and monitored by a health professional, is the best decision. Start with your GP, who along with a psychiatrist, is qualified to prescribe hormone or other medication. Your GP can also refer you to a qualified, experienced psychologist for counselling, and some sessions will be covered by Medicare.

See the 'More info for help with depression & anxiety' section on page 183.

DIY depression help ideas

- exercise (see the 'Exercise section' in Chapter 3, It's Your Approach)
- feet on grass, sand, and in sea or river
- walking in nature
- get a lot of air around you
- look at clouds, if possible through trees
- audiobooks, music, dancing
- team sports or games, in person or online
- connection with people: a reading, walking, swimming or gaming group, the dog park.

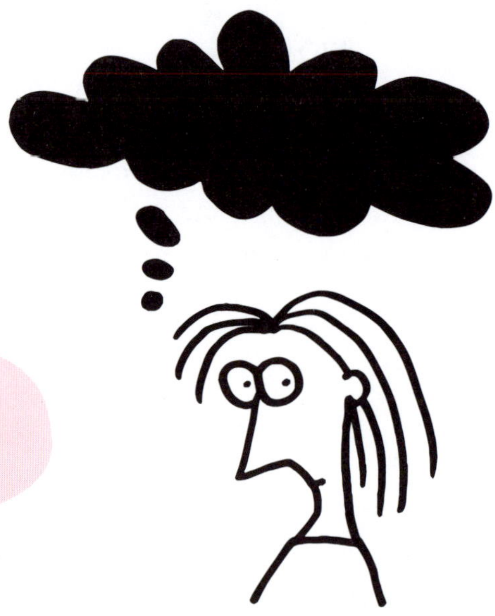

If I don't do my daily dancing I find myself slipping into, not quite depression, but certainly sadness. I drag myself back to dancing and immediately feel good again. Magic! Jo, 56

The Der Factor

> Feeling of mental overload. Menopause so often coincides with teenagers and ageing parents. Ann, 53

It seems obvious of course, but important that research has confirmed the idea that older women are more likely to feel depressed if they are financially insecure, lonely, have debilitating menopause symptoms including hot flushes, wee problems and vaginal dryness that might be getting in the way of good sex. Tackling those things, if possible, will help: hints elsewhere in the book.

Antidepressant medication

Over and over I hear stories from women in their 40s and 50s who went to their GP with all the symptoms of perimenopausal brain-related symptoms, and the possibility of a fall in estrogen levels is never mentioned.

Lots of us have been prescribed various forms of antidepressants, and many of those medications also used to be anti-anxiety. Carefully prescribed antidepressants can be great tools to help calibrate mental health. But many women can come to realise they shouldn't have been on antidepressants at all, or, had they known, they could have at least questioned their doctor about the possibility of being prescribed MHT instead.

To make things worse, many women who did just that were scoffed at or told by doctors they were too young for perimenopause, or that falling or erratic estrogen wasn't a factor for them unless they had changes in their period, or hot flushes – which isn't true.

Menopause specialists now know that if perimenopausal brain symptoms are suspected, many women who are prescribed MHT find that after 3 to 6 weeks their brain fog, self-loathing and general mental malaise lifts almost miraculously. If it doesn't help, back to the doctor for another chat.

Perimenopausal women who can't take MHT because of a history with cancer, or another reason, can often be prescribed a class of antidepressant and anti-anxiety medication that also combats hot flushes, called SSRIs – selective serotonin re-uptake inhibitors, and SNRIs – serotonin and norepinephrine re-uptake inhibitors.

>

SSRI & SNRI prescriptions for depression & anxiety

There's conflicting evidence about the use of these medications. They can be really useful for some people, not seem to have any effect, or be more of a problem than a solution for others. Many safety and dosage studies for medications have been done only on men. Studying the different doses that might be required in menopause compared to other times of life is virtually unheard of.

SSRIs, for example, were originally tested on white men, many of whom were of very different weight and fat distribution than a woman, say, of South Asian heritage. One of the consequences of this is that recommended doses of these drugs, as well as other sleeping and anti-anxiety medications, can be unsuitably high for women.

While many people owe a manageable, happy life to these medications, perhaps millions of people have probably been prescribed these drugs when they may not be the best thing for them; the dose is not appropriate, and patients are given no warning of common side effects such as libido loss, reduced effect over time, or about the likely difficulties when they want to stop taking it.

Withdrawal should be supervised, gradual and incremental, sometimes by shaving slivers off pills, to create smaller doses stepping down over weeks or months. Common withdrawal symptoms can include the bzzzt feeling of a mild electric shock in the brain ('brain zaps'), stomach upset and nausea, tiredness, sleep problems, dizziness, feeling cranky. And eventually for many, relief.

Online communities and advice have sprung up where people who've been through withdrawal give advice on getting off SSRIs and benzodiazepine medication: despite this being something that affects millions of people, there is usually little or no official pharmaceutical or medical advice on how to do it safely.

The agreed best-practice approach now is that going on antidepressant medication shouldn't be a first-line response to mood symptoms in likely perimenopause. While in some cases this medication is necessary and useful, for most people it's wise to consider some other approaches first that have proven useful effects, including MHT prescription, counselling and cognitive behaviour strategies, and exercise.

Find a GP and or specialist doctor who is clued into all of this and who will be a partner with you in your care. They should regularly review your progress and dosage for your weight, symptoms, and hormonal circumstances. A psychologist can be really helpful in talking to you about antidepressant use, but only a GP or other medical specialist can prescribe them and check whether they're OK for you, including whether they could affect other medication you're on.

When I take my antidepressants I feel like 'me'. I'm still the same person, but I can cope, I laugh, cry, get annoyed, but I don't get the raging bursts of anger, the mood swings or the self-doubt, thinking I have no friends or no one would miss me. Bec, 50

Progestogens versus your brain

Some progestogens, especially the progestins variety, are associated with feeling blue and being irritable: standard premenstrual sort of symptoms. (Off you pop to Chapter 2, It's Your Hormones, for all the lowdown.) Especially if you used to suffer from premenstrual mood swings, or found that progestins in the Pill or IVF treatments affected your mood in the past, talk to your doctor. Ask about taking a form of MHT that uses a less suspect progestogen such as micronised progesterone in pill form, or a suitable progestogen-emitting IUD, along with estrogen in a patch or gel.

If you're on the Pill, ask for one that has been shown to be 'mood neutral'and press the point. If your GP doesn't know, or says that isn't a thing, ask them to do the research, or you could get a new doctor.

The interplay of hormone levels and impact on mood can be awfully complex and have completely different effects on people: breastfeeding changes in dopamine and prolactin can be blamed for low feelings, but another hormone that's activated, oxytocin, is associated with good feelings. One day we may be able to dial up exact levels of different hormones to create a perfect cocktail for people that suits them. Until then, it's a bit of a soup of suspicions, assumptions, and a drip-feed of evidence, building knowledge brick by brick.

Anxiety

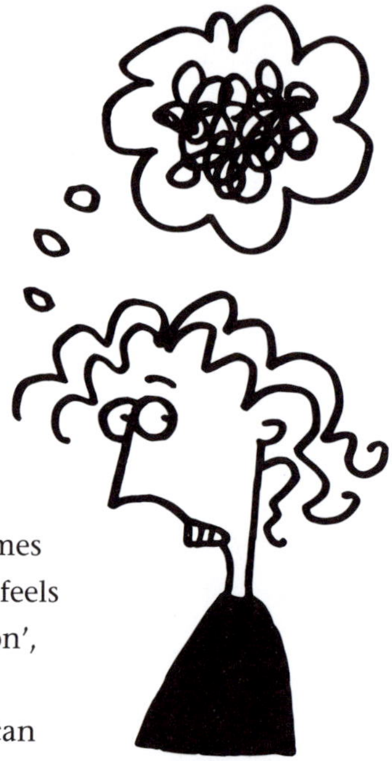

Feeling anxious is one of the major perimenopause symptoms according to respondents to the Survey. About 85 per cent of almost 8000 women said it affected them to some degree and about half said it was tough, or truly terrible for them; only 14 per cent said they didn't feel anxious as a perimenopause symptom.

Anxiety is kind of the equally evil twin of depression. Sometimes they arrive together, or on alternating unwelcome visits. If anxiety feels like a problem for you, please read the earlier section on 'Depression', as info on self-help and medication is pretty similar.

Lots of us experience anxiety feelings in perimenopause. It can be anything from a non-specific morbid dread, waking up worrying, spikes of anxiety when you think about tasks or expectations, to frightening panic attacks. When (if) the physical changes of menopause hit you, they can be easily mistaken for severe anxiety.

A hot flush can feel like a panic attack or an intensely mortifying embarrassment. The common, harmless heartbeat skittering or beat changes we're so rarely warned about, which is caused by a fall or fluctuation in estrogen, can make you wonder if you're going to have a heart attack. (For more on hot flushery and heart bizzo, see Chapter 5, It's Your Body.)

All the weapons I had in place to deal with anxiety failed me during menopause. I had to start again to learn to combat it. I found less empathy from the medical profession this time around, though. Pat, 56

As cheesy as it sounds, I upped my yoga practice from once a week to nearly daily. Sometimes it's only 7 mins, but it's helped with feeling generally calmer at times. Al, 49

What's worse is having anxiety about the possibility of a panic attack, which then ultimately brings them on. Caro, 49

Anxiety and mild panic attacks doing my job in sales that I'm super confident in. Louise, 54

Anxiety flared up about a year before the physical symptoms started. Dawn, 52

MORE INFO for help with depression & anxiety

Talk to your GP about needing help, queries about MHT and other medication and referral to specialists who may be able to help, whether gynaecologists, endocrinologists, physiotherapists, psychologists or psychiatrists.

If you get info from a general mental health website on a condition like anxiety or depression, even from a respectable organisation, it may not even mention menopause as a likely cause, or MHT as a possible fix.

Relaxation and meditation apps and podcasts can help with mood swings and sleeping issues.

beyondblue.org.au
24-hour helpline: 1300 224 636
This independent mental health charity specialises in depression-related challenges and conditions. They have fact sheets, checklists, practical suggestions, online chat or email help.

lifeline.org.au
24-hour crisis line: 13 11 14
The confidential, anonymous service for severe mental health feelings and suicidal thoughts.

butterfly.org.au
Helpline: 1800 33 4673
The Butterfly Foundation specialises in eating disorders and eating behaviour problems, as well as body image issues.

sane.org
This is the service to help with diagnosed mental illnesses and disorders, and complex related issues such as psychosis, trauma and obsessive-compulsive disorders. Contains fact sheets, guides, and support for families, friends and carers.

I am no longer the same person. I feel I can't go out anymore as I am a loose cannon waiting to go off. Liz, 46

Getting out walking my dog in fresh air at a good pace gave me peace. Gillian, 58

Art making helped! Jo, 63

Sometimes it's like having a tiny demon living inside your body. She makes you say and do things. Kitty, 49

I'm scared to have my GP record the mental health symptoms as it has previously affected income protection insurance outcome. I don't want to risk it at my age. Kylie, 50

Thoughts of self-harm, suicide or despair

It's rare and you probably won't feel scarily terrible. But if you do, or if you have any thoughts about how it would be better if you weren't here, or of hurting yourself, or that you'll never feel better, that's disordered hormones or misbehaving brain chemicals speaking. Promise me, please, that you'll reach out for help. There are ways to make friends with your mind again, to quieten, manage or banish those thoughts, and for you to feel calmer, worthy, loved, needed and optimistic. Tell friends and relatives you've thought about it, talk to a hotline, talk to your GP.

MORE INFO on despair

lifeline.org.au
Crisis line: 13 11 14
Texting service: 0477 13 11 14
Anonymous, immediate support and advice for anyone feeling they're at a crisis point, or might soon be.

respect.gov.au
Advice line: 1800 737 732
Anonymous help, support and counselling about controlling, coercive and/or violent relationships.

Irritation & rage

I made my husband wear his slippers in the house because I couldn't stand the sound of his shoes on the floorboards! Gail, 52

Lots of perimenopausal women say they feel inexplicable, sudden or escalating feelings of being fed up, irritated and even a sense of rage. It's only more recently that women are realising that this isn't a failure to cope, but a result of hormonal changes and unrelieved outside pressures.

Extreme rage and anger was and is debilitating . . . seeing a psychologist to help with coping strategies. Marriage is in turmoil after 30 years. Mood swings off the scale. Scary. Melissa, 53

Hating on life in general – family, kids, people, everything and everyone tbh. Lina, 53

I had a very, very low tolerance threshold for bulls$@t. Lisa, 54

Somewhat startling results from this Survey showed that about half of the women who responded to a question about being easily annoyed said this was tough or truly terrible for them in perimenopause. Less than 8 per cent said they didn't recognise it as a symptom at all. Almost 13 per cent said they experienced it but it wasn't bad, and nearly a third said it was sometimes annoying.

I turned into someone else and I didn't like her. Marian, 61

A question about whether they recognised rage as a symptom was a runner-up. Almost 28 per cent never experienced it; more than two-thirds did. Just over 14 per cent were unfussed, nearly a quarter were sometimes annoyed by it; one in five of those found it tough and about 14 per cent thought it was terrible.

People who feel more cross and fed up during perimenopause say it's not just at home, it can be expressed as road rage, or frustration at work, or just a general sense of feeling irritated or furious at things that in the past would have been annoyances that were soon brushed off or forgotten.

Just over a quarter of Survey respondents to the relevant question said they felt impatient with their partner during perimenopause and that made things tough, and almost 25 per cent found it truly terrible. Overall they were less likely to be impatient with their children, but about one in five found that tough, and nearly under one in ten found it awful.

I don't get the mention of anger issues as a perimenopause symptom - any anger/rage I experience is 100 per cent justifiable – have you seen what it is like for older women to survive!! Felicia, 60

I feel like I am at my most powerful and confident in having control of my life and then next minute I have lost control — my body is controlling me with hot flushes, mood swings, scattered memory, easily annoyed, sleep disruption and anxiety. Kirsty, 48

Doctors believe that the same hormonal carry-on that can cause the premenstrual blues has a role in moods during perimenopause. They usually favour boosting estrogen in perimenopause balanced with a progesterone rather than progestins (see Chapter 2, It's Your Hormones, for more). Rage and irritation can be a manifestation of depression and/or anxiety, so have a read of the sections on those earlier in this chapter.

> Perimenopause seemed to intensify the anxiety and depressive episodes related to my ADHD. I was either incredibly sad or in a rage.
> Julie, 62

It's certainly worth looking at some situations that are understandably pissing you off. Why SHOULD you do all the planning, cooking and cleaning in a house that's filled with other grown-ups? Or do all the work at your office but get paid less than a younger man? Maybe you're exhausted by hormone-caused lack of sleep; your alcohol use has crept up; there's a crazy burden at work and at home; and the cumulative experiences of a lifetime. See if you can take a step back and ask which is which.

> At times when I am giving one of the kids a bollocking, I think, 'What am I doing, I don't feel like that and why can't I stop.' I feel like an alien has taken over my mind. Annette, 51

Severe hormonal mental disorders

Premenstrual dysphoric disorder (PMDD) is a condition that turns some women's period cycles into a recurring nightmare of awful depressive and physical symptoms. It wasn't even recognised by doctors until a couple of decades ago. For some women, medication-induced menopause or a hysterectomy that creates early menopause is the answer.

The 4-day post-birth 'baby blues', post-natal depression, and depressive premenstrual feelings are believed to be linked to a plummet in allopregnanolone, a brain chemical in the steroid class, that helps to balance and mitigate feelings of anxiety and depression. You know what I'm going to say next, don't you? There's not enough research to understand this yet.

If you have a history of misbehaving hormones, such as bad premenstrual symptoms or even PMDD, you're probably at higher risk of perimenopausal and menopausal depression or mood problems. If you're frightened or shocked by your perimenopausal feelings of depression, self-harm or even suicide, get some help straightaway. Don't muck around. Call a helpline. (See 'More info for help with depression & anxiety' on page 183, see your GP, get a referral to a gynaecologist, endocrinologist and/or a psychiatrist.)

Sleep

Perimenopausal women are plagued by sleep problems, which can contribute to family disharmony and even resignations from work. Sleep problems are estimated (guessed) to affect around half of women in perimenopause, or more. For most women it goes away once they're in menopause and past the symptoms stage – but that could be anywhere between 4 and 15 years.

(You might as well get a Post-it note, write 'There isn't enough research on this' and stick it to every page of this section you read. Oh, just stick one to your forehead in backwardsy writing so you see it in the mirror.)

What IS known is that sleep problems are tormenting. Severe insomnia can make you feel desperate and unable to cope, and makes your metabolism slow down.

I *do* wish people wouldn't use the phrase 'sleep hygiene', which sounds pompous and a bit weird to me, as if you need a sponge bath while you're unconscious. I simply shan't.

Of the Survey respondents who answered questions about sleep, more than 90 per cent said they had some sort of sleep difficulties in perimenopause. More than a third said they had difficulty getting to sleep, almost two-thirds said they woke during the night and stayed awake for long periods, and half said they were bedevilled by waking with night sweats. Almost a third said they took something to help them get to sleep, whether prescription or otherwise.

And it was almost a 50–50 split between those who thought alcohol affected their sleep patterns,

Why is so little known about women over 40 experiencing insomnia when nearly every single fucking woman over 40 experiences sleep issues??? Elissa, 45

It's crazy-making.
Gigi, 51

I feel that if I could sleep in, I could manage the insomnia disruption and function properly, but gotta get kids to school, me to work – it just doesn't fit. Lack of sleep is so common among my friends, it's scary. We're like zombie mums. Good old Elissa, 45, again

If I could sleep I would be able to cope with everything better and have my normal energy level.
Deryn, 58

Exercise has been said to help combat menopausal symptoms. I think it's more [about] getting out in fresh air and activating the melatonin that does it. Susan, 57

and those who didn't – it's a medically known association. It's entirely possible ('WHERE'S THE RESEARCH?!' I shout into my pillow) that moderate to mildish perimenopausal symptoms would be, let's say, 78.95 times easier to deal with if we were getting enough SLEEP.

Melatonin made the biggest difference to my overall wellbeing . . . prescribed by doctor got me back to sleep. J, 55

Trouble falling asleep

Reduced estrogen may have an effect on melatonin hormone levels, which generally boss your sleep patterns. A hotter body (phwoaarr) and peaks of hot flushes may get in the way of getting to sleep soon after turning off the light. Hundreds of women in the Survey said they were taking melatonin. It was the most commonly named tablet taken for sleep reasons, followed by MHT, herbal tablets, prescribed sleeping tablets and antidepressant/anti-anxiety medication.

I discovered podcasts, which help with anxiety-related sleeplessness that started around menopause. Margaret, 54

Weird, catastrophic, doomsday type thoughts just before going to sleep. Leigh, 50

I wear a crystal to help me sleep and have a chamomile tea to relax. Natasha, 45

I found a weighted blanket really – REALLY – helped. Carolyn, 54

Waking up at the wrong times

Contributing factors can include night-time hot flushes, aka sweats, and any alcohol drinks you had during the day or night; they're all common causes of waking during the night or too early in the morning. Anxiety, a sense of hypervigilance and a busy mind can stop you falling back to sleep quickly.

My darkest times were the dead of night, but I needed some sort of reassurance that what I was experiencing was totally normal, and that I would be OK. Cathi, 55

At its worst, I missed work mostly because I was afraid to drive. Ali, 56

I am awake between 2.30–4 am every single night. It's torture! Gayle, 48

I just get so tired I feel like giving up. Karyn, 48

What helps perimenopausal sleep problems

Thousands of respondents to the Survey for this book said that some form of activity, from exercise classes to dancing, helped with their sleep problems as well as their mental health generally. People have found one, some or all of these helpful:

* MHT, which should curb night sweats and flushes
* meditation, music or sleep-inducing apps or podcasts
* bedclothes that are easy to throw off and on, i.e. layers of cotton and wool blankets rather than one big doona
* sorting out, if you can, a good mattress, pillows and blockout curtains
* regulated bedtime and wake-up time, especially one that is more suited to your natural inclination (not easy for you, dear shift-workers)
* having sleep rituals
* prescribed doses of melatonin hormone supplements
* exercising during the day in a way that makes you physically tired, but not within a couple of hours of bedtime.

I alternate between melatonin, herbal pills and medical pills. Marie, 58

There are lots of podcasts and apps for meditation and sleep, some of them featuring the sexy rumbling voice of a Shakespearean actor who you can imagine in flannelette jarmies. Few such Shakespearean night-denizens will talk about the possible hormonal cause for perimenopausal folk, but they can still be helpful.

I have trained myself to read then meditate to get back to sleep – getting rid of alcohol in my diet really helped my sleep issues. Rosie, 50

Cut down caffeine. Nat, 54

On MHT I still wake 50 per cent of the nights, but the quality of sleep is far superior. Sadie, 50

The hot flushes and night sweats really affected my sleep, waking me up regularly and then prevented me from going back to sleep. HRT provided a quick relief. Nikki, 55

Use sleep music. Installed split system air conditioning above bed, a godsend. Deb, 57

Went to a sleep psychologist for Cognitive Behaviour Therapy. That and HRT eventually improved it to the extent where I sleep OK 4–5 nights a week. Tracey, 52

Now I wake between 5–6 am like clockwork. I want to sleep in. Jen, 49

What doesn't help

> I pretty much always have a hot flush just when I'm about to fall asleep. Sleep disturbance is a massive problem for me. RT, 61

You know these but I'm writing them down anyway. The annoying thing is that you can fight these truisms for months or even years ('But I like reading my tablet in bed!' 'I'm too cool for a bedtime!'). And then when you're ready, for many people they do actually work, which is both really annoying and a relief.

> Anxiety and insomnia seem to be good friends, everything is worse at 4 am. Had to discipline myself to wait until 9 am before I act on any decision made at 4 am. Kate, 60

Avoid:

- alcohol – it will wake you up in the night, or too early
- caffeine drinks and chocolate (no bucket of tiramisu for you at 9 pm)
- any digital screen use in the couple of hours before sleeptime
- not having a bedtime
- reading ludicrous romance books until the wee hours fighting sleepiness all the way but enough about me
- snoring partners – they must either be banished from your bedroom or sort themselves out with medical treatment. If you're the one who snores, get treatment for that.

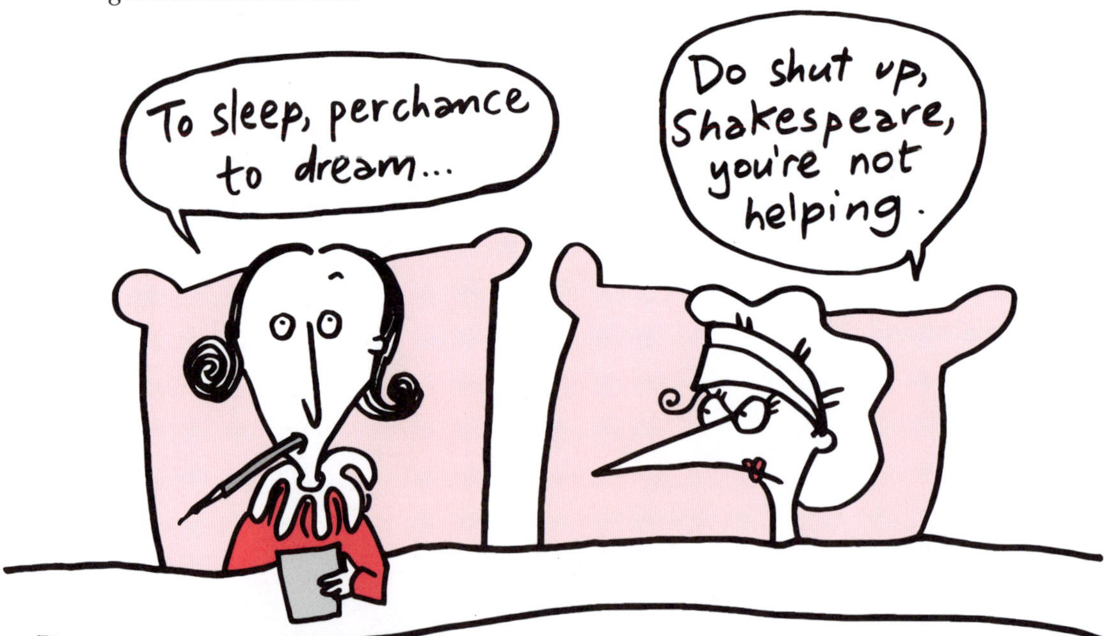
To sleep, perchance to dream...
Do shut up, Shakespeare, you're not helping.

Sleeping pills

Many doctors and specialists believe that careful doses of melatonin can help with sleep problems, but you should talk about this with your GP. Over-the-counter sleep medications can't be used long-term (i.e. one packet after another). More heavy-duty prescription sleeping tablets have a range of risks, including sometimes being prescribed to women at double the dose they need. Prescription sleeping pills are known to be a danger for addiction (aka dependence). Don't go on alone out of habit: regularly check in with your health professionals about doses and your needs.

Herbal supplements – have requested sleeping tablets and doctors will not prescribe them for fear of addiction. Amanda, 49

I developed an addiction to Valium. It took me 2 years to wean off and a further 2 years of withdrawal side effects. MHT solved my insomnia issues. Robyn, 62

Who's Who in mental health practitioners

GP Your local doctor can help by ruling out a physical reason for a mental health problem (for example, the side effects of a medicine prescribed for something else), and refer you to a psychologist, psychiatrist or other specialist. If the doctor suggests medication, always ask what the aim is, whether the dose is appropriate for you, whether MHT should be tried first and when and how you should come of it.

A **natural therapist** cannot diagnose a mental health condition. A doctor and naturopath should each know what the other is prescribing. A natural therapist can help with lifestyle advice, and vitamin, mineral and herbal supplements. Alternative treatments cannot take the place of prescribed psychiatric medication needed by people with a serious mental illness.

A **psychiatrist** is a medical doctor who specialises in the brain and mental health. They have done at least 5–7 years of basic medical and surgical training, plus specialist training and experience in psychiatry. As well as skills in anatomy, drug knowledge and diagnosis, a psychiatrist will have extensive experience in psychotherapy, talking with and listening to patients.

>

Many psychiatrists have subspecialties, which include anxiety, eating disorders, or trauma. Other medical doctors can refer patients to a psychiatrist. Psychiatrists can be involved in ongoing care and prescribing medication, and often work in tandem with psychologists. The Royal Australian and New Zealand College of Psychiatrists site is **ranzcp.org**.

Psychologists must have done a 4-year university course, then 2 years of monitored experience with patients or a master's degree that includes supervised time with clients. They are bound by a code of ethics. Psychologists can't prescribe medication. You don't have to have a referral from a GP to go to a psychologist, but a GP is likely to have useful contacts, and can get you a Medicare rebate for several visits.

The Australian Psychological Society site **psychology.org.au** has info on qualifications and lots of fact sheets on mental health issues – choose 'Topics'. The advice line (1800 333 497) can help you find a qualified psychologist.

The Psychology Board of Australia site **psychologyboard.gov.au** will tell you if your psychologist is registered. Choose 'Practitioner search'.

Anyone can call themselves a **counsellor**. Make sure you understand the credentials of your counsellor. Look for reputable training and qualifications, experience in your special area (say, eating disorders, or anxiety). The Australian Counselling Association **theaca.net.au** is a membership body with a voluntary code of ethics, info on approved courses, and a complaints procedure.

A **psychotherapist**, usually a psychologist or psychiatrist, will use different therapies and talk with you about your problem, feelings or illness, maybe about things like your childhood, and help you with your hopes and plans for the future. Anyone can call themselves a psychotherapist, so check qualifications. The Psychotherapy and Counselling Federation of Australia **pacfa.org.au** has a section on qualifications and how to find a therapist.

A **cognitive behavioural therapist** uses a popular technique employed by many psychiatrists, psychologists, psychotherapists and counsellors to help people identify triggers for feelings and new ways to respond to them.

Alcohol & other addictive behaviours

This section looks at self-soothing attempts like drinking, illegal and prescription drug use, gambling and social media use, and other factors that can feel like coping mechanisms and be fine for some people, but can lead to dependence, addiction and major problems for others. See the 'More info' section coming up for help with any dependence or addiction issues.

Alcohol

When I was still writing this book, and women would say something like, 'Hurry up and finish the book, menopause is a nightmare,' a lot of them would add immediately, 'Thank God for wine, eh?'

Many of us say we use alcohol to try to deal with anxiety, menopause symptoms and sleep problems.

Only 15 per cent of respondents to the Survey said they saw alcohol as something they used to help with menopause symptoms, but almost 40 per cent said they'd changed their alcohol habits in perimenopause. Some drank more, some less.

Over a third of women who answered alcohol questions said they didn't drink at all; just under 14 per cent said they had one drink a, night; almost 9 per cent had two on a usual night; under 5 per cent drank half a bottle of wine or drank more than two drinks several nights a week; under 17 per cent drank several nights a week; and 11 per cent said they regularly had more than three drinks on a Friday and Saturday night. Most of us drank wine.

Annoyingly, all the optimistic 'red wine plus dark chocolate is a healthy diet' chat in the world won't make it so. Alcohol isn't medicine.

Drinking wine made hot flushes worse, but I need wine to cope with the crankiness. Anne, 50

I am completely unmotivated. The only thing that makes me feel good is drinking because it disconnects my brain from my heart. Yvonne, 48

Grog was not so good – it was the easy go-to fixer but the effects were awful. I started to get hangovers which I'd never had before and I would feel the effects on my mood for days. I could not use grog as an elixir or fixer. Rebecca, 58

Alcohol makes the flushes much worse. I stopped drinking altogether, even though . . . I really wanted a glass of wine of an evening! Caroline, 54

I self-medicated with wine and long chats on the phone to my sister when coping became difficult. Jen, 52

I certainly did drink more alcohol when I had perimenopausal symptoms . . . so I became a half-a-bottle-to-a-bottle-of-wine a night kind of lady. I don't regret it. It got me through. Lisa, 56

Drinking more per session but less often. Not drinking to blackout anymore. Auntie Anarchy, 54

I drink more to mask the pain of it all, I think. Kaz, 47

Wine . . . for energy at 5 pm. Beck, 52

In the responses to the Survey, hundreds of women volunteered the information (not in answer to a question about alcohol) that drinking made their hot flushes and mental symptoms worse, and really messed with their sleep patterns. A lot of women said they drank less during perimenopause; a lot said they drank more.

The problem with 'moderate' drinking

The mantra that everything in moderation is good for you doesn't work if your definition of moderate is a bit dodgy. (Or, indeed, if you're being moderate with flaming chainsaws or arsenic, but that's another book, probably). Decades ago I went to meet a boyfriend's parents, and I hope they never noticed how far my eyebrows had disappeared into my hairline. The door from the living room to the kitchen had been removed, and they had two giant fridges: one for food and one with two large tanks inside for red and white wine (their house had become a delivery point between two local pubs).

Each tank had its own metal hose with a trigger nozzle that was used to deliver wine into glasses that were the size of cereal bowls. The wine was squirted in to a level so high that it rose a millimetre or so above the top of the glass, creating a trembling curve for which the scientific name is a convex meniscus. I'd estimate that each of those glasses of wine contained three to four standard drinks. They explained they 'only had two to three glasses a night'.

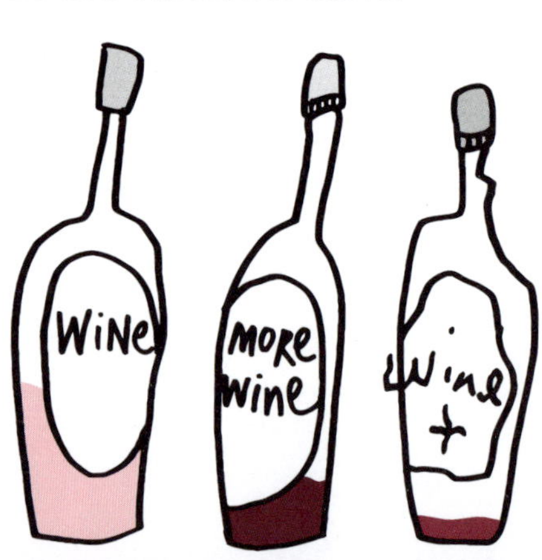

But isn't a more moderate daily intake alcohol good for you? Isn't the Mediterranean diet life prolonging, so every night you should eat olives and pizza and drink barrels of red wine? News sites love a 'study' allegedly showing that alcohol is fine, if not practically a health food. Unfortunately, no amount of iffy studies are going to change some settled truths.

Alcohol to relieve my menopause symptoms did not work. Stix, 59

I realised that I no longer gave a shit if my liver failed, so now I drink on social occasions. That said, one can of 14-per-cent alcohol sparkling rosé (noice, classy!) is all it takes to get me pissed. #blessed. Lee, 56

Recently decided to stop having a glass of wine or two every night because I sleep better and feel better without it. Bron, 59

Since perimenopause started I can't drink wine (migraines), champagne (migraines) and if I drink more than two drinks I'm a mess the next day. Kate, 49

I don't really drink often because of its links to breast cancer, and I have enough trouble with weight without adding extra alcohol calories. Miss it, though. Lisa, 54

Drinking alcohol now makes my face, neck, and chest very red. Sassy, 49

Now that I think about it, I do have a drink while cooking dinner, and have probably been doing it for awhile, but didn't relate it [to perimenopause]. Janelle, 50

Having a drink after work with my husband was a special time. We'd sit and chat, talk about our day. I've switched to soda water with the occasional drink now. Nat, 54

Drinking alcohol at night makes the sweats worse. I know when I'm doing it that I'm going to pay for it. Alice, 52

Drinking, cancer & other risks

Drinking any amount of alcohol raises your risk of getting most known cancers, including breast cancer, and heart and liver disease, and hastens the loss of calcium from bones. Drinking a lot of alcohol raises the risk of cancer a lot. If you add smoking and alcohol together, or alcohol plus being significantly above a healthy weight range, it increases the risk to a dangerous level.

An accepted British study cited by many health workers, which followed 1.28 million women in past decades, has shown startling results about alcohol and the risk of breast cancer. It estimated that, statistically, the average woman who identified as a one-drink-a-day person was at an 11 to 12 per cent higher risk of breast cancer than a woman who doesn't drink at all. Those who had two drinks a day doubled their statistical risk to 22–24 per cent. It's important to say that most women *don't* get breast cancer – but for those with other risk factors, including being above a recommended weight range, not exercising and a family history, you might want to take that all into account. Alcohol is believed to be the cause of 5 to 11 per cent of breast cancer cases.

Drinking a 'moderate' amount of alcohol (remembering that this means different things to different people) doesn't seem as protective against heart disease as once thought. Drinking is also a known, significant risk factor for depression.

Alcohol is known to raise estrogen levels in the blood, but it is hard to measure and doctors say the risks cancel out any possible benefit, not least because alcohol creates a higher risk of breast cancer than extra estrogen does. You're much better off dealing with hormone levels using medication.

Despite clickbait reporting, doctors, mental health specialists and researchers say 'moderate drinking' being beneficial is not a reliable study finding. Mainly because the people who drink 'moderately' are more likely to have more money and better healthcare and healthier lifestyle to start with. Such studies also have varying and results-confusing definitions of moderate and often classify former drinkers as non-drinkers. Most alcohol studies are on white men.

I consider myself a high-functioning alcoholic, which I only half joke about. It's becoming an issue I'm in denial about.
Lisa, 48

Just drank alcohol to cope with issues in my life. Big mistake. Became a full-blown alcoholic. Went into a rehab for 11 months. Have been clean for nearly 17 months. Yay me!!! Jo, 64

Meta-analysis studies that distil the results of lots of drinking research are full of statistical palaver so confusing that even your pancreas looks puzzled: but here's what we do know.

There's no proven health advantage of light, moderate or heavy drinking.

Heavy and binge drinking is proven dangerous, and light occasional drinking is probably not a problem for most people.

> In the main throes of menopause between 45 and 50 I was drinking up to two bottles a night sometimes. I'm not proud of that. Theresa, 57

Safe drinking levels

Safe drinking levels set by national health authorities are lower for women than men, but due to pressure not to seem sexist, recommended numbers of standard drinks are often announced as the same for men and women: for example, the recommendations to have less than 10 drinks a week, some alcohol-free days and not to drink more than four drinks a day.

Every addiction specialist and doctor in the field of menopause or psychiatry that I spoke to thinks four drinks a night, regularly or often, is a dangerous or seriously unhelpful level for perimenopausal and menopausal women. Frankly if I had four drinks most nights I may as well sleep under the coffee table. But I can see that if I built up to that level over time, it might *feel* normal even if it was doing me harm.

> I drink a lot more. I drink every day now, sometimes also in the middle of the night if I'm awake for hours and want to sleep. Sandra, 58

> Alcohol became a coping mechanism so I quit more than a year ago now. Kristie, 54

> Out with friends I drink till I'm drunk, but we all kinda do. Ema, 51

> I drink more than I should, but it helps take the edge off my desire to stab people. Janine, 48

What is a standard drink, anyway?

I crave the 'relaxed' feeling two glasses of wine gives me. I never used to. Claudia, 45

I was a little chastened to realise that:

* 1 stubby or can of full-strength beer = nearly 1.5 standard drinks.
* 1 low-alcohol stubby or can of beer = about 8/10ths of a standard drink.
* 1 common restaurant/bar glass of red or white wine (150 ml) = just over 1.5 standard drinks. So drinking 4 glasses on a night out is actually 6 standard serves.
* 1 common restaurant glass of bubbly = almost 1.5 standard drinks.
* 1 ready-mixed long-neck of spirits plus mixer (e.g. gin and tonic) = between 1.5 and 2 drinks, depending on bottle size.

Any standard drink in Australia has 10 grams of alcohol in it. If you have baking equipment you can do a little experiment. Give or take, depending on individual brands, 10 grams of alcohol is in:

* about 100 ml of wine
* about 30 ml of gin, vodka, or whiskey. (A one-fluid-ounce jigger is about equal to 30 ml.)

What changed my habits was realising I was drinking too much in pandemic lockdown way back then. I don't have a jigger (nor a cocktail-onion fork), and when I measured how much I usually slosh in while making one gin and tonic it came to about 2.5 standard serves of alcohol. And if I put ice in the glass first, I had noooo idea how strong I was making it.

I also realised that if I had a bottle of gin, I just drank some most nights until the bottle was gone, but I can have a litre bottle of vermouth in the pantry and use a couple of teaspoons in a Nigella recipe a month and it will last approximately 10,000 years.

So I'm not the sort of person who could have a little selection of bottles on a cocktail trolley; I'd just drink it all by Saturday. It's a good thing to know. I don't buy bottles of gin and mix my own anymore; if I want some I buy ready-mixed bottles, which tell me on the label what they are.

I'm drinking more and on more occasions. JJ, 64

Alcohol & perimenopause

Stuff to know:

* Drinking more alcohol is a common feature of perimenopause.
* A common pattern is to move from drinking one drink in the evening to two or three glasses, and from occasional use to most nights.
* The increase in alcohol use can be a major factor in unwanted weight gain.
* People think a drink or more will help them get to sleep, but the older you get, the more alcohol messes with your ability to stay asleep.
* The older you get, the worse the hangovers are.
* Binge drinking and heavy drinking are known risk factors for depression and anxiety.
* Alcohol use during perimenopause can affect heart rhythm.
* Alcohol companies target women in their 40s and 50s with specific marketing evoking friendship and freedom.

Alcohol was the worst for the mental symptoms. I stopped drinking alcohol completely and noticed a huge improvement in my mental and physical health.
Mim, 57

After just two sips my face is aflame and itchy. Now I just smell my husband's wine glass when we're out for dinner. Weird, hey?
Kelli, 48

More research is needed (arggghhhh) to find out why women feel temporarily as if alcohol is helping them wind down, and reduce their anxiety – something to do with neurotransmitters and brain chemicals – while it has an ongoing depressive effect.

What doesn't help change drinking habits

* Some women are going to private clinics and even holiday destination, fancy-hotel-like rehab programs, but coming back home without ongoing support and strategies.
* Be wary if a GP's go-to solution for your worries about drinking is to prescribe antidepressants.
* It's rare for people to change ingrained or addictive habits without help.

I realised that my teenagers needed to see someone with a healthy respect for alcohol! **Isabel, 52**

I'm really falling out of love with my old friend alcohol. **Kali, 46**

I nearly fell off the wagon during perimenopause when I would feel overwhelmed. I took up knitting instead: yes, sad, I know, but it serves me better than getting shit-faced. **Suzette, 53**

I drink. I didn't for the first 45 years of my life. **Elise, 58**

I realised that my terrible migraines were mainly caused by alcohol, i.e. they were very severe hangovers even from small amounts. **Harriette, 51**

Seem to have developed an alcohol intolerance. Massive flushes after drinking and get really bad headaches after one glass. **Liz, 56**

What can help change drinking habits

We often don't reach out for help with drinking because we're ashamed of being seen as out of control, or a messy woman, or a bad mother. Being seen as able to cope, multitask and stay organised and focus is often a badge of honour among women. It can seem shameful to say you need help, when it's actually courageous. The sooner you reach out to a friend, specialist website or doctor, the better.

A good GP will be glad to help you if you want to cut down your drinking, or stop. Some are not well-trained to help, or it feels like they're judgey and dismissive, or they don't connect your mental health problems with menopause. Ask for recommendations for a good doctor and switch, or check out 'More info' on page 202.

If you feel stuck in a pattern, or recreating a pattern from your past, a qualified psychologist can help you work out why and how to change.

Tips to be in more control of alcohol

If you can, don't have a stash in the house, so you have to go out to buy something to drink. And maybe try these:

* Have a day, or a week, or weeks or months 'off' alcohol.
* Stick ice-cubes in a small glass of white wine and effectively water it down halfway.
* Choose alcohol-free options, especially if you're having alcohol a few times a week. Invent yourself a mocktail or find a new fave signature drink to suit yourself – whether a go-to sophisticated soda and bitters with a lime twist or a party-pink sparkler.

- Give yourself a one-drink or two-drink limit per day.
- Buy half-bottles.
- Wait 20–30 minutes between drinks.
- Have 1–2 non-alcoholic drinks to every alcoholic drink.
- If you realise it's hard to cut back, that's an important time to think about getting help, even anonymously. An aim might be to easily be able to not drink for a month.
- Recognise that for most of us in the grip of a habit or addiction like this, stopping by yourself is hard, or impossible, and also unnecessary.

If you're struggling to cut back, see 'More info on help with alcohol', coming up, for where to get help. If you drink every day, or drink several drinks a day, or have other health problems, it might be dangerous to stop suddenly without help. Start with your GP or one of the helplines.

I feel it takes the edge off my mood and hot flushes . . . but now alcohol has made me not a very nice person. And then I make choices that I regret and am ashamed of. **Melissa, 46**

I have a lot of 40-something friends who battle with the booze. I don't drink because I would be one of them. **Heidi Rose, 47**

I have quit drinking altogether (260 days and counting!) and feel sooo much better. **Rachel, 45**

Sober 21 years in AA. So incredibly grateful I did not have to sort out my drinking and menopause at the same time! **Helen, 55**

Be a drinking pal

Help friends who aren't drinking: don't challenge or cajole them when they don't want to drink. Be cool about offering or ordering something non-alcoholic but festive or mocktaily. If someone confides in you about a drinking problem, say you admire their courage, support them to get help and offer to research some starting places.

MORE INFO on help with alcohol

hellosundaymorning.com
Hello Sunday Morning is an Australian independent website providing support, advice and camaraderie if you want to reduce or stop drinking. Includes personal stories, recommended books and docos. The free Daybreak app provides help and support to change habits.

***High Sobriety: My Year Without Booze* by Jill Stark**
A respected journalist combines empathy, personal experience, research, and practical suggestions about drinking and mental health.

fare.org.au
Choose 'Resources and Support' on the main page of this lobby and support group, the Foundation for Alcohol Research and Education.

turningpoint.org.au
Has online self-help courses you can go through privately; home & email counselling, SMS supports; tactics to resist pressure to drink. Backed by the federal health department and the Turning Point centre for research, treatment & training. You can do a self-assessment. From the drop-down 'Treatment & Support' menu, choose 'self-assessments', then choose 'alcohol'.

Gambling, gaming & social media

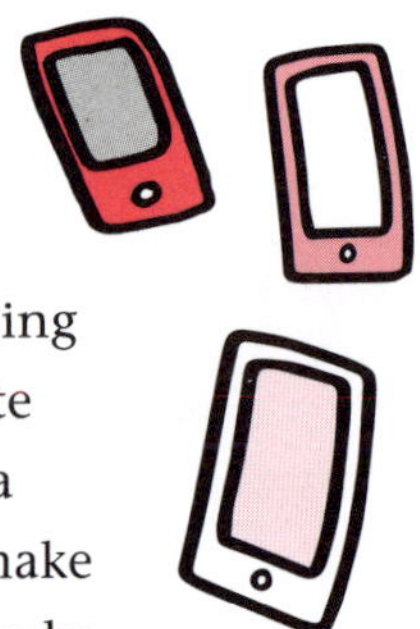

Many women have a gambling problem that spikes during perimenopause and beyond, whether it's online, poker machines, wagering apps or something else. Others might find themselves feeling obsessed with gaming, or scrolling social media, which can stimulate reward-feeling or calm-feeling brain chemicals. Knowing you have a problem can evoke really strong feelings of distress and shame, or make you feel too embarrassed to tell anyone – but it can happen to anybody. Reach out for help: see the 'More info' section opposite.

It's OK to have days where everything sucks and you just want to stay in bed. Everyone has things that make their life difficult at times. Kate, 49

Prescribed medication & other drugs

You can be dependent on, or addicted to (whatever your preferred terminology) all sorts of things that carry a health risk for you, ranging from sleeping tablets to cannabis products.

Weed can be another thing women use to try to help with perimenopause symptoms. This can be a particular problem during menopause too, because smoking is a bad idea for your heart and various other health reasons in perimenopause and beyond. Edibles can be a better bet, but can also have side effects. No studies exist that put topical cannabis-related products above estrogen for skin or vaginal use. Other factors to consider include reliable dosage, a quality-controlled source, and local laws.

Many of us have experienced becoming dependent on prescribed medications for sleep or anxiety or depression, or may misuse them, or use somebody else's prescription. If this sounds like it's become a problem for you, reach out to one of the services in the 'More info' section coming up and/or talk to your GP.

* MORE INFO on addictive behaviours

All these services can provide help and advice; you can choose to be totally anonymous. Some people find useful help at Alcoholics Anonymous, Narcotics Anonymous and Gamblers Anonymous. Others may prefer a service or program that doesn't embrace a notion of a 'higher power' or the guidelines for '12 steps'.

beyondblue.org.au
Helpline: 1300 224 636
24-hour chatline from the website, plus fact sheets on all sorts of problems and solutions. Search 'alcohol', 'benzodiazepine', 'gambling', or 'cannabis' on this independent mental health site. Beyond Blue is largely funded by donations.

psychology.org.au
The Australian Psychological Society represents trained and qualified psychologists. Use their online 'Find a psych' service to search by location and type of issue you'd like to work on. (Your GP may also have a recommendation.)

>

counsellingonline.org.au
Online self-help courses you can go through privately by yourself, plus home or email counselling, SMS support sign-ups, tactics to resist social pressure to drink, and more. Funded by the federal health department and Turning Point addiction research, treatment and training centre.

smartrecoveryaustralia.com.au
Support for addiction recovery from a non-religious no-12-step alternative to Alcoholics Anonymous, with peer-support, by a coalition of drug and alcohol services, available online or in person.

gamblinghelponline.org.au
Hotline: 1800 858 858
Federal health department funded service with support, advice, calculators, recovery stories and more.

Addicted Australia
A documentary following the lives of real people struggling with addiction and dependence who find a 6-month treatment program. Expert help brings hope and transformation to their lives. (SBS On Demand)

yourhealthinmind.org
Locate a specialist psychiatrist in addiction, alcohol or gambling using the the national directory of qualified psychiatrists of the Royal Australian and New Zealand College of Psychiatrists (RANZCP). Use the 'Find a psychiatrist' search function. You can search by your location, too.

rethinkaddiction.org.au
A national campaign to reduce the stigma and shame of addiction and dependence. Includes shared stories, and an online support referral page.

I resigned from one job thinking I could no longer do it but I look back now and realise it was the anxiety. Kim, 51

If I'd known about the benefits of healthy diet, exercise, mindfulness, fasting, limited alcohol – then I'd have done all of them. Jo, 59

I'm undertaking a massive phase of change that might take many more years to emerge from. I want to focus on tending to my body's needs. Polly, 44

My mental health has been all over the place. Being an empty nester is part of it. Wendy, 57

The takeaway on your mind

Perimenopause can scramble emotions and vandalise your mental health. Contributing factors include hormones, brain chemistry, psychology and Doing Too Much. Different medical and psychological options can combat brain fog, depression, anxiety and recurring or new mental health palaver. Be aware of possible symptoms, and be careful with yourself. You can tackle sleep problems, and a dependence on alcohol or other things that aren't helping or make things worse.

That's all good news and here's more: so many of us feel that once we've vanquished the symptoms of perimenopause and any hang-around problems, we feel freer, more confident and suitably scary when required.

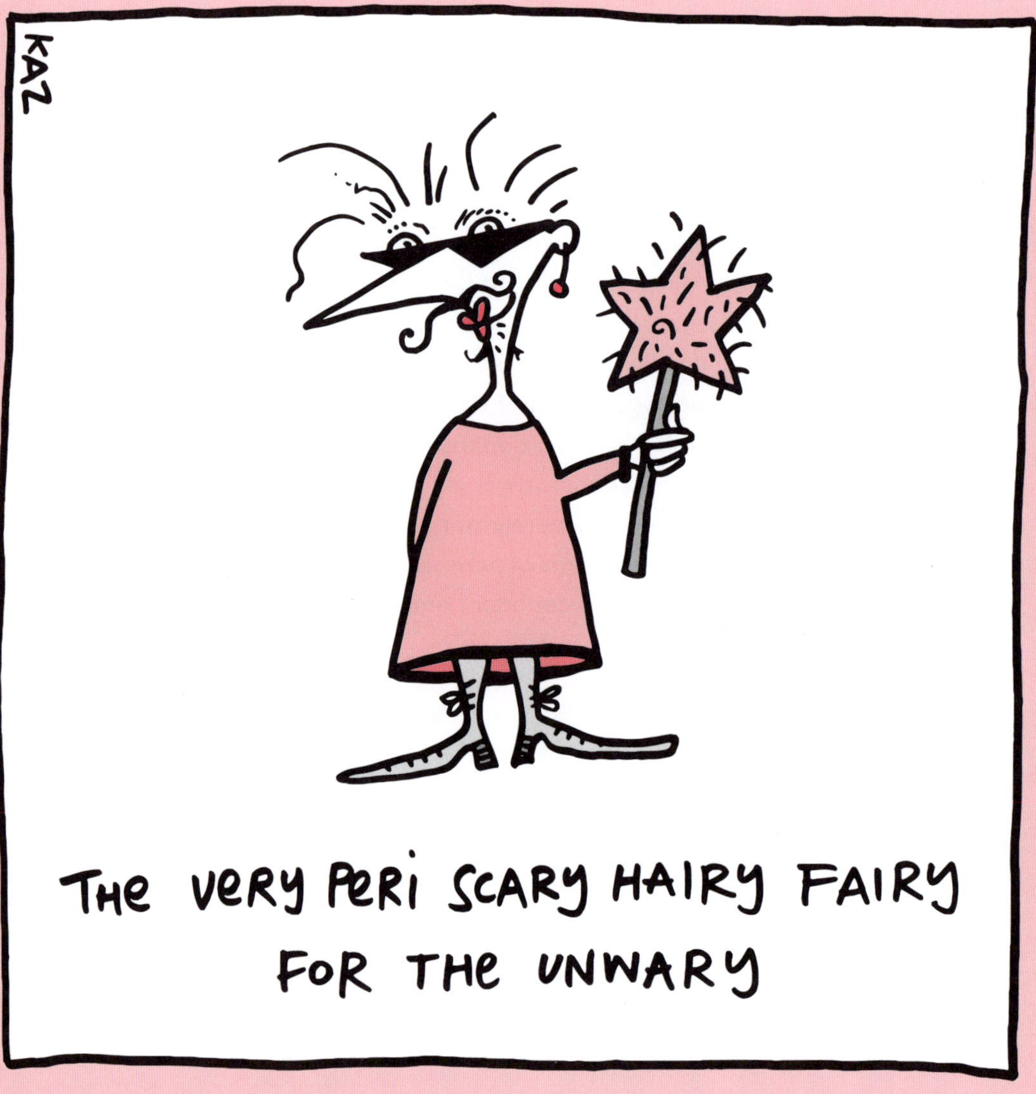
KAZ
THE VERY PERI SCARY HAIRY FAIRY
FOR THE UNWARY

5

It's Your Body

There are approximately seventy eleventy million possible variations on symptoms of menopause (give or take). You won't get them all, but you might get variations on some of them.

News and product-selling sites have started to bombard us on articles about perimenopause, but the common body symptoms issues they talk about are usually just hot flushes with a nod to a whispered 'lack of libido'. Hardly anything is said about the least glamorous or hardest-to-sort out symptoms, like Mysteriously Irritable Vulva, madly heavy periods, and beardy nipple hair. This chapter will wade into the known, and the lesser known, physical symptoms, not to mention the ones we had noooo idea had anything to do with hormones.

So many women answering the Menopause Survey for this book said they knew nothing about perimenopause before they were in it, or just thought it would happen when they were old, or thought the only symptom was hot flushes. Strap yourselves in, lovelies.

See the list of possible menopause symptoms on pages 36–37. And the 'Who's Who in medical & other practitioners' and 'Who's Who in natural practitioners' lists in Chapter 3, It's Your Approach, for info on the difference in training and focus between doctors, specialists and other health practitioners.

We've got you covered

For the mental symptoms of pre-perimenopause and perimenopause, like bursting into tears and being unaccountably furious, see Chapter 4, It's Your Mind.

For physical changes that a lot of us tend to think of as appearance-related, such as hair loss, grey hair and body hair, wrinkles, and fingernails, see Chapter 7, It's How You Look. The 'Exercise' and 'Eating & weight' sections are in Chapter 3, It's Your Approach, and physical hormonal changes that affect that aspect of your life are in Chapter 6, It's Your Sex Life. We could have put all those physical symptoms in this chapter, but frankly, we needed the room.

Because some of the symptoms of perimenopause are similar to those in other illnesses, googling can result in self-diagnosis of just about anything else you can think of. I popped some perimenopausal symptoms into the government health department site and it told me I might have a virus. The internet, as always, is no substitute for talking to a qualified medical person.

Instead of just searching the entire internet for a symptom, please bookmark the trusted, independent, not-selling-you-anything menopause society websites on pages 36–37, and use their search functions for the latest and best info on symptoms, or look something up in this book's Index.

Anyway, ta-daaaa. Here come all the possible symptoms. If you do get some, you might be slightly annoyed by them, or if you're unlucky, you will plunge into despair because of them. The timing might span a couple of years, or well over a decade. The good news is: there's stuff here about what you can do about them to make your life much easier.

I went to a new GP once and mentioned that I seemed to be the only person I know who doesn't feel the cold. His response was 'Hahahaha menopause'. That was all he said on the subject.

Jennifer, 55

I changed GPs and I mentioned the hot flushes and itching skin were keeping me awake. She put me on medication . . . which works. I'm amazed. 15yrs since my symptoms began and this is the first time anyone mentioned there was anything I could do about it!!!! Maria, 58

Strange periods

> My periods were torrential, needing sanitary protection changes every 20 minutes. Iron levels were less than half of the minimum. Merilyn, 56

What the actual hell, you are entitled to ask, is going on with my period? Any or all of these things: it's irregular, spotty, seems to have disappeared, heavy bleeding one month then not the next, unpredictably arrives with longer or shorter cycles, 'flooding' and visible stains from soaking through pads or tampons, clots, no cramps, worse-than-usual cramps, no premenstrual symptoms; full-on premenstrual symptoms, periods lasting more than a week. Your period blood might be more watery and light, or dark coloured.

All this period palaver is due to the unpredictable, erratic or falling levels of estrogen and progesterone in perimenopause.

If your ovaries are trying to compensate for falling levels by pumping out more estrogen one month, or if your progesterone levels fall further one month in proportion to estrogen levels, you'll get a build-up of extra lining in the uterus, which then has to come out as a period. So it's a period with way more blood than usual, and perhaps clots as well.

If your ovaries try to keep responding to your brain glands trying to run a menstrual cycle, one ovary might even have the equivalent of a closing down, everything-must-go sale, and release two eggs at once, which may also increase the build-up of uterine lining, making for a heavier period. Conversely, there may be no egg and a very light period.

> I had three periods that went for 9 weeks each. Camille, 45

> I was losing heaps of blood every three weeks. Dr Google didn't give me a clear answer about heavy bleeding . . . I was too busy to go to the doctor. It was scary and debilitating. Tiffany, 48

> Chairing a board meeting. No sign of a period for 18 months. Realised with horror I was bleeding heavily. Had to stay sat. Room full of blokes. Looked like a ritual sacrifice had occurred when I finally got up. Lotta, 58

> Hysterectomy definitely helped – couldn't have continued for another year with (all) the blood loss. Tonia, 56

Many women say unpredictable heavy bleeding can be an absolute nightmare for them at work, or social occasions, or travelling. They've said it was a factor in them quitting work, and refusing invitations to events with friends or family.

Heavy periods can also result in iron-deficiency anaemia, causing you to feel tired, washed out and maybe even dizzy or faint. It's important to check your iron levels.

In the Survey for this book, women identified heavy periods, including ones with clots, flooding and going on for weeks, as a real problem during perimenopause. More women rated heavy periods as terrible or tough to endure, than women rated hot flushes that way.

> Having a Mirena IUD has helped me a lot. I have had it now for 18 months. It has stopped the heavy periods. Jodie, 48

More than two-thirds of 7522 women identified heavy periods as a symptom: almost 10 per cent had them and weren't bothered, over 17 per cent were sometimes annoyed, 18.5 per cent found it tough and a little over 23 per cent had a truly terrible time with them.

More than 70 per cent of women answering the relevant question experienced erratic periods, about 42 per cent weren't much fussed by them, a bit over a quarter said it was sometimes annoying, about 14 per cent said it was tough, and just under 8 per cent had a terrible time. Hardly anyone minded much about getting lighter periods: almost 50 per cent said it didn't happen to them, about 42 per cent did and didn't care much, and only a handful found it annoying.

Stuff that can help with irregular periods

Most doctors would suggest imposing a settled level of hormones with a progestogen-emitting IUD, or prescribed the Pill or MHT.

> When I don't have my period, I seem to be spotting. I am lucky to get 2–3 weeks between periods. WHAT THE HELL??? I thought they were supposed to go away!!! Fiona, 47

> I had irregular periods and when I went on a plane I would get one. Gillian, 58

What can help with heavy periods

These things:

- Get a 'why' medical diagnosis.
- A progestogen-emitting IUD, the Pill or MHT prescribed by a doctor.
- Having more emergency supplies such as pads, tampons, period undies, wet wipes and plastic bags, spare undies and even spare trousers at home, at work, or in the car.
- Doubling up with two period products during a heavy bleeding: e.g. a super tampon *and* a pad.
- Take a reliable multivitamin with an iron component (this doesn't alter your bleeding symptoms but will replace any significant iron loss during big bleeds).
- An endometrial ablation (removal of the top layer of the endometrium).

I've started wearing period undies all the time because I'm so worried I will suddenly get my period. Gemma, 50

I had a Mirena inserted to address the erratic periods, and it has been so amazing not to have to worry about that anymore. I used to skip my period for 2 or 3 months and then bleed for weeks. HP, 49

Fibroids

Fibroids are non-cancerous growths on the uterus that can cause heavy bleeding. They're more common as you get older but before the time of medically diagnosed menopause. Most fibroids are harmless and most will shrink down in menopause, because they're 'fed' by estrogen and progesterone.

Many can be treated or kept to a smaller size with medication; some can be removed with surgery. Sometimes they'll cause the need for a hysterectomy, the removal of the uterus. Fibroids are identified using an ultrasound and treatment needs to be determined by a gynaecologist.

Don't assume any unusual bleeding for you is menopausal, or is due to harmless fibroids. Any of that should be investigated in the rarer case of something more dangerous. Uterine tissue can be inspected by ultrasound, or a tube-telescope up into the uterus, or in fewer cases, by a surgical curette procedure using anaesthetic, in which an instrument is used to scrape cells off the lining of the uterus (endometrium) to be analysed by a pathology lab.

Keep using contraception

However bonkers it seems, if you are having any period-like bleeding, or have had some in the last year or so, you may be able to get pregnant.

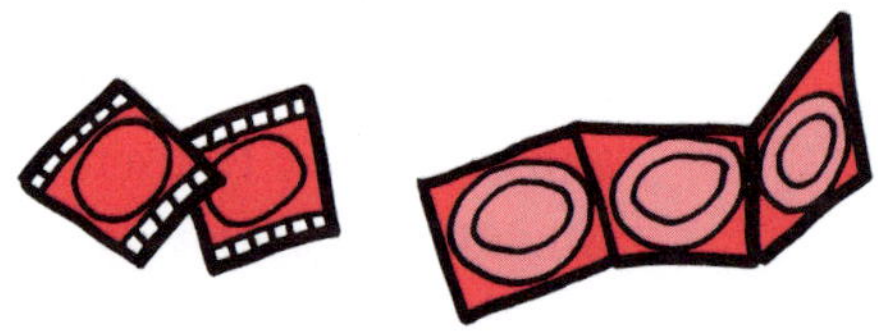

Vasomotor symptoms

A lot of perimenopause symptoms are classed by doctors as 'vasomotor'.

It's pronounced 'vayz-uh-motor' (or 'vayse-ommitta' in the US). The symptoms are the ones caused by the hypothalamus region of your brain, which controls how your heart and blood vessels pump blood around your body (arteries take blood out from the heart, and veins send it back through). The word comes from the Latin word for a container, *vas*, and for moving, *moto*.

So vasomotor symptoms include all the ones related to blood and blood pressure, such as hot flushes and night sweats, red-looking skin like blushing, heart-rate changes including speeding up or irregular beats, feelings of tingling or little electric shocks, and hormone-related headaches and migraines.

Hot flushes

Hot flushes are the splashy, big-shot symptom of perimenopause, the best-known vasomotor symptom, perhaps the first you notice and recognise as related to perimenopause, and often, the only one other people can see that you're experiencing.

Most women get some experience of hot flushes in their perimenopause. It can happen at the start, middle, or end of perimenopause; or it can continue for months or years past the final period when you're technically *in* menopause, also sometimes known as post-menopause. They can be mild or ghastly, or rare or happen once or 20 times a day. Hot flushes are not imaginary or caused by a psychological

> The hot flushes were the worst; every hour on the hour for about a year. I became so hot, sweat dripped off the ends of my hair. I still get at least one hot flush a day.
> **Jennifer, 67**

reason, and most women in perimenopause will experience them.

A hot flush can typically last only a minute, or five minutes: for some of us, it's a momentary sense of heat, like walking into a giant oven and out again. Others hardly notice them. For others, hot flushes are violent, intense, extreme, sudden events.

The average length of time to experience come-and-go hot flushes is about 4–5 years, and unlucky ladies might be having them for 12 years or more. Some women themselves say they've experienced hot flushes for at least 15 years, or more.

You can have hot flushes without any other signs of perimenopause. You can get hot flushes if you still get periods, or if you haven't had a period for years. Many women in perimenopause may not have lots of hot flushes but may have a varied but higher temperature for days, weeks, even months. This can make temperatures feel way too hot for you in workplaces and a shared bed.

Risk factors for more severe hot flushes

If you're well above your healthy weight range, or you smoke, you're probably more likely to get hot flushes. They're extra tough on people already under stress, and who have depression or anxiety about financial problems. We know African American women may experience more severe ones, and Japanese women who ate a consistent, traditional high-soy diet all the years before their first periods may have the fewest. There's scant medical research on the experience of First Nations women and the range of known physical menopause symptoms.

My nan's word for a hot flush is a 'foofy'. Kelli, 48

[I've been] carrying a fan. Elegant and useful. Tracy, 60

Rolling hot flushes every 30 minutes made it pretty tough to work. Trying to chair a meeting with sweat rolling down my face was undermining. Never sure whether mental symptoms were really sleep deprivation. Rose, 60

I could go and lie in the snow in my bra and knickers and be happy for about 40 mins. Melissa, 49

The hot flushes were mostly in my feet. More than half the women I know had worse ones in their feet. I went to bed with an ice pack. Ness, 51

A younger woman at my work was so unkind to me about my hot flushes. It was awful. Jules, 55

In the Survey for this book, more than 12 per cent of women who answered questions about hot flushes said they were truly terrible, and about 21 per cent said they found it really tough. About 26 per cent found it sometimes annoying, almost 19 per cent said they noticed it but it wasn't bad, and about 18 per cent said they hadn't noticed any.

> While my hot flushes kept me awake at night, I used the time to read research papers on the effectiveness of various treatments, then settled on one in conjunction with my GP.
> Vanessa, 54

> One young man at work would joke about me getting hot when he was around. I'd laugh but inside, not funny. At one stage the hot flushes were so significant they would stop me mid-sentence . . . 10 of these a day.
> Karen, 55

> It had been WEEKS of having them every day by the time it dawned on me.
> Stacy, 52

What a hot flush feels like physically

It feels like a bloom of intense heat from the inside. Your body temperature shoots up. A lot of people describe it as feeling like it starts in the middle of you and then rushes up to your head. Others reckon it starts in the head and floods down.

Real heat will radiate from you, and anyone who touches your skin will feel it. It can help to throw off a jacket, or stand in front of a fan, but that won't stop a hot flush on the spot: your body will keep generating heat from inside, and you have to just wait for it to subside.

Your brain will then tell your body to cool down, so it makes your heart pump faster to send hot blood from your core out to your skin and extremities to radiate heat off and away (including your scalp). It will also break you out in a sweat to cool you down.

The sweating from a hot flush can feel like nothing much; or with severe ones, it can be a sudden event, as if your skin turned on sprinklers: sweat can roll down and drip from your scalp and nose, bloom under your arms and breasts, on your back, between your buttocks. Some people feel chilled afterward, wet from sweating.

What a hot flush can feel like emotionally

An unwelcome hot flush can feel intensely difficult if, at that same moment, you're focused at work or in a social situation where a flush can feel like embarrassment, or you worry it will be perceived that you're embarrassed, worried, flustered, nervous, not coping, unsure of yourself or even what looks like a physical 'tell' that you're lying.

This can be really acute while you're public speaking or addressing a meeting, or greeting a customer, and feel like it's undermining your authority as, say, a teacher or a nurse giving instructions.

A hot flush produces the same physiological results as a panic attack or flash of embarrassment, and can therefore trigger an involuntary flight, fight, freeze or dread response. Feeling at their mercy can really stomp on your confidence and sense of self.

If a hot flush trips into feelings of sudden anxiety or panic, or you're not in a supportive workplace or safe-feeling social situation, it can then make you feel all of the things a flush can be mistaken for, which prolongs the sweating or hot feeling, and raises your heart rate: a sort of vicious circle. A hot flush is literally the opposite of being cool or chill.

I had anxiety every time I had a hot flush as it would start off (just before a flush) with a feeling that something was terribly wrong, and I felt like I was going to die. It took me a couple of years to realise. Tony, 59

I had hot flushes for years and years, but the truly horrible sense of dread disappeared after some psychotherapy. Jaki, 67

A feeling of pervasive dread was the physiological effect of hot flushes as my brain was getting the message that there was danger. Jen, 53

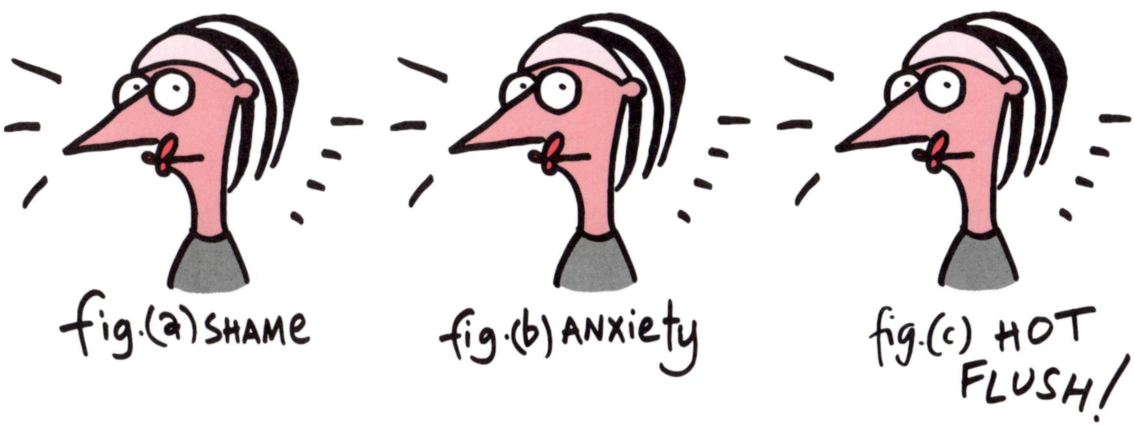

If it feels like this for you, it might take superhuman willpower in the moment to reframe hot flushes, as some women recommend, as power surges. But with informed people around you who are not dickheads, you can move the dial to 'No big deal' or 'Hello, here comes one of these again', rather than, 'Oh no, no, not now'.

I had a hot flush and my glasses fogged up completely! My friend and I laughed and she fanned me with the menu.
Liz, 45

What causes a hot flush

Absurdly, we don't know exactly why hot flushes happen – we know they're caused by a drop in estrogen. It's believed that even a small estrogen fall, if it's fast, can create an intense hot flush. We don't know why the body dilates your blood vessels and sends more blood pumping around so that your temperature spikes.

In other words we don't know if the body is saying, 'You've lost some estrogen, we'll try and make you hot for a useful reason', or, more likely, if it's just a side effect of your hormones being too erratic for comfort. We don't know how much the lack of follicle stimulating hormone has to do with it, but it's definitely something (yes, I think you're right, this *would* be a good time to discuss public funding for physical and mental symptom menopause research with your local member of every goddamned-arsed parliament).

Normally, men's body temperature is hotter than women's, which accounts for the thermostat in many offices, other workplaces and shops being set hotter for an average white man in the 1960s.

Don't be fooled by any nonsense saying that your body sweating is telling you that you have to purge toxins so you need our detox tea or special cleansing diet. To get technical for a moment, that's utter bollocks.

Getting help for hot flushes

If a GP says you're too young for hot flushes without taking a further history and asking you a lot of questions, and tells you those symptoms are psychological or you should just put up with them because they're to be expected, but they're making you miserable, or uncomfortable, or you don't want them,

I told my GP about the terrible fierce hot flushes all the time that made life impossible, and he said, 'Oh well, you're not going to die. Is anything else bothering you?' (A woman explaining to an endocrinologist why she needed extra help.)

insist on treatment options being presented to you, or find another GP.

Right now, around the world, women are spending billions on 'menopause' products that will not lessen or cure their hot flushes (more on what works and what doesn't, coming up).

> Tried herbal medicine . . . didn't help at all. Terrie, 54

> My doc prescribed an old-fashioned blood pressure medication for my hot flushes. It made them bearable and helped with my blood pressure. Noemi, 60

> My acupuncturist has given me some foul-tasting herbs that have been very effective against hot flushes and, to a lesser extent, night sweats. Amanda, 48

Management of hot flushes

The most important thing to realise about hot flushes is that no woman has the same experience. Everyone has their own mix of intensity and frequency of flushes, often in unpredictable ways. It's not run to a 28-day cycle (not that all periods are, either), and it might happen every day for a week or a month, then nothing for weeks, then happen every day for a week, then nothing for 3 months. Or just feel like it's both unpredictable and happening all the time.

So here's what none of us get to say to anyone else, 'It's so terrible, you have to take MHT' or 'What's the big deal, I hardly noticed them' or 'a homeopathic treatment will cure them' (homeopathy can't work because it has no active ingredients).

If your workplace is reasonable, hot flushes can be handled with a matter-of-fact approach. Stories abound of women in meetings or behind counters throwing off cardigans, then shirts and sitting in a singlet or T-shirt till they put it all back on again – but that won't be possible or allowed in every workplace.

Older actresses have reported having to stop filming, flush away for a few minutes, then resume after a make-up artist sponges their faces and redoes their face. Maybe pretending you're Meryl Streep will help. I mean, it probably will in any other situation, too.

Things that can help hot flushes

For several years I took an antidepressant (SSRI), and I know it worked because when I went off it, I went from 3–4 hot flushes per night to 8–10. Then I went on HRT and am down to 1–2 hot flushes per night. Tania, 53

You might try:

* **Riding it out**. If you're lucky, they won't feel severe, or go on for more than a few months. But if they're getting in your way, or awful, this may not feel like an option at all.
* **Being busy**, distracted and not feeling under scrutiny. In other words, if it doesn't matter if you're having a hot flush you may not notice a milder sort of flush. (If a perimenopausal woman flushes in the forest . . . will she shout at you if you point it out?)
* **MHT**. The best-known reliable treatment that works and is considered generally safe. It can take a few weeks to a couple of months to kick in. As always, women with a uterus need to take progesterone with it and it's often not recommended for women who've had an experience with an estrogen-related cancer of the breast, endometrium or a history of blood clots or stroke. (See 'MHT' in Chapter 2, It's Your Hormones.)
* **Other prescribed medication** can be useful for women who can't take estrogen medication: ask a switched-on GP, endocrinologist, gynaecologist or your oncologist. Newly developed medicines, as well as SSRI and SNRI antidepressants (serotonin and norepinephrine re-uptake inhibitors) can help with hot flushes but may not be suitable for you. It's best to talk to your doctor about the latest developments and what's best for you.
* **Some antidepressants**, in low doses, can reduce hot flushes and sweats. But they are also associated with a loss of libido and it can be complicated to stop taking them, so talk to your doctor about that before starting.
* **Keeping a diary** of flushes to see if there's a pattern, or when they feel worse. Knowing how many there are might help you decide if you can deal with them or want to get medical help. Tracker apps and monitoring devices can also do this, but they can be used to sell your data too, so you'll be the target of hard-sell ads.

I first experienced it in my late 20s. I vividly remember getting hot flushes that felt like my head was going to explode and putting my head in the freezer. Andrea, 54

What won't help hot flushes

It's part of life, after all, all women go through it, suck it up, princess. Myrtle, 58

This stuff:

* Smoking and caffeine, because they restrict your blood vessels, too, which can make your brain go: quick, send more blood around and flush up, baby!
* Binge-drinking and everyday drinking is thought to make hot flushes worse (I mean, it probably just makes everything worse, to be fair, unlike pretending to be Meryl Streep).

Do 'natural' products work against hot flushes?

A lot of studies have been done on 'natural' treatments, and so far no acceptable independent research shows their product's formulation and recommended dose cures moderate to severe hot flushes. Some may work on mild symptoms.

No 'herbal' or plant based over-the-counter stuff, without a prescription, is known to work or, importantly, is regulated by authorities in terms of exact doses, ingredients and effects.

This is so hard to get our heads around but is absolutely true: just because something is legally sold, and on a shelf in a chain chemist, or online, does not mean it will 'work' for you. Although we are supposed to be protected by consumer and health legislation, in practice, billions of dollars of supplements are sold in Australia that don't do much of anything at all, and certainly don't help hot flushes.

Sadly for those of us who'd rather buy something 'natural', in so many cases, particularly when it comes to hot flushes worrying enough to want treatment for, it's just a waste of money.

Sage for sweats helped for a while and now HRT is fab!! Bronwen, 54

Avoid homeopathic products: they can't work and have no active ingredients, and steer clear of so-called bio-identical hormone creams and 'natural' progesterone creams. See the 'Progestogens' section in Chapter 2, It's Your Hormones, for more on why.

Reliable studies show no useful anti-hot flush or hormonal effect from eating or drinking soy products or from any compounded hormone or other hormone supplement that isn't a ready-made prescription product that is registered and approved by health authorities in specific doses.

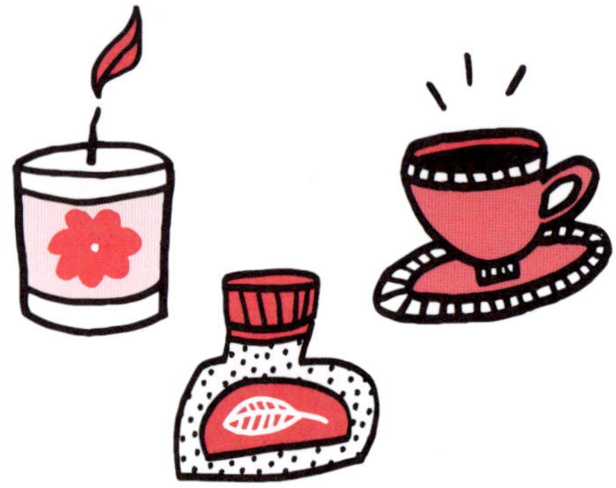

After researching this book, I wouldn't buy any menopause supplement products not on prescription. Even if labels and marketing blurbs say 'hormones' or 'menopause' on the label, it may do nothing whatsoever to your hormone levels.

Look out for the word 'supports': that's unprovable, vague, and often used because there's no acceptable scientific studies with any evidence that the specific formulation does anything at all to hormones or has any effect on hot flushes. Same-same for 'boosts', 'designed to regulate', 'balances' or 'helps to balance' hormones. Meaningless. (Of course, seek your own medical advice about individual products.)

Also, beware of products which are supported on websites and in ads with testimonials. 'Kirsty of Kingaroy says: Since I've been taking "Faffer Hormone Pills" I'm happier, sleep well, have no hot flushes, have slimmed down, am icily calm, now working as a *Vogue* model and have slept with Idris Elba twice'.

Usually the testimonials list some or all the known symptoms of menopause as something being cured. Again, these quotes are unprovable; it might even be something wholeheartedly believed but not a result of taking the supplement.

Studies generally show no useful or significant effect on severe hot flushes from phytoestrogens such as red clover products and black cohosh products. Some black cohosh products have been implicated in liver damage and failure. These products are not on prescription or regulated in the same way. (See the 'Phytoestrogens' section in Chapter 2, It's Your Hormones.)

Some products may not have reliable amounts in recommended doses and may not be what the label says, or have dangerous additives. This is of particular concern with Ayurvedic as well as other unregulated products.

Most doctors, faced with a patient wanting to take 'natural' products will not argue, even when they know it won't work and know in most cases it's unlikely to do harm. Doctors don't want to get into fights with patients.

I learned to wear black as it hides the sweat better. It's not a fashion choice; it's one of dignity. Jen, 49

I'm still taking [an SSRI] and really notice the hot flushes if I miss a day. Sonya, 55

Non-medical things that can help in other ways

You can:

* Be open about it at work and at home, if it's safe for you.
* Throw off a jacket and belt out 'I Will Survive' at the top of your lungs in a staff meeting.
* Compare hints and stories with friends.
* Have some control over heat levels in an office or other workplace, home and bedroom, using a fan or a water spray.
* Lose or gain some weight if you're above or below a healthy weight range for you.

Mental health & hot flushes

As mentioned, because a hot flush feels like anxiety or embarrassment and is often accompanied at the start by a heart rate acceleration, your brain can recognise it as alarm or something really unpleasant. For many women, it's like being forced to hold up a sign saying, 'I'm older than you think I am', or 'I can't control this thing about myself'.

The out-of-control-feeling aspect of hot flushes can trigger previous mental health issues, which you may have been managing well for years: a blast from the past of, say, depression, anxiety, trauma, OCD or eating disorders. (See Chapter 4, It's Your Mind.)

If you can use cognitive behaviour techniques, and/or chats with friends and co-workers so you don't feel ashamed of something that doesn't need to be kept hidden, you'll be much better off. But there are some feelings and situations that you may not be able to control: don't suffer in silence, reach out for help.

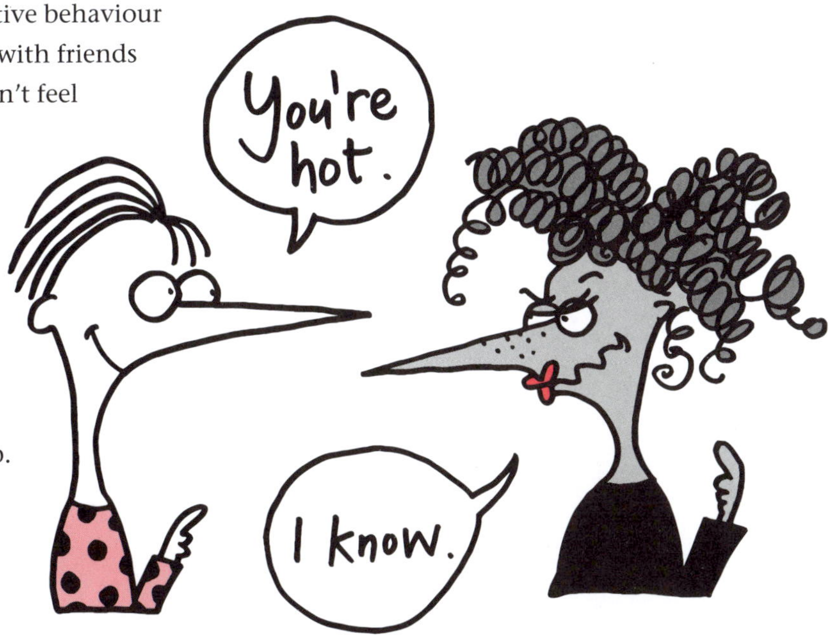

Night sweats

BOOM! You're boiled hot on the inside, there's a literal fire burning within you. You throw the doona off, and you're freezing at the same time. Can't describe how this feels, but it's fucking horrible. **Sam, 51**

A night sweat is just a hot flush in its pyjamas. But when you get a hot flush in your sleep, you might wake up to feeling roasted under a doona, or even in the nuddy. Then, when the nocturnal flush is over, you can be wet with sweat and suddenly feel damp and chilled. This can be a big ingredient in the insomnia recipe.

Most women in the Survey said they had night sweats and hot flushes, meaning many women don't identify a night sweat as a hot flush. Almost exactly a third said night sweats were tough; more than one in ten said it was really bad. About a third were occasionally annoyed; almost 14 per cent said they were no big deal; and just over one in five never had them.

Night sweats are different. Wake up multiple times a night completely soaked, PJs, bed, hair. Cannot share a bed with my partner. The smell is horrendous. It's like a bucket of water has been tipped on you. **Annie, 48**

Helpful hints for night sweats

* Hurl any wet bedclothes into the corner to deal with in the morning, towel yourself down and get into a new nightie or T-shirt, whatever you might wear to bed. As this can happen several times a night, have some spares, perhaps a ballgown and a cocktail frock.
* Try bed layers: sheet, cotton blanket, other blanket or light doona so they're easy to throw off, or fold back. Some companies sell a doona that's warmer on one side of the bed, for a partner.
* In severe cases, a waterproof mattress cover is a bonus.

I had a routine of making sure I had towels handy, plus extra nightwear, so I could dry off, change, put a towel under me and one over me (wet sheets!) and get back to sleep. Nothing else helped, and it was best just to minimise emotional disturbance by taking a practical approach. **Maria, 58**

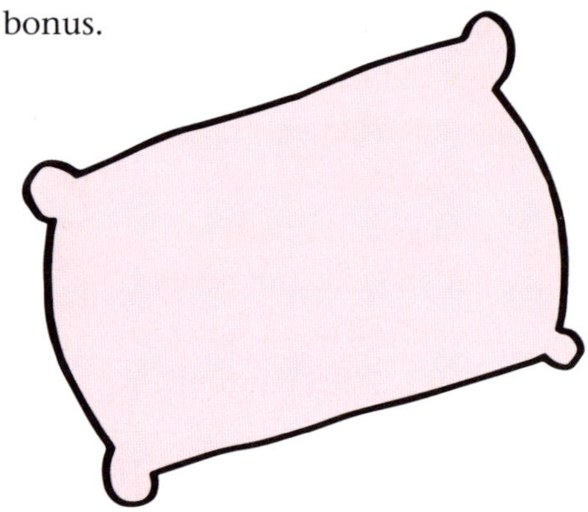

Sweats & scentsibilities

Perimenopause can give rise to weirdness about smells, in the same way that 'pregnancy hormones' can cause a greater sensitivity to smells, and elicit stronger reactions.

Conversely, you may also be overusing perfumes because you've built up a tolerance to the smell. Looking at you, ill-advised patchouli fiends and people given a vat of Miss Dior every Chrissie.

If you're plagued by sweaty hot flushes, you might worry that you have offensive smelling sweat. A hefty underarm antiperspirant deodorant (look for 'sports' or 'men's' brands – I know, ridiculous – or for heavy duty, unscented ones). For rough times, carry sensitive wipes and an antiperspirant to reapply. Deodorants won't stop you sweating. An antiperspirant that contains aluminium will help.

Antiperspirants under your arms won't stop sweat from elsewhere if your body dumps heat out of itself in other places: head, gusset, under the bosomry, etc.

Because MHT will reduce/cure hot flushes and bring down a generally elevated hormonally based temperature, people on MHT may notice they sweat less.

Headaches & migraines

> I had counselling in a pain clinic as I experienced hideous, life-changing migraines. Francesca, 59

Headaches and migraines can get worse in perimenopause, especially if you used to get premenstrual headaches. These headaches can be utterly unpredictable in perimenopause because your hormones levels are all over the place. Guess what, they don't know exactly why. The theory is that the quicker the rate estrogen levels fall in your body, the more likely it will affect blood vessel flow in a way that triggers a hormonal headache.

Everyone's different, but tension headaches tend to feel like a tightening around the forehead, and hormone-related migraines can throb, often on one side, and be accompanied by sensitivity to light, seeing auras, a sense of smelling something, and feeling nauseous. To complicate things, you may be getting more tension headaches and not as many hormonal ones, or vice versa.

Women are about twice as likely as men to experience migraines and of course estrogen levels can go up and down like a yo-yo in perimenopause, causing repeated migraines when estrogen falls again. Once in full-on settled menopause, migraines should stop. But we're not sure how relevant progestogens and brain chemicals are, too.

For some unlucky people, MHT makes migraines worse. Patches and gels may be a lower risk for this than estrogen in pills.

People often take painkillers for hormonal headaches that don't affect their cause and have side effects, so a diagnosis is good. Women who have a hysterectomy that triggers menopausal symptoms are often not told about the connection to headaches.

The Pill, or prescribed MHT, is generally suggested, to smooth out hormone levels. For those who can't take MHT or if MHT makes migraines worse, a visit to a headache specialist or endocrinologist should get you expert advice on other available treatments. A headache diary or medical history can help a doctor help diagnose hormone-related headaches.

Menopausal migraines means you may be at higher risk of stroke and other cardiovascular problems; the risk is much higher if you also smoke.

Only 36 per cent of women who answered the question in this book's Survey said they had no perimenopausal headaches: of the rest, around 34 per cent say it wasn't a big deal for them or sometimes annoying; it was tough for about 12 per cent and awful for just over 7 per cent.

All the sounds and smells became overwhelming and I also think my fragrance allergies are becoming worse. One whiff of the wrong perfume or scented candle can give me an intense headache. Maria, 49

Developed hormonal migraines for the first time – 1–3 times weekly. Required medication daily. Even required hospitalisation. Not one migraine post-menopause. Jenny, 62

Things that can make migraines worse

The triggers can be different for everyone, but can include delayed meals, getting dehydrated, sleep problems, bright lights, too much coffee, colas or energy drinks, alcohol, being run down, and smelling or eating things that you're intolerant to, such as food additives or types of food.

Heartbeat changes

Harmless changes in heartbeat regularity that might feel like palpitations can be triggered by a fall in estrogen. Because it's not a better-known perimenopausal symptom, many women, and their doctors, haven't realised that erratic heart behaviour can be connected to your estrogen levels.

For hundreds of years, right up to today, women have been wrongly diagnosed with panic attacks, too much caffeine, stress, and some version of the all-purpose imaginary symptoms or 'hysteria' when it may have been totally real, estrogen fall-related, un-scary heart-rate changes in perimenopause.

It can be a double whammy of wrong assumptions: from 'You're too young for any perimenopause symptoms' and 'It can't be that, you still have periods' to 'Well, this is obviously a psychological symptom'.

Of course, any heart carry-on or change in heartbeat habits should be mentioned to a doctor and totally checked out. Heart rate misbehaviour combined with hot flushes can sometimes indicate a thyroid problem or other condition. Many women describe what feels like a tremor inside them, in different parts of the body.

About 30 per cent of Survey respondents to heart questions said heartbeat changes in perimenopause were sometimes annoying; 10 per cent said it was tough and 3.5 per cent said it was awful. About 40 per cent didn't have any, and almost 18 per cent experienced them but weren't much bothered.

> Your Survey has prompted me to research my infrequent ventricular ectopic heartbeats in relation to perimenopause. My cardiologist and GP did not mention a possible connection.
> Andrea, 54

Heart risks

Estrogen keeps our blood vessels supple and helps to protect against inflammation or higher blood pressure. From the time of perimenopause onwards, the lower level of estrogen raises our risk of higher blood pressure and cardiovascular disease. Cardiovascular disease includes heart failure, heart pains, heart attack, heart disease and stroke. Heart disease and stroke kills many more women than breast cancer in this country.

From perimenopause you're likely to have a few extra heart risk factors. MHT may be helpful, and doesn't cause heart disease. Talk to your GP about medication options to reduce your risk, especially if your grandparents or parents had a history of heart disease or stroke. If you do take MHT, you still need to be vigilant.

Women's specific warning signals and symptoms of a heart attack are different to men's, and their signs of stroke are often not recognised. This can be more deadly for women. Symptoms women are more likely to have can be mistaken for simple nausea, fatigue, shortness of breath or indigestion.

Other risk factors aside from menopause for heart problems and stroke include high blood pressure, high cholesterol (cholesterol levels rise in menopause), smoking, being above a healthy weight range, lack of exercise, alcohol, and some medical conditions such as polycystic ovarian syndrome (PCOS) and autoimmune disorders. If you had high blood pressure or diabetes during a pregnancy, you have a higher risk of heart problems around after menopause.

Aboriginal and Torres Strait Islander women already have almost double the risk of heart disease, so if you're over 35, get regular check-ups and be vigilant, especially in menopause. Everyone else should talk with their doctor about when to start regular checks. You'll probably need blood pressure, heart rate, diabetes and cholesterol level checks.

I changed GPs but they weren't much better. I feel like no one was interested in my symptoms at all until I had a stroke. Leonie, 45

I know that it's important for women to do weight bearing exercise as it decreases their risk of osteoporosis and heart disease. Caz, 50

DIY ways to reduce heart risks

* If you want MHT, ask your doctor about whether it's safe for you.
* If you smoke, ask for help to quit.
* Aim for some sort of huffy-puffier exercise. (See the 'Exercise' section in Chapter 3, It's Your Approach.)
* Have a plan to reduce stress. (Ha. Aha. Ha.)
* Lose weight if you're above a healthy weight range.
* Ask your GP if you need medication to reduce high blood pressure and cholesterol levels, and check that dosage is appropriate for you as an individual (most heart drug trials are done on men).

MORE INFO on heart risks & stroke

mchri.org.au/guidelines-resources/community
The Monash Centre for Health Reseach and Implementation backs a coalition of health experts and women advisors who produce apps and advice on heart health, PCOS and early menopause.

jeanhailes.org.au
Search 'cardiovascular' or 'symptoms of heart attack and stroke' on this independent women's health website.

Bones

A bone density scan identified early menopausal bone density loss. This led to spinal surgery due to weak bones. Amanda, 58

Bits of what your bones are made of (technically that's known as . . . um, bone) keep being reabsorbed and disappear, and get replaced all your life. The retreat of bone is kept in check, and the replacement goes strongly while you have a higher level of estrogen in your body. This protective process is helped with healthy levels of vitamin D and calcium and exercise during which you carry your own weight (i.e. walking versus swimming, where the water holds you up).

When your estrogen falls much lower, your bones start to reabsorb too much of themselves, more quickly, and don't regenerate the way they used to.

The result is called reduced bone density (aka osteopenia), or in the more severe stage, osteoporosis: the loss of strong bone tissue, with a higher risk of fractures and broken bones as you progress into menopause.

Bone density tests using a special sort of X-ray can help doctors make a diagnosis of bone loss, but many women are proactively choosing to help protect their bones by taking MHT (or the Pill in early menopause, switching to MHT at the age perimenopause might be expected).

Half of women older than 60 have bone loss. The peak time of faster bone loss is in the perimenopause time, which continues until about 3 years after being in full menopause (meaning 4 years after your last period).

Lack of estrogen all through your life, a history of eating deprivation and diets, weight-restricting elite sports and a calcium or vitamin D deficiency can all contribute to osteoporosis.

Risks and associations for bone problems

These things:

* low or erratic estrogen levels
* 'early menopause', including Primary Ovarian Insufficiency (POI)
* smoking
* binge or heavy habit drinking
* a history of dieting
* a big caffeine habit (coffee's worse than tea)
* more than two standard alcohol drinks a day
* family history of weaker bones
* getting older
* vitamin D, protein or calcium deficiency
* being below a healthy weight range for you
* an athletics career
* a history of missed periods
* hormone imbalances
* low muscle use
* no exercise
* lack of strength
* falls
* thyroid and autoimmune problems
* known side effects of medications, including some steroids.

> Weight lifting improved bone density (with HRT), also improved back pain and bladder confidence. Jo, 61

> My mother has severe osteoporosis so I'm glad to have got HRT at 49 a year after I went into menopause. Anna, 49

> I must take [osteoporosis medication] for the rest of my life or my bones will crumble. Two shots a year costs approx. $1200. Not subsidised by the government. It is fucking outrageous. Katie, 51

> I do High Intensity Interval Training and weights when I can as I have osteoporosis at 48, which is just the saddest thing! I want to have functional mobility till I die. R, 48

Help for osteoporosis

Your doctor might suggest:

* a bone scan so you know what you're dealing with
* a blood test for relevant deficiencies
* MHT with the usual caveats of estrogen being paired with progesterone if you have a uterus; and no MHT if you have a history of certain medical conditions

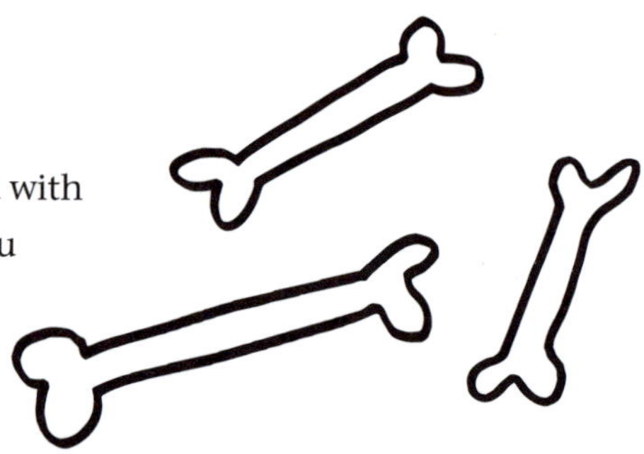

* non-hormonal bone-boosting or protecting medications (they can be a pain in the stomach, so ask your doctor for hints to reduce the chance of heartburn and nausea)
* vitamin D and calcium supplements
* a referral for good professional help with eating behaviour or nutrition.

DIY help for bone density loss

Keep up multi-directional weight-bearing exercise: activities and sports in which you carry your own weight, including dancing, walking, trapeze or weight and resistance exercise as well as, or instead of, swimming and cycling and being carried triumphantly about by an acrobat.

Vitamin D

Get your vitamin D levels tested every 2 or 3 years and take a supplement if you need to. For years I have crossly tried to find out the difference between recommended length of time of sun exposure to best convert enough vitamin D with or without sunscreen, for people with dark skin. It is always a total pain in the arse, nobody ever seems to know and just keep repeating recommendations about time, and sunscreen, which always seem to be for white women – but the ones in Cairns summer, or Norway winter? Veiled folk or the bikini-ed?

Closest I can get: if you're white and have lots of exposed bits of yourself, a few minutes to 20 minutes of sunshine a day can help boost vitamin D. For others, especially those who winter in southern climates, it might be easier to take a supplement. And stop using winter as a verb.

MORE INFO on bones

healthybonesaustralia.org.au
Formerly Osteoporosis Australia, with fact sheets.

menopause.org.au
Search 'bones' or 'osteoporosis' on the Australasian Menopause Society site.

jeanhailes.org.au
Info on medical and nutritional advice to prevent bone loss or encourage bone regeneration as much as possible.

Breasts

I woke up one morning, not long after I turned 50, with gigantic bosoms. Then I started thickening around the middle. Now I am a busty column with a bad attitude. Maudy, 56

Bosom time.

How does menopause affect breasts?

After menopause, your breasts say goodbye to all the glands that would have supported breastfeeding if needed, and will be mostly fat tissue from here on. You might have experienced tender or explodey-feeling breasts before periods in the past, as rising progesterone and estrogen at that time of your cycle started to prepare your breasts in case they were needed in about 9 months for breastfeeding.

So as hormones are all over the place in perimenopause, unpredictable bosom oddness can come and go: a sore, full, tight or tender feeling, or sensations of burning, fizziness or even slightly stabbiness. These can also be an early sign of pregnancy, or be caused by some common medications.

Almost half of the women answering the breasts question in the Menopause Survey for this book said they had noticed breast changes in perimenopause. (And of course, others said they didn't have their breasts any more after a mastectomy.)

Wearing a tight, supportive bra like a crop top or sports bra can relieve some annoying sensations. Underarm lymph nodes stimulated by a vaccination can sometimes cause a big lump near a breast up towards your underarm, on the side you got the jab, but if it doesn't disappear in a week or so, take your bosoms to a GP or gynaecologist for a check-up.

My main symptom so far has been stabbing breast pain. It was worrying at first because I thought it was a heart attack. Victoria, 46

I do mourn my previously rather lovely breasts that did a great job feeding three kids and bringing much pleasure to me and my husband. Sigh. Maria, 58

Worries about breast cancer

Do monthly self-checks on your breasts. Benign (non-cancerous lumps) are more common in menopause, but so is breast cancer: always call the GP and get a diagnosis immediately if you notice a lump. If an office manager says there is no appointment within the next two days, say it's a breast lump and you need an appointment ASAP. Your GP will give you a fast referral for a scan. If you are at all worried, insist.

The McGrath Foundation site **mcgrathfoundation.com.au** and Breast Cancer Network Australia site **bcna.org.au** both have instructions on how to do a breast check and info on awareness.

This stuff all needs to be checked by a GP immediately: any dimpling, puckering, nipple discharge, rash, changes to one breast different to the other.

You should be having a breast check mammogram every 2 years (it's free after the age of 50, but they stop sending reminders after the age of 70; you can keep reminding yourself).

MHT doesn't cause cancer, despite wrong-town studies and scares in the past. It increases your risk by a much smaller amount than having regular wines, for example.

But if you've already had a diagnosis of breast cancer, ovarian cancer or uterus (womb) cancer, then MHT may not be recommended for you. That's because when taken as a general oral pill, it can deliver estrogen to those areas of your body that have had cancer, which can 'feed' on estrogen. It's probable, though, that you can safely take topical estrogen vaginal cream, if that useful for you, because it won't go anywhere near your breast or uterus receptors.

The nuances of the risks and reasons are explained in the MHT section and cancer risks sections in Chapter 2, It's Your Hormones. Sadly, even some GPs have yet to catch up with the latest knowledge about MHT and risks.

The older you get, the higher your statistical risk of getting breast cancer. Less than 5 per cent of women will die from breast cancer, partly because screening and advances in medical knowledge means we catch it earlier, and treat it better.

If you've been diagnosed with breast cancer

Speak to your oncologist and GP about your treatment options for perimenopause and menopause symptoms. There's heaps you can do instead of taking estrogen.

> If I'd not changed GPs and been taken seriously enough/sent for tests . . . I would likely not be alive.
> Kate, 62

Mouth weirdness

For heaven's sake, if you can believe it, perimenopause can also cause changes in taste, red, bleeding or receding gums, dry or itchy mouth and tongue, sensitivity to hot and cold food and drinks, 'burning mouth syndrome', and the loss of teeth.

The usual culprit is an estrogen fall, so MHT can be suggested, although it's really not a stellar solution to any skin-related problems. Other approaches include putting up with it and throwing crockery.

See your dentist regularly after perimenopause starts because what else are you going to spend your millions on? You can chuck a teacup now.

> How do you explain to someone that a food you have loved for 40 years now tastes foul? Dana, 49

Tummy troubles

Digestion changes in perimenopause can include acid reflux, bloating, constipation and fartiness. Possibly caused by a slower metabolism, slowed by having less estrogen. Those of us with experience of endometriosis know that uterine cramps can affect the bowel next door, causing constipation and diarrhoea at certain times, so it stands to reason there might be some neighbourhood carry-on during perimenopause.

Researchers have also suggested that higher stress in perimenopause might suppress healthy gut bacteria, but that may also be an excuse to sell you probiotics that don't work. Estrogen seems to affect the gallbladder but, staggeringly, there isn't enough research on that yet. I really would like to tell you that the cure for this is drinking cocktails and eating a lot of chocolate frogs, but it isn't and here we are.

Mention any of these, if they're a problem for you, next time you visit a doctor for something else, drink water and eat vegetables and for heaven's sake try not to fart near microphones.

> One thing I did forget to mention is that my flatulence is through the roof – not a fear, but a reality that I haven't seen mentioned anywhere. Jeanette, 48

Joint aches & pain

Yep, this is a known symptom too: see Chapter 3, It's Your Approach, for the lowdown on joint pain, aches and exercise, or look up 'joint pain' in the Index. Many women in the Survey said they developed more tendon, carpal tunnel and repetitive strain injury (RSI) issues in perimenopause.

Weeing

I simply refuse to call this section incontinence, or genitourinary syndrome of menopause, and you can't make me. Instead I'm going to close my eyes and point at a statistic: the majority of women over 50 have some sort of unwanted, sneaky accidental-weeing situation happening.

Or, it happens to one in four women. Or half. Or more than 70 per cent of mothers. And at least one in ten women under 30. You can make up any statistic you like, because there isn't enough research on this, definitions of 'incontinence' vary, women are embarrassed to talk about it; published statistics wander all over the shop. Whatever. It's a hell of a lot of us.

As I scrolled down the thousands and thousands of responses from women in the Survey telling me about unwanted or unpredictable weeing, it was agonisingly clear that so many of us feel mortified, secretive, and really distressed by it.

Of those who responded to relevant questions in the Survey, almost 60 per cent said they recognised unexpected weeing as a symptom. Other answers showed nearly 38 per cent experienced weeing when laughing, about two-thirds experienced weeing when sneezing; more than half when coughing, and more than a third when physically active. About 6 per cent reported weeing during sex.

I'm constantly on the alert to plan life around toilets. **Trish, 60**

A boss complained to me about how often I went to the toilet. **Kirsty, 44**

I honestly feel ashamed and embarrassed, especially in front of my husband. I just joined online support groups and find it is so common but I still hate it. **Jacinta, 63**

Felt betrayed by my body. Went from being a woman to a person with an undercarriage. Thankfully, a continence nurse was helpful and encouraging. **Julia, 60**

Feels terrible, but I've had 3 kids and put a lot of my pelvic floor issues down to that. **Kellie, 51**

I feel defeated, scared to laugh in public or go out to many places with lots of walking or exciting places, for fear of not making it to the toilet or there not being enough toilets at the event. **Hannah, 52**

I feel embarrassed and middle aged. Also I didn't realise this would happen even if I didn't have children! **Flip, 52**

About 60 per cent also said they experienced sudden urges to wee. About one in five women found weeing symptoms tough or truly terrible.

As for how it makes us feel, the leaky wee or having sudden or more urges to wee, the one word hundreds of women used was embarrassed; hundreds more said annoyed, or frustrated, or old, many others said angry, hopeless, humiliated, worried, vulnerable, anxious, embarrassed, dirty, like an old lady, like I'm losing control of my body, disgusting, vulnerable, insecure, horrified, not sexy, accepting, awful, restricted in wanting to go out of the house, sad, scared, stressed and surprised, cranky, gross, crap happy to wear pads, or not; smelly, unattractive, uncomfortable, and weak.

Thank goodness, I can laugh with the girls about it. **Tully, 58**

Others said it didn't worry them too much, it felt normal, OK, minor and manageable.

Some wee problems are caused by having a weak, misbehaving or ungoverned pelvic floor, some are caused by bladder problems, caused or worsened by your ligaments, tissues and even blood vessels being less usefully plump and strong as your estrogen levels fall. Urogenital specialists and surgeons tend to think bladder problems that can be helped with surgery and medications are overlooked and only the pelvic floor is emphasised; whereas pelvic floor physiotherapists worry that some problems can be fixed by education, exercises, and pessaries, and surgery should be suggested only as a last option.

The constant weeing at night is the worst. **Julie, 64**

Probably the most important thing to do, then, is get a diagnosis for a wee problem, which can be expensive and time consuming. But if you have a problem to do with leaks, or sudden urges, or weeing what seems like all day long, you deserve to have help to fix it, and so you shall.

First we pause to introduce you to your bladder.

Meet the bladder

Oh hi. Your bladder sits up inside you, connected to the outside world by a tube going through your pelvic floor called the urethra, which opens to the outside world between your clitoris and the vagina. (From the front to the back, the order of the useful things nestled in your vulva between your labia goes: clitoris, urethra, vagina; then you leave the vulva, and encounter the perineum, then anus.)

The bladder is a muscle, and you can think of it like a deflated party balloon when it's empty, and a slightly inflated balloon when it's full. When it's full, the bladder sends a message to your brain, and your brain tells you to go to the loo. But if your brain tells you often that you need to go when your bladder isn't actually full, that's an overactive bladder. And if it releases early before you can get to the loo, that's urge incontinence.

While some online info announces that lady-bladders hold say 300 to 400 mL, which is one-and-a-half to two cups of wee, and men are more likely to have a capacity of up to 700 mL, surgeons tell me there isn't much difference, with about a half-litre capacity for both. It's impossible to prove, anyway. Feeling fuller, or going more often, may not so much be reliant on how much liquid is in your bladder, but more by physical problems, or different feelings, sensitivities, and habits.

Ahem, there hasn't been enough research into bladder function in women to really know what's going on as we get older. We mostly know quite a lot about anaesthetised rats and their wee.

We do know that our bladders probably stay about the same size as we get older, but muscles get weaker. The power of the flow can be less strong, and you can have some wee left in your bladder after you go to the loo – so you already have a head start to feeling it's full again. More body weight in general can also squish the bladder a bit so it feels fuller quicker.

Any bladder problem needs a diagnosis: see your GP and get a referral to a urologist if necessary. Medications for bladder problems may become cheaper over the next few years as more generic products become available. See 'More info' sections on the pelvic floor, and specific bladder problems and medical treatments coming up.

The main wee problems

Wee leakage and other problems tend to really kick in during your 40s and 50s. The two main problems are:

* **Stress urinary incontinence: accidental wee leakage.** This sneaky wee is caused by your bladder being squeezed by the stress of coughing, jumping, laughing, lifting or sneezing, and you can't engage your pelvic floor muscle response efficiently to clamp and stop it. And/or the scrunchie-like 'sphincter' that does the actual clamping has become weak. 'Stress incontinence' is not caused by psychological stress – although if your body's response to a boost

Had minor leakage until I worked on pelvic floor exercises and now no problem, yay.
Karin, 62

of anxiety is to want to wee, and your clamp isn't working well, leaks can happen. Some women assumed to have stress incontinence actually have urge incontinence.

* **Urgency urinary incontinence, aka irritable or overactive bladder.** You feel like you really need to go all the time, during the day and night. More than eight times a day or more than once overnight is obviously very inconvenient. Sometimes your brain will trigger your bladder too early, or too often, and you think you need to go, or feel 'busting' when you're not, really. This is called an overactive bladder and leads to doing lots of smaller wees more often.

For some women, a sudden uncontrollable urge can happen with a mental association, such as getting home and putting their key in the door. Urge incontinence can also be associated with anxiety.

Let's get to how wee problems might affect you, and what you can do about it.

I take [medication] about twice a week. Much improved. Ema, 51

Constantly mentally clocking time and distance ratio to the nearest bathroom. Shell, 50

Have tried to reduce my coffee and alcohol intake which is incredibly boring. Kirsten, 53

Haven't done anything due to embarrassment. Jan, 47

Risk factors for wee leaks

It's normal and common to have one or more of these associated risk factors and to have pelvic floor problems, but that doesn't mean they're fine or can be ignored:

* **Being in perimenopause or menopause**
* **You're a woman or non-binary or trans person who was assigned female at birth**, especially in perimenopause or menopause.
* **Being in a higher weight range**: extra pressure from above can weigh down the pelvic floor. It can also push down and squish together organs, putting more pressure on your bladder.

* **One or more full-term or late-term pregnancies**: the extra weight of pregnancy puts strain on the pelvic floor, which can stay weaker afterwards. At least one in three women who've given birth know what it's like to wet themselves.
* **Vaginal birth**: pushing can strain the pelvic floor, and much more rarely, a physically traumatic birth can tear a part of the pelvic floor from its moorings, causing irreparable internal damage that leads to prolapse.
* **Gynaecological surgery or injury**, or radiation to the pelvic area.
* **Lower back pain**.
* **Movement or exercise triggers** including sneezing, laughing, lifting, dancing, jumping, lifting weights or other exercise, or coughing. This is especially hard for people with a chronic cough, hay fever, asthma, and who smoke.

> I had some childbirth-related injuries to my pelvic floor that only just became apparent after 20 years.
> Fiona, 54

* **High impact exercise** in young and older women, including cycling, spin classes, trampolining and running, horseriding and significant weightlifting. This can happen even with accredited classes, and to elite athletes. No exercise should regularly result in a vulva or perineum nerves that feel numb, severely irritated, or like 'pins and needles'. Seek help with positioning, saddle padding and other variants, such as how long you do the activity. Remind any exercise instructor to help you protect your pelvic floor.
* **A history of constipation** or a habit of 'straining' when you poo.
* **Not exercising generally**. Moving around in different ways makes your muscles do useful things and keep working well.
* **Recurrent urinary tract infections (UTIs)**.
* **Some medical conditions** including multiple sclerosis, Parkinson's disease, Ehlers-Danlos syndrome, stroke, spinal injury, diabetes.
* **Being elderly** and having dementia.
* **A weaker pelvic floor**.

All right, back up, what *is* my pelvic floor?

Yes, you do need to know about this, despite the woman who raised her voice during a lunch I went to and said, 'Do I HAVE to do pelvic floor exercises?!' You don't have to do anything, I said. 'But do I HAVE TO?!!' she shouted. 'Can't you make them more INTERESTING?' Lady, I write books, I don't do vajazzling with Christmas lights.

Almost all of the generic skeletons you see in posters on a doctor's wall or online are of a man's skeleton, with narrower pelvises. I have never seen a GP who had a plastic model of a woman's pelvis complete with pelvic floor. And every one of them should.

Imagine – because it's true – that your hipbones cradle a space for a sort of bowl-shape between them. On the back side is your spine, curling in towards your bottom and ending in the coccyx: on the sides, your hipbones wrap round your sides towards the front.

But the bowl-shape itself is holding stuff. It houses our lower body organs, which all sit on a lining on the flat bottom of the bowl. That lining underneath everything is called the pelvic floor. It stretches horizontally across below, like a trampoline, and holds up your bladder, uterus and intestines. Things like the pancreas are higher up, outside the bowl-shape. I don't know what a pancreas is, you'll need another book for that.

What does my pelvic floor actually look like?

We've all got one but hardly any of us have laid eyes on one. Diagrams and pictures online and in anatomy texts range from orange-tinged pictures that look like a 1970s recipe with rampant vertical bananas representing the urethra, vagina or rectum, and indecipherable cross-section diagrams.

When I asked some learned professors to describe it they said things like 'The muscles are attached along the inner walls of the true pelvis to a condensed area of the obturator fascia, known as the tendinous arch of levator ani muscle.' (Sometimes when you speak to doctors it's like they've rocked up in a scuba outfit and you're in a netball uniform.)

Anyway, I grabbed some metaphorical lapels and best I can do is: it's a trampoliney sort of flat, red steak in a rough oval shape, about 1 cm thick, with lines of white tissue streaked through it. I asked if the tissue is muscle and no and . . . (loses consciousness).

If you could crane your head forward, and then look down with X-ray vision, this sketch below is kind of what you'd see of the pelvic floor. It's very roughly a sideways oval within your pelvis. It's anchored all around: attached to the pubic bone inside you at the front, and at your coccyx or tailbone at the back, and also attached around the curved sides.

One of the kind urologists consulted for the book is concerned that I haven't indicated that the urethral meatus is within the vaginal hiatus (wut) so fair warning: this is not a perfectly accurate medical diagram! It's just a very general way for you to picture your own anatomy.

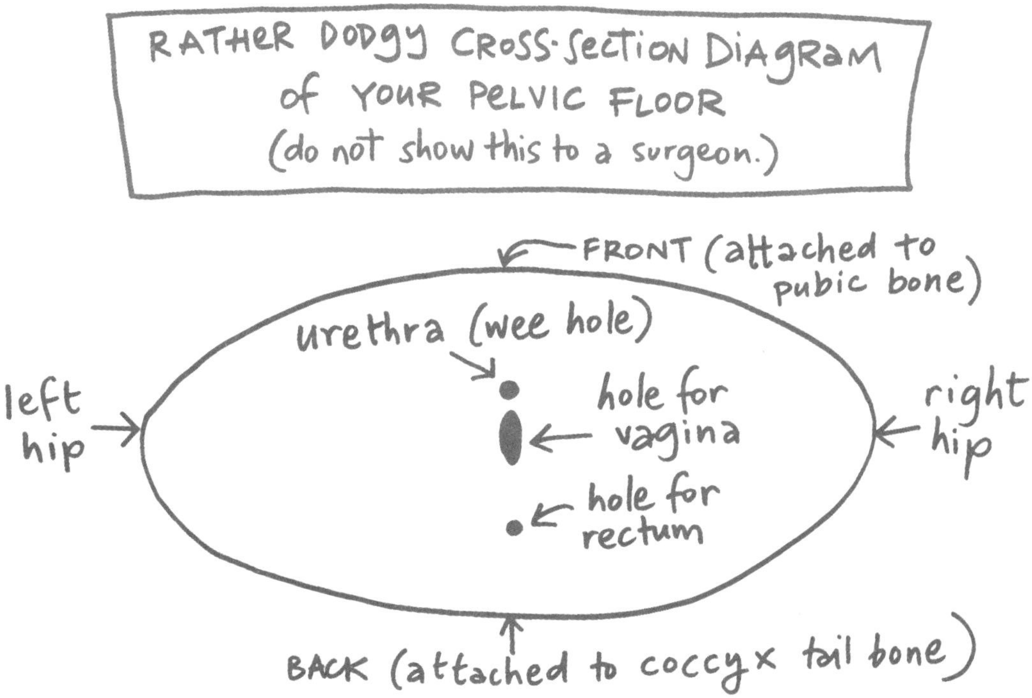

The pelvic floor isn't one flat oval muscle, it's a network of different ones, all connected as part of the 'floor', tethering it and allowing separate bits to work independently. It has three main holes in it, where tubes have to go through. The tubes are organs that lead to the outside, down between your legs: from the bladder to the outside through the tube called the urethra; the tube from the cervix at the bottom of your uterus to the vaginal entrance called (hurrah) the vagina, and the tube from your intestines down to your anus, called the rectum.

Each one of these tubes has a kind of muscly scrunchie around it, so that when you squeeze your pelvic floor muscles, the scrunchie-sphincters also squeeze around the tubes. By doing this, you can cut off or control the flow of wee from your bladder, squeeze your vaginal walls together and let them go again, and control the urge to poo.

If you imagine a side-view of the pelvic floor, think of it like a horizontal mini-trampoline inside, with three tubes in a row from front to back, poking through it vertically, like drinking straws, or skinny chimneys, extending above your pelvic floor, and also below. At the point they all go through the trampoline, they go through a hole surrounded by a muscular scrunchie. Each of the tubes connects to an organ above, travels through its own hole in your pelvic floor and ends at an opening on the outside of your body. The largest one is the vagina, and the smallest one is the urethra.

What does the pelvic floor do?

If your pelvic floor muscles are weak or there is too much downward pressure due to weight from above, it sags more like a hammock instead of being a taut trampoline, and the scrunchies get weak and don't snap back to squeeze as well. For many women, it's the weeing control that they have the first, or the most difficulty with. The worst case scenario for many of us can be incontinence, ranging from sneaky wee if you sneeze, cough, laugh or jump, to no control at all.

So one of the main jobs for the pelvic floor is to control continence and allow you to squeeze anything tight inside your vagina (fingers, vibrators, a stray penis). The other main job is to help keep various ligaments and gently packed organs in place, and keep your bladder and uterus from 'prolapsing'.

Gravity, lack of muscle tone, some medical conditions, pressure from extra body weight above and ligaments weakened by lack of estrogen can combine to push down or allow the sinking of an organ to where it's not supposed to be, which is called a prolapse. (See the 'Prolapses' section, coming up after the wee section.)

How to find your pelvic floor

Sit on your hands in a way that you can feel your lower pelvic bones. Squeeze your vagina, or squeeze as if you want to stop weeing. Or cough, or sing. Can you feel a movement like a contraction? Your pelvic floor just kicked in and contracted.

Strengthening your pelvic floor

Our pelvic floor is literally our bottom line: it's crucial. We need to maintain as much control as we can get over our pelvic floor as we get older so we can guard against sneezy wee or otherwise unexpected pants-wetting. The good news is that for most women this all that's needed, totally doable, and free, using exercises.

Contrary to lot of info received online and from friends or relatives, it's not just about practising the squeezing and tightening of your pelvic floor muscles. It's about being able to relax *or* tighten: it's about controlling them. Many of us have pelvic floor muscles that are too often tightened when not needed, or kind of 'stuck' halfway tightened, or for various reasons including over-exercise of the pelvic floor muscles, the pelvic floor can become 'dysfunctional', which adds to wee problems going to the loo, or having penetrative sex.

What are 'Kegels'?

Once upon a time, yet another male doctor named a female body part or gynaecological procedure or implement after himself; in this case Arnold Kegel, who developed the idea of pelvic floor exercises in the late 1940s. So US resources usually refer to 'Kegels' as the exercises, and even the muscles themselves as 'Kegels', and this is now a common global word. Had women been able to go to medical school centuries earlier, as the men did, we would probably have worked out about exercising the pelvic floor in approximately 900 BC. So that's enough of Dr bloody Kegel.

How to combat sneaky wee: pelvic floor exercises

In the absence of a separate medical bladder problem, the best defence against sneaky weeing is pelvic floor exercises. Most of us know the feeling of squeezing our pelvic floor muscles to try not to wee if we're busting for the loo, and many perimenopausal women know it also helps to brace yourself if you cough, to try to avoid an anticipated wee leak.

> The best thing about fellow menopause workmates is we would sit and do them at work, then laugh uncontrollably and wee a little in our pants.
> Blondie, 64

But just tightening up now and then is not enough. It's not about how violently you can squeeze, and doing too many can be a problem, too. Pelvic floor exercises are not just about raising one eyebrow, smiling enigmatically, and tightening your vagina on the bus. Some can be done lying down, some standing or sitting.

First, you will need a diagnosis of your problem, and you may need to start by learning breathing and other techniques to fully relax the pelvic floor and sphincter-scrunchies. And then learn how to control, and tighten them, and relax them again.

If you're like most ladyfolk, you won't find doing the exercises difficult, but it can be hard to remember to do them, or be disciplined about doing them every day. A lot of people do them as part of yoga, or another exercises routine. You may have tried ones you read about online, but found they haven't worked, and given up. A lot of women start to wear continence pads as backup for unexpected leaks.

Frankly, most of us don't seek out professional help on how to do them unless we've developed a problem and have a greater incentive. You may need to learn individual techniques while a pelvic floor specialist checks what it's actually doing to your pelvic floor. One doctor told me that about a third of their new patients have been doing pelvic floor exercises correctly for them, about a third have been doing them in a way that doesn't help, and about a third have been accidentally doing ones that make their problem worse.

Always get info on how to do pelvic floor exercises from one of the independent health organisations in 'More info on pelvic floor exercises,' coming up soon in this chapter. If you have leak problems, see your GP, a gynaecologist, a urologist and/or a physio with a pelvic floor specialty who can set you on the right path.

A 63-year-old woman who answered the Survey for this book said she puts a Valium up her vagina to relax her pelvic floor. *This is not a DIY situation.* A specific, related kind of relaxant can be prescribed as a pessary by a doctor for pelvic floor spasm, pelvic pain and other conditions.

I didn't know I could do anything [about this]. **Siobhan, 55**

Pelvic floor exercises helped . . . I have improved strength but the problem has become a sudden unexpected urge to wee. **Fiona, 56**

Drink less coffee, trying hard to practices continence strategies, including those for anxious bladder. Never knew this had anything to do with menopause! **Ali, 49**

I am a teacher and leaving class [to wee] is a challenge. **Nic, 49**

A pelvic floor assessment by a physio

Your specialist physio should have recognised tertiary qualifications in physiotherapy, plus extra qualifications in the pelvic floor specialty. You can't just go to any physio who usually sees knee injuries.

After some discussion of your problems or needs, your specialist physio will need to insert one or two of their fingers, or a narrow probe, into your vagina, to do some checks. They'll feel how hard, and where, you can squeeze while their fingers are still inside and they'll check there's no prolapsing carry-on from any other organ.

It's intimate, and a bit odd to be chatting away while that's all going on, but the physio should be very professional, matter-of-fact, and kind. They should ask for your consent and explain what will happen before examining you. Do tell your physio if you still deal with trauma from an assault, or anything else that will help them make the situation the best they can for you.

Your physio will get you to practise the exercises (relaxing and tightening) so they can feel if it's doing useful things to your pelvic floor, and give you some instructions on how to practise them from now on. If you've been annoyed by leaking, you might be asked to keep a wee or incontinence diary for a few days or a week, to record frequency (how often you wee) and volume (how much liquid you drink, and how much you wee). You can take home a plastic, eventually disposable, mini-potty with measurements on it, which sits inside your normal toilet seat – you wee into that and record the amount. The glamour never ends.

Saw a pelvic floor physio, diagnosed a bladder prolapse, probably from giving birth, and just started using a pessary. Changed my life, brilliant. No one ever talks about this. Emma, 46

Consulted a women's health physio who recommended pelvic floor exercises, which worked very quickly to improve my symptoms. Billie, 51

My pelvic floor physio told me my pelvic floor was too tight so I needed the opposite of what people assume. Neeta, 60

My pelvic floor muscles go into spasm on arousal – extremely painful so I avoid sex. Jo, 60

Always carry spare knickers. **Sally, 54**

What else helps to stop sneaky wee?

All of the following suggestions can be combined with a pelvic floor squeezy exercises program for strengthening pelvic floor muscles that's approved by a specialist physio. Don't take any herbal or other treatment for a bladder problem without a diagnosis and approval from a doctor or specialist physio, and telling them what you're taking.

Tens of thousands of Australian women wear incontinence pads or liners and absorbent undies, which manage, but don't stop, unexpected weeing.

See the list of 'Risk factors for wee leaks' earlier in this section, and avoid the ones you can. And:

* If you are carrying extra, unwanted weight, try to lose some. (Not with short-term dieting; see the 'Eating & weight' section in Chapter 3.) More weight from above the bladder and the pelvic floor can makes things more difficult.
* A prescribed estrogen cream or pessary gently delivered to the top of the vagina using a little plastic plunger-applicator can help. This is considered safe for women with a breast cancer history because it's localised to the vaginal area but, as always, check with your doctor. A couple of plunge-ups a week might be enough, not only to combat vaginal dryness, but also to strengthen bits nearby which hold up and help the pelvic floor and bladder behave themselves.
* Estrogen is known to strengthen connecting and supporting ligaments and tissue which have estrogen receptors, near the bladder. It can help the bladder behave itself and is protective against UTIs. (Do bits of estrogen just dance through the vaginal wall and throw themselves onto the pelvic floor ligaments? This is why I am not a qualified doctor, isn't it?)

I use estrogen cream to the vulva. **Sam, 53**
(Sam, check with your doctor: that cream should almost certainly go inside your vagina next to the cervix.)

Cross my legs and pray. **Tina, 53**

I found regular weight sessions at the gym and doing pelvic floor exercises really helped. Eventually I could crack walnuts. **Keryn, 55**

After many years my GP finally prescribed vaginal estrogen, which worked like magic. **Jo, 48**

I use an in-vagina exercise tool. **Eunice, 53**

I wear period underwear and incontinence pads. **Dana**

I did a pelvic strengthening course with an exercise physiologist and it made a world of difference. Toots, 56

My co-workers are used to me yelling out, 'I'm going to wet my pants!' as a lot of my job involves heavy lifting. Hilary, 50

Medication and panty liners. And Pilates. Judy, 59

Do you know, it hasn't actually occurred to me to do anything. Kim, 48

Fitted for an estrogen (vaginal pessary) ring. About 95 per cent successful. Jane, 47

* Get all recommended vaccinations every year because the less you sneeze and cough the better; use hand sanitiser and keep up with any asthma management plan.
* Lower back pain can trigger pelvic floor problems, so get help for that.
* Wee before an exercise session, but try not to do lots of 'just in case' wees when you don't feel you need to go because it can 'train' your bladder to want to empty way before it's full each time.
* Some gynaecologists and physios suggest you use a tampon in the lower half of the vagina while exercising, which can help support the bladder.
* Ask any instructor or gym whether suggested exercises are 'pelvic floor friendly' and assess whether this info seems reliable.
* High-impact exercises can make wee leeks worse for some women. A change of routines or pelvic floor exercises might help.
* During danger periods (hay-fever days, exercise classes) wear an incontinence pad. Place them on your knickers a little further forward than you would put a period pad.
* Eat fruit and veggies every day, and drink enough water, which helps avoid constipation.
* Spread drinks across the day, about 1.5–2 litres in total. Don't avoid drinking water to dehydrate yourself, this will make it worse.
* Try to do at least half an hour of exercise a day (I know, it's easy to say).

I wear black when exercising. Jessica, 41

A herbal product is legally sold under the name of Urox, and included in the 'Happy Bladder' pills brand. This use is approved by the Therapeutic Goods Association only if you've been given a medical diagnosis of an overactive bladder, with the added advice to go back to a doctor if symptoms continue.

Urox is allowed to be marketed as 'maintaining or supporting healthy bladder function'. Sellers of the herbal formulation say it supports the collagen and tissues in the bladder area and helps bladder muscle messaging and control. A research study connected to the manufacturer with men and women participants concluded it reduced overactive bladder and incontinence symptoms. Medical doctors differ on whether it's useful for overactive bladder.

What *doesn't* help stop sneaky weeing

The marketers are coming for you and your pelvic floor. It's a billion-dollar business. Embarrassed women buy stuff online and advertisers target key search words to get their results up high in the list. All sorts of herbal and other treatments are being sold with claims to help the pelvic floor or wee problems and without any evidence.

Beware of:

* Kegel or pelvic floor exercise apps and weights, 'trainers', pessaries, balls or similar in-vagina devices and doodads – without the supervision or a diagnosis from a qualified specialist pelvic floor physiotherapist. These trainers, timers and alert systems can make a problem worse and cause pain.
* Online-bought or sight-unseen pessaries, spacers or silicone 3-D shapes that stay at the top of your vagina for weeks or months, without diagnosis and professional advice from a medical or physio specialist.
* Paying for vibrating or 'pulsing' or magnetic field chairs or devices purporting to exercise your pelvic floor while you sit. Research on this is mixed but ultimately there's no proof they work. Also, we do know that paying for various vibrations and pulses isn't better

The more weight I gained, the worse it got. Pixie, 60

Avoid trampolines! Gina, 58

Avoid drinking water if I have to go somewhere. Kathy, 51

What do I do about it? Laugh and wee more! Jo, 66

Avoid the star jumps. Annie, 57

Once it was tampons, now it's panty liners. Stashed into every handbag, glovebox and backpack. Alex, 53

than doing your own pelvic floor exercises for free. These 'electro-magnetic treatments' providers say they won't do them on anyone with a history of endometriosis or with an IUD, possibly because these services haven't been tested on people with them or because they're known to increase pain triggers.

* Almost all herbal or vitamin supplements, collagen and similar supplements. They don't specifically target or help the pelvic floor.

MORE INFO on pelvic floor exercises

Ask your GP, gynaecologist, urologist or local physiotherapy clinic to recommend a good continence or pelvic floor specialist nurse or physio. They will almost certainly be women. You won't need a referral, you can just make an appointment yourself.

pelvicfloorfirst.org.au
Helpline: 1800 330 066
Specialist nurses funded by the Australian Department of Health through the non-profit Continence Foundation of Australia. Choose 'Exercises for women' for advice and explanations, then 'Resources and videos', for more. There are diaries and questionnaires to help you assess your need for help.

yourpelvicfloor.org
This International Urogynaecological Association site has fact sheets on incontinence issues, prolapse and surgery procedures. Ignore 'Find a provider' and choose 'Resources' for downloads.

continence.org.au
The Continence Foundation of Australia. Choose 'Get Help' for lists of professional specialists closest to you.

jeanhailes.org.au
Search 'pelvic floor exercises' for some specific instructions.

mayoclinic.org
On the homepage of this US medical site, search 'Bladder control' for an article on self-help, including 'bladder training' and irritating drinks and food to avoid, and search 'Kegel exercises' for instructions.

Overactive bladder

Some things are known to contribute to the problem, including UTIs and caffeinated drinks. It's more common in menopause, the older you get, or if you have some medical conditions including diabetes, a history of stroke, vaginal prolapse, or multiple sclerosis, or if you are carrying a lot of extra, unnecessary weight. See your GP or a urologist for a proper diagnosis of overactive bladder. There are many useful medications, 'bladder training' techniques and procedures.

Medical treatments for bladder problems

For urge urinary incontinence (feeling like you need to go and not being able to control it), first treatments usually include medications that calm the bladder, weeing behaviour instructions, a recommendation for individual pelvic floor exercises or nerve paralysing and muscle relaxing injections.

For stress incontinence (the coughing, laughing or jumping kind), some doctors recommend injecting a bulking substance directly into the urethra which can help it grow stronger: this very often requires a second injection for a full, more lasting effect.

In real problem cases of stress urinary incontinence, when other solutions haven't worked, surgery to help strengthen the ligaments is recommended. This is by means of using a 'sling' under your urethra made of medical mesh tape, or a graft of your own tissue, to help hoist up and support the bladder. Sometimes an alternative, no-mesh, stitching technique is used. The operations are performed under general anaesthetic, usually with a couple of nights in hospital and about 6 weeks gentle recovery at home.

You may want a second specialist opinion or try other ideas before agreeing to any medical or surgical procedures, which can of course be prohibitively expensive.

I change undies 2–3 times a day. Putting off going to doctor about it. It's not THAT bad. Nina, 55

I am too embarrassed to speak to the doctor about this. Janine, 57

I got a treatment recommended by my doctor called MonaLisa Touch, which was meant to . . . increase elasticity of the bladder. Expensive and uncomfortable procedure that did sweet FA! Jane, 57

(Quite right, Jane. See Chapter 6, It's Your Sex Life, for more on this nonsense.)

You need a very experienced surgical specialist who can satisfactorily explain the risks of complications and side effects as well as the possible benefits, including known rates of ongoing pain during sex. You may be concerned about the use of mesh, having heard of ghastly complications from vaginal sling mesh surgery. There's more on that in the 'Prolapses' section, coming up. Not all surgery involving mesh is the same. This is another reason to make sure you have an experienced surgeon who can explain everything you need to know before you decide whether you want mesh surgery.

Do not get 'vaginal laser surgery' or a 'vaginal rejuvenation' laser procedure. There is no evidence it will help a bladder problem or anything else, and it's ludicrously expensive. Please see my rant against it in Chapter 6, It's Your Sex Life.

> I see a urogynaecologist to figure out if/when surgery will be most effective. Betsy, 63

> Went to gynaecologist and saw a women's health physio. Had a pessary inserted for prolapse. Tried all-natural, less invasive solutions, but after 18 months ended up having prolapse surgery. Naomi, 46

MORE INFO on bladder problems

Here's where to get trusted info for an unlucky dip of bladder problems.

yourpelvicfloor.org
Search for 'Patient Information Leaflets' for useful, updated International Urogynaecological Association fact sheets on many conditions, medications and surgery related to continence, prolapse, cystitis, UTIs, overactive bladder, the pelvic floor, birth injury repairs, and urethral carbuncles. (Lordy.)

continence.org.au
Find fact sheets and advice or check out financial aid for buying pads.

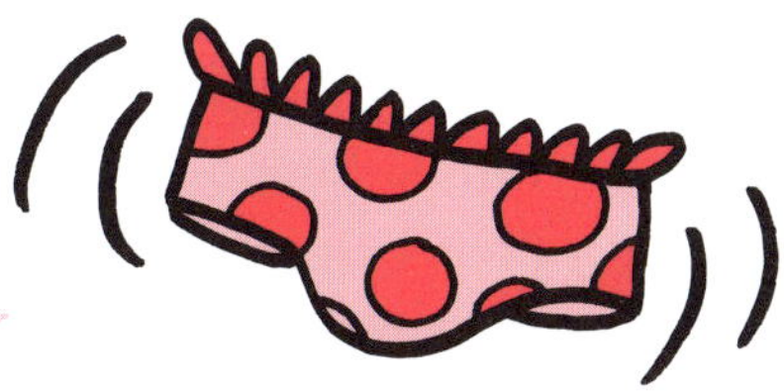

Urinary tract infections (UTIs)

As they get older, some women develop a tendency for recurrent UTIs. In later age, sometimes the only outward symptom can be confusion and delirium. It's important to get a doctor to diagnose the UTI. Most properly diagnosed UTIs are quickly righted by a course of antibiotics. We're more susceptible than men because germs don't have as far to go up a female urethra to cause problems in the bladder. Guard against UTIs by weeing often and regularly. Repeated studies show that no useful cranberry juice ingredients are delivered to the bladder so it's no more useful than water. Also, never ignore blood in your wee, make an appointment with your GP.

Actually went to my doctor, had a urine test, diagnosed with a UTI. A small course of antibiotics helped.
Debbie, 62

How to go to the toilet

I know, you've been doing it for decades. But these hints will help. For a start, have a mind-boggle at this: the height and placement of home and public toilets, made for an average, taller man, are designed against the health and comfort needs of women, as well as children. So:

* When weeing, tilt the top half of your body forward – you can put your elbows on your knees and even give a little wiggle. This empties your bladder more fully, which means it doesn't fill up as fast. Utilise any 'while-weeing' exercises a physio give you.
* Use a 'squatty potty', otherwise known as a 'poo stool'. Not a potty at all, just a small plastic stool about, say, 15–20 cm tall to put both feet up on when you poo: it puts your body in the best position for doing it without straining, which can weaken the pelvic floor. I suggest you call your squatty potty something more dignified, like Sir Algernon Dalrymple.

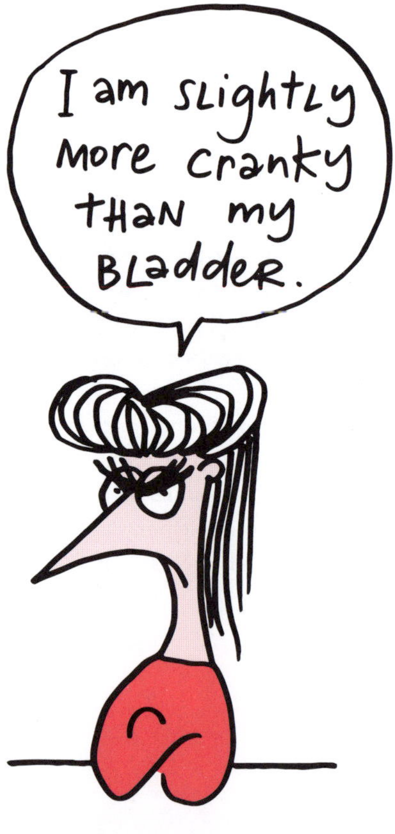

How much water to drink a day

Be guided by how thirsty you are, how hot it is, and how much sweating you've been doing, not a googled website article or a social media 'nutritionist'. You don't need a magic number of litres to aim for.

Which food & drinks irritate or help your bladder

Websites and social media stories endlessly tell you to give up caffeine, alcohol and the bubbles in fizzy drinks and spicy foods because they can irritate the bladder and cause urge or stress incontinence. But some people eat curries every day for their whole life, and most urologists wouldn't even mention fizzy drinks to you unless they know you drink 6 litres of Passiona a day.

Nobody seems to know exactly why they make your individual bladder cranky but coffee, tea, caffeine drinks and alcohol drinks can make you feel fuller, which create a more urgent need to empty, and the need to go extra times in the night. They're diuretics, which just means they make you wee more than the same amount of water would.

Carbonated or fizzy drinks are often mentioned but there doesn't seem to be much research on why: once through the stomach and in the bladder, they might tickle nerves or otherwise be a trigger. Caffeine is considered the major villain, especially in coffee but also tea, colas and energy drinks. Nobody seems to know why citrus or soy is in these lists.

In extreme cases of alcohol-related bladder palaver, being very drunk or 'pissed' (hence the term) can cause you to miss the signals that you need to wee, which then happens involuntarily as your bladder is full of the high-volume amounts of fluid.

The upshot is: beware of generalised advice and info in articles about wee problems online. The best way to find out what irritates your bladder or might be associated is to do some experiments to identify your own trigger foods or drinks.

Prolapses

It's really common for older women to have some sort of organ prolapse. Your pelvic floor is helping to hold up your bladder, uterus (womb) and parts of the rectum (bowel) and vagina. With a weaker pelvic floor and supporting ligaments and blood vessels that are depleted by less estrogen in peri- and menopause, all these organs can drop or droop from their position and press on the walls of the vagina from outside it, causing a bulge inside the vagina. That's called a vaginal prolapse.

The bladder can protrude into the front of the vaginal wall, the rectum can bulge into the back, and the uterus can drop downwards into the vagina. These all have their own technical prolapse names.

In centuries past, a uterus coming down was called a 'falling womb'. Some women who've had their uterus removed find that the top of the vagina itself begins to fold down within itself.

The organs can't fall out of your body but they can slowly collapse out of place. Some prolapses never cause symptoms, others interfere with easy weeing and pooing. Sometimes, they are easily felt and symptoms include a heavy or dragging feeling in the vagina, a feeling of a bulge or lump in the vagina, weeing problems, bowel problems, and/or a weird feeling during penetrative sex.

A prolapse can cause a lump you can feel in the top of the vagina, which presses towards the urethra or the other way towards the bowel, making it harder for wee and poo to travel past the lump and out of your body easily. Estrogen tends to keep ligaments and other tethering factors strong, so less estrogen (menopause) can mean a higher risk of prolapse.

In the olden days (say, 100 years ago and before) to hold back a prolapse, women wore strange leather belts with long strings that joined to rubber tubes attached to the bottom of a rubber funnel, which was placed up inside the vagina. Others are still advised of a desperate, Middle Ages-y 'home remedy' – putting a potato or pomegranate as high as it will go into the vagina. Social media posts have reported (or propagated an urban myth) that some women have sprouted potato vines and leaves up there. (Regardless of gardening prospects, don't.)

> I'd had a prolapse since my first pregnancy but thought it was normal because nobody ever talks about it. Yvette, 46

Risk factors for prolapses

* gravity
* getting older
* full-term pregnancy
* traumatic vaginal birth
* history of giving birth to a big baby
* menopause
* being above a healthy weight range
* hysterectomy
* heavy lifting, coughing, sneezing, very vigorous exercise; anything that puts pressure on the pelvic floor
* constipation.

I saw a pelvic physio who was fantastic. Still doing daily pelvic floor exercises to help with this issue and it's improved heaps. Truly wonderful woman I felt safe with and who could accurately diagnose an anterior prolapse and, luckily for me, improve it significantly. Helen, 48

Lots of us are embarrassed to talk about incontinence or unexplained bulgy bits but please talk to your doctor about any symptoms or difficulties, as they can get worse. It's routine and common for a good GP, gynaecologist or urologist to diagnose a prolapse, probably through a discussion of symptoms, an ultrasound, use of ye olde speculum to gently lever open your vaginal entrance a little bit, a peering up there by a doctor, and/or a hand or narrow probe being put up the vagina.

Treatment for prolapses

Treatment can include strengthening the pelvic floor using prescribed exercises, avoiding bladder irritants, fitting a ring that sits at the top of the vagina, at the cervix, to hold things up (you can't feel it when it's in place), losing some extra weight, using estrogen pessaries or cream which are deposited at the top of the vagina to help strengthen ligaments and the pelvic floor in the general area, and surgery. (Estrogen cream in the vagina is usually fine for women who've had breast or endometrial cancer, but check with your doctor.)

Pessaries that stay in the vagina and 'hold up' the cervix can also be used – no more the DIY potatoes and pomegranates of the past – which include rings, usually made of silicone, which can be left in place for a day, a week or months. They can be taken out by you, or a doctor or specialist pelvic floor physio who can teach you how to DIY clean and reinsert, and either must be taken out during penetrative sex or are okay left in place, depending on the type: work out with your specialist which one you need.

Different shapes and sizes make a big difference to the management of various kinds of prolapse. Don't buy vaginal pessaries online.

Routine vaginal repair surgery can be recommended, using stitches on the front or back wall of the vagina to help it better support itself. Many women were advised in the past to have surgery to implant a medical-grade mesh, to strengthen vaginal walls against a prolapse, or the hold of the pelvic floor around the urethra tube. Complications from this surgery, often after months or years, are estimated by some to affect 1–2 women in 100 for the urinary operation and 10 in 100 women for vaginal prolapse. In many of those cases, the effects were catastrophic trauma, pain and complications.

US and Australian health authorities have effectively banned the use of this surgical mesh for prolapse repair and billions of dollars has been paid in compensation worldwide. Women with mesh inside them that isn't causing problems should not do anything.

Meanwhile, many specialist Australian surgeons still use surgical mesh under urethras for some stress incontinence problems, saying it's safe, and that they would happily have this themselves. They also believe that it can be safe for vaginal prolapse itself, but used in the abdomen, not in the vagina.

Women who require urinary-related surgery need to know that their doctor is fully trained, very experienced, and a specialist. They will need to inform themselves fully of possible risks and benefits.

MORE INFO on prolapses & transvaginal mesh

jeanhailes.org.au
Search 'prolapse and incontinence' on this independent, holistic and medical women's health site.

Continence Foundation of Australia
The nationwide number 1800 33 00 66 will connect you with a specialist nurse advisor.

safetyandquality.gov.au
The Australian Commission on Safety and Quality in Health Care has several fact sheets on mesh complications and removal. Search 'transvaginal mesh' on its main page.

Surgery

> I got prolapse surgery (pelvic mesh omg!). It worked for a while and then my incontinence started again when I gained weight. Now that I've lost the weight and I'm a bit fitter, I seem to have reasonable control.
> Rachel, 50

Many women are more likely to need gynaecological surgery after the age of 40 or 50. Be proactive in asking for help and information. As public hospital waiting lists for important surgeries can be long, ask what you can do to help yourself while you're waiting.

Most surgeons see you on the operating table and then maybe 6 weeks later, in some cases not even that. Very few of them have any idea what it's like for women day-to-day, recovering. They routinely describe likely pain as 'discomfort', and underestimate when you will 'feel yourself again' or be able to walk, and for how long without feeling terrible afterwards.

> I had a repair about 10 years ago. Changed my life.
> Jo, 46

Some surgeons are even flick-passing post-operative care for gynaecological operations, telling patients to get their abdominal wound stitches removed by a local GP or practice nurse. I would get another surgeon if one told me this.

The Australian Commission on Safety and Quality in Health Care reported on hysterectomies several years ago at the time of writing. It noted that the rate of hysterectomies per patients is much higher in regional areas. As that should not be the case, getting a second opinion might be a sensible idea. Hysterectomy rates have fallen over the last decades as some more popular treatments for conditions like heavy bleeding are better known by doctors, and a more conservative approach is generally taken for non-cancerous conditions.

Hints for when you need surgery

* Think about getting a second opinion.
* Find a specialist in the exact operation or problem you're having.
* Ask surgeons for sources of reliable information online about the kind of operation you've been advised to have.
* Ask your surgeon how many of these operations they've done before, and what the known risks and benefits are.
* Raise any worries.

* Ask the surgeon to tell you what sorts of scars to expect, if any.
* If you are in hospital after an operation and they want to discharge you but you don't feel strong enough to go home, and don't have someone to look after you there, say you will stay another night. If they say you're cleared to go home, ask by whom and to see them. Put it on record that you want to stay another night. Better to stay longer in hospital than to go home wobbly. (Don't tell them I said this.)

Hysterectomy

This isn't a book on hysterectomies; a small but very significant percentage of women need one – many thousands every year in Australia. But here's a few things to know. Your recovery time may well be longer than the surgeon tells you: post-op fact sheets are notorious for underestimating effects.

You should always question if, and why, a surgeon plans to remove your ovaries, especially if you are under 50 years old. The more safe, body-made estrogen production you can carry on with, the better.

Hysterectomy patients who also have an oophorectomy (removal of ovaries) may not be warned about sudden menopausal symptoms to expect once their ovaries are gone, or what medication they should start taking to help protect their bones and heart. Ask about this.

Other post-hysterectomy and oophorectomy possible side effects are often not raised with you by doctors, including changes to your sex life, and the positions that were previously easiest for you to orgasm.

One 54-year-old woman wrote in the Survey that she'd had a hysterectomy 20 years ago and was waiting to experience menopause symptoms. It's likely that operation took her ovaries as well, and that she has already been in menopause for 20 years

I had a hysterectomy at the age of 38 and he took out everything except my ovaries. I hit menopause at the age of 48 and at 51 it is slowing down. Denise, 51

After seeing the doctor and psychologist, I was able to identify that I was going through grief and loss of a hysterectomy. I don't have children, and I had chosen not to have children, yet my body and mind were grieving the loss of my womb. Really odd to go through! Tanya, 55

and wasn't offered medication to protect her bones and heart. I hope she goes to a specialist to get more information now.

Not least because I know many people end up needing to have a hysterectomy and how many find it distressing. I have no patience for arguments about whether having a uterus makes you a 'real woman', or any other such palaver, good DAY to you.

After the hysterectomy I suffered memory problems. I didn't know this was a side effect. Nancy, 52

I had a complete hysterectomy at 61 because of fibroids. Up until then I still menstruated!! Sue, 66

After recovering from my hysterectomy, the first thing I did was splash out on new white bedding. I love it. I don't miss that constant anxiety or having to sit on towels, lest I flood. Jo, 47

MORE INFO on hysterectomies

healthdirect.gov.au
Search for a fact sheet on this federal government health department site using 'hysterectomy', which then links to various different types of surgery.

jeanhailes.org.au
Search 'hysterectomy' on this dedicated women's health site.

Drier & itchy skin

The other night out at dinner with friends, all women over 50, my friend Annie took a mini-tube of moisturiser out of her bag, rubbed it all over her hands and squished it between her fingers, and without a word of explanation passed it to the next friend. It silently did the rounds and then it was popped back in her bag. We're thirsty ladies.

This section covers the almost universal problems of dry, itchy and irritated skin all over, including the vulva and vagina, and then we shall leap gingerly onto

> When I next saw the GP and asked her AGAIN, she admitted that after our first conversation she checked and found out it was a symptom. No solution offered except over-the-counter hay fever medication. Sue, 51

what menopause does to nails. For dry vagina chat that specifically relates to your sex life, see Chapter 6, It's Your Sex Life. For wrinkles, age spots, grey hair, hair loss, body hair, and other appearance-related palaver related to skin, see Chapter 7, It's How You Look.

A few things conspire to make your skin drier: less estrogen makes your skin thinner and less plump, and therefore more prone to irritation and rashes, and more vulnerable to the effects of low humidity, including air-conditioned and heated environments, dry, cold weather and low-humidity hot weather. And ageing means your body doesn't make as much of two useful proteins any more: the plumping agent collagen and stretchy elastin.

About four in five women reported to the Survey for this book that they noticed drier skin in perimenopause. About half said it varied from sometimes annoying to terrible. A whopping two-thirds of respondents who answered the relevant question said they had itchy skin as a symptom.

You can try to treat dry skin from the 'inside' with prescribed estrogen supplements, but doctors disagree on whether this helps and there's plenty of anecdotal evidence from women taking MHT who say it seems to do nothing for their dry skin or itches. There are no estrogen receptors on outer skin for estrogen cream to be able to glom onto and do anything useful. So what *can* you do?

> I use [a non-drowsy antihistamine] for the itching, particularly at night to allow me to get off to sleep – a bit easier to ignore. Tania, 59

> 'Dry eye' is one symptom of menopause that is not well known. A doctor kept diagnosing conjunctivitis. Now I put in drops 3–7 times a day. Kerri-Ann, 61

> Skin stopped itching when I started using soap-free body lotion. Dee, 51

> [Put a] cold washer on itchy crawling skin. Tracey, 59

What helps dry skin

You need to do two main things: protect and nourish your skin, and stop annoying it. So:

* Use a non-irritating face and body moisturiser for dry skin from a pharmacy: it's a more rich, dense-feeling cream which is harder to rub off and is better at preventing the evaporative effects of heat and dry air.
* Choose a moisturiser with a minimum of ingredients that you can afford that feels nice and nourishing, and tends to stay put for a while. This creates a temporary barrier on the skin but won't change the skin itself. Paraffin, shea butter, glycerol or hyaluronic acid all bind and trap water.
* Have short, lukewarm (not hot) showers, pat dry and use a pump-pack of body moisturiser that's easy and habit-forming to use after each shower. If you don't buy in a pump-pack, you can decant into one.
* Look for dry-skin specialist brands for non-perfumed, non-soap cleansing bars and body washes.
* Feel free to peel the label off the better, cheaper cleansers and moisturisers and write a fancy brand-name on it with a Sharpie.
* Be aware that no cream is getting lower than the outer layer of your skin.
* If you use perfume, pay attention to where it goes and whether your skin in showing signs of irritation. Necks are particularly vulnerable to later-life perfume annoyance.
* Don't let dry skin go unattended, as it can lead to dermatitis, which leads to cracked skin, which can end up with infections.
* The only dermatologists I've ever heard who disagree with the above points tend to be selling their own, or someone else's, brand-name product.

What doesn't help dry skin

These things:

* More expensive moisturisers are not necessarily better, and in some blind tests cheaper barrier creams perform better. Because of perfumes and extra ingredients, they can be major irritants.

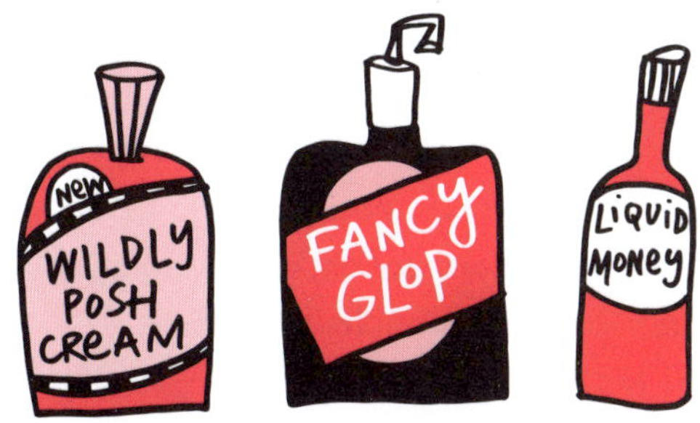

'Make your own labels...'

* Supplements and moisturisers or creams including collagen and other oils may be no better, or be worse than standard moisturisers. Body-made collagen and oils help keep the skin more elastic, but there's nothing (except advertising and hope) to say that taking supplements in a pill, or slathering them on with a cream, gets to your skin in a way that changes it in the slightest. There's more in Chapter 7, It's How You Look, about why claimed collagen or elastin in creams can't get into your skin and change it.
* Supplements of vitamins, seaweed, 'superfoods', miracle botanical ingredients and so on. The advertising implication that they 'support' clearer or 'better' skin means nothing.
* Yes, vitamins and minerals are essential for healthy skin. That doesn't mean vitamins and minerals in a cream or supplement will make your skin any better.

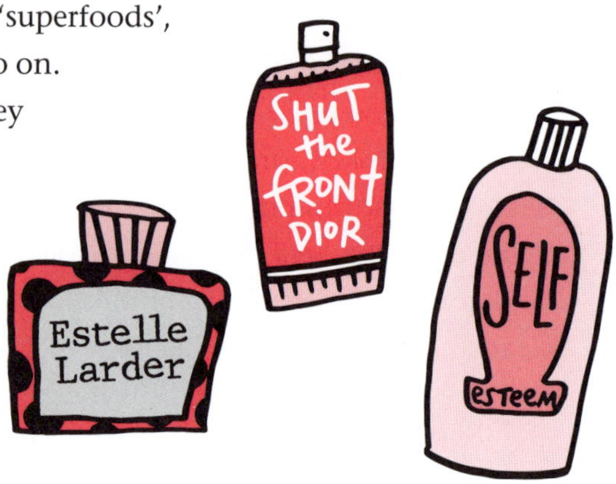

Of course, the go-to list of birthday presents for older women gets smaller when we take off perfumed body washes and moisturisers. We're now down to books, candles, and, um . . . dessert.

Go easy on the exfoliants

Exfoliants scrub and scratch away at the top layer of skin, causing surface damage that then encourages new, softer-looking skin to grow and re-cover the area. If you overdo it – more than once a week, or with too much vigour, or use a product with unforgiving materials such as pulverised nut shell – results can be less easily described as a glow, and more accurately as low-level swelling or inflammation, encouraging rashes, itchiness and even a more hospitable environment for infection.

Dry feet

Many heel balms are cheaper if you buy them as 10 per cent urea cream. Yes, because it's made of wee. (Sort of.) Urea can be an irritant on thinner skin, which is why it's recommended only for tougher areas such as heels, hands and elbows.

I remember a fashion column by an industry reporter years ago when she complained that her cork-soled Birkenstock sandals had started to suck moisture out of her feet. Instead, she had got older, her skin was drier, and walking with your heels out (in clogs or sandals) and going barefoot, especially in summer, on hot baked ground or concrete or sand, causes more evaporation and abrasion.

Dry, blown heat indoors during winter or drying your tootsies in front of the heater or fire will do that too.

If dry heels progress to deep cracking, infections can follow.

What helps dry feet & heels

Moisturise your feet and heels using cream that's at least 10–20 per cent urea. You can do this before bed, cover with cling wrap (or beeswax wrap, you dear planet-lover) and wear socks over the top. This ensures some moisturising of feet, and also socks.

What doesn't help dry feet & heels

* Don't wash feet or anywhere else all the time with soap; use soap substitute.
* Don't use harsh foot peels and full-on exfoliants. They will make you feel smooth but don't add moisture to your skin.
* Foot soaks and long baths, especially in hot water, dry you out more.
* Use gentle pumice stone or foot files. Harsh, sharps ones upset your skin and that's drying too.

Itchy skin

The perimenopausal and menopausal itchy skin symptom has bamboozled and driven many of us a bit bonkers. We wonder if we're imagining it. Why have clothes labels suddenly started itching like mad? Have we got bloody lice again? Scratching or rubbing the skin can make things worse.

In later years, if you're over 65, doctors often diagnose it as 'pruritus', which is just Latin for itchy, for God's sake. It's caused simply by having drier and thinner skin as we get older and have less estrogen. Again, MHT seems to be not much help.

Things to help itchy skin

Strategies for combating or eliminating scratchy irritants:

- Cut out size and brand labels from clothes, try replacing hook-and-eye bras to stretchy no-fastening ones.
- Try wearing your nightclothes inside-out to avoid scratchy seams.
- Previous tolerable fabrics like a low-wool percentage blend may now be a problem: switch to fleece or other fabrics, or wear a scarf and cotton tops underneath to stop a woollen jumper touching bare skin anywhere.
- Buy 'sensitive', unscented and anti-allergenic laundry soap or powder for your clothes, especially undies.
- Choose a non-soap cleanser for face and body.
- Use a non-perfumed, few-ingredient moisturiser.
- In persistent, difficult cases, use extra-strength moisturisers recommended by a pharmacist.
- Try a prescribed antihistamine cream or medication if all else fails.

Things that won't help itchy skin

Topical estrogen cream won't help except inside the vagina, where it will combat irritating effects of bacteria and acid–alkaline imbalances. No natural supplements are proven go-tos. Vitamin and mineral supplements won't help unless you have a diagnosed deficiency.

> The itching is beyond belief and no one told me anything about it. I put up with it for years! Donna, 58

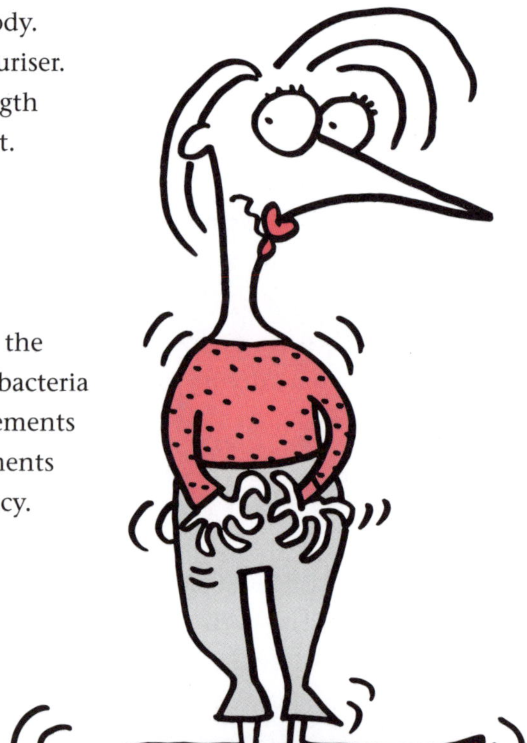

Creepy crawliness

One odd itchiness symptom for some people is the literally creepy phenomenon of formication: the sensation of ants crawling on your skin, otherwise experienced as little prickles, or like bubbles hitting the skin. (Formica is Latin for ant.)

Many women have this symptom and never connect it to menopause. I didn't until I researched this book. Some people describe their symptoms online and are told they're hallucinating, or the sensation is psychological. Doctors believe it's a by-product of perimenopausal itchiness caused by thinner skin. Call it micro-irritations, if that helps.

Some women don't feel a difference between itchiness or formication; others experience them as distinct. It can feel worse at night, in bed, hotter under bedclothes, and when you may be more hyper-aware of sensations and not distracted. Some doctors reckon that levels of dopamine play a role, but they're not yet sure how it works.

You and your doctor will need to rule out other reasons for the sensation, including dry skin conditions such as eczema, a developing allergy or intolerance, a reaction to medication or non-prescription drugs, or an underlying condition, from anxiety to a neurological problem.

I hate the feeling that bugs are crawling on me.
Terry, 51

The Mysteriously Irritable Vulva

Ah yes, The Mysteriously Irritable Vulva: one of Agatha Christie's lesser known works and a common annoyance of perimenopause. Your undies might start feeling constantly wet – and not in the erotic romance novel way: 'Tork handled me with his manly man-hands and suddenly my lady-pantily-panties were soaked' but in a 'Good God, this is uncomfortable' way. 'Hey, wasn't I supposed to have a dry vagina?', you ask yourself, probably not out loud in the supermarket.

Or you may realise you often seem to be dealing with a maddening vulval itch that can't elegantly be attended to in public. Some vulvas can go past irritated to simply furious. Men seem to have been blithely adjusting their scrotum through their pants in public since forever, but women don't tend to madly scratch away at their undercarriage during a conversation, however tempting it feels.

It's relief for peri- and menopausal women to know it's normal to get vulval itch but that doesn't mean we have to put up with it.

In peri- or menopause a common culprit is a vaginal infection or imbalance caused by lowered estrogen. Our bodies are constantly covered with and harbouring millions of microscopic bacteria, most of it protective and necessary. One of the places bacterial flora happily frolic about is in a healthy vagina – sometimes doctors call it an ecosystem or microbiome.

Your vaginal fluid usually has a pH level within a normal range, which is a little bit acidic. This normal acidy-pH level, which protects women against infections, can be altered by having less estrogen in the perimenopause and menopause, by penetrative sex with someone, or something, and by douching or washing inside the vagina with commercial products, including unnecessary perfumes and soaps. If the vagina gets into a more alkaline (less acidic) state it causes, problems and encourages infections.

The vaginal cream definitely helped. It relieved the itching and pain during sex. Patricia, 66

I didn't know my itchy vulva was due to menopause!!! Why is this never talked about? MellyEllen

Seeing a vulval dermatologist – she is my new fave person! Kaz, 52

HRT helped but I still have itchy vulva. Only thing that works is steroid cream. Jacqui, 57

Possible reasons for itchy vulva

* Discharge caused by microbiome imbalance, less estrogen and a more alkaline environment (see above).
* Thrush and other yeast infections; rarer in perimenopause.
* Common vaginitis, a term which covers several vaginal infections caused by bacteria or a fungus *(honestly)* that cause itch and burning. These include bacterial vaginosis, trichomoniasis, aerobic vaginitis, and various candida funguses including thrush. Depending on the infection, symptoms can include a fishy smell and/or changes in the colour and consistency of vaginal fluid, and cause painful sex.

- Irritating, possibly unnoticed discharge caused by a sexually transmitted infection, including chlamydia or gonorrhoea.
- Dermatitis, also known as eczema: usually characterised by inflammation, itch and maybe scaliness and flakiness.
- Any grumbling infection wrongly treated. Many of the treatments for vaginal infections are the wrong ones, or the right ones but not prescribed to be used often enough or for long enough to really eradicate it. See 'Thrush', on page 268.

There's an unlucky dip of possible other causes of and contributors to an itchy vulva:

- Less estrogen causing thinner skin on the vulva, and less fat and collagen padding underneath making it more vulnerable to irritants.
- Irritation caused by blunt ends of shaved or cut pubic hair.
- Glue, perfumes and additives in panty liners, soaps, douches, etc.
- Pubic hair removal methods, including shaving, waxing, depilatory creams, exfoliators and moisturisers.
- Friction irritancy caused by sweat, sex, vibrator use, bicycle seats, wet swimsuits, horseriding saddles, synthetic fabric, thong and string undies, so-called talcum or other powders, and even menstrual blood or wee, especially if using a pad designed for periods instead of incontinence situations.
- Pool chlorine.
- Scars from childhood genital cutting, and genital piercings.

A gyno diagnosed me with chronic thrush. She said I needed a long course of antifungals plus maintenance dose for the next 6 months, but no GP will a) prescribe or b) EVEN FUCKING SWAB MY VAGINA TO TEST FOR THRUSH! Jen, 54

My perineum is itchy and sore all the time. I use steroid cream every day to cope with the itch/pain cycle. Hilary, 51

Soaking one's ladybits in a borax solution has been a game-changer for me. It soothes everything down. Eden, 61

Nappy rash cream helped stinging vulva from wee. Claire, 64

Getting a diagnosis of a vagina-caused vulva problem

Your GP must examine you to make a diagnosis of a vulva or vagina problem. They should know the symptoms of different possibilities. If it's not blindingly obvious from an inspection, a nurse or doctor will take a swab from inside your vagina with a kind of long cotton bud, and send it off to a pathology lab. They should ask for your vaginal pH level to be tested: if it's higher than a usual range, it can indicate a vulnerability to infection.

If your GP diagnoses a perimenopausal or menopausal itchy vulva as being thrush without examining you, or even after examination, ask if they've ruled out lichen sclerosus or lichen planus (see the box on the page opposite), because although far more rare, they can cause severe damage and scarring.

Fixing a vagina pH imbalance

Many problems are fixed by adjusting the pH balance in your vagina, which has become too alkaline because of a fall in estrogen.

A vaginal infection that triumphs over the body's immune system and normal vaginal pH can continue to change the pH levels. (This is *not* a DIY stick-something-else-up-there-like-garlic-or-garden-furniture situation.)

After perimenopause hits, many women plunge prescription estrogen cream or pessaries, or other acidic gel medication, up to their cervix twice a week, or the first week of every month for a year, to keep their vaginal bacteria balance in check.

Despite suggestive advertising and advocates, no douche, supplement, or other 'natural' or 'detox' so-called remedy or food is known to alter the in-vagina pH balance.

The go-to treatments are an in-vagina estrogen cream, usually twice a week, and if the problem persists, a consistent use of boric acid pessaries (basically, adding safe acid), which have to be made by a compounding pharmacist.

If you're given boric acid vaginal pessaries, they may look exactly like a capsule you usually swallow. *But do be careful.* Boric acid is safe and does its job when delivered into the vagina, but if it's swallowed it can override stomach acids and put a hole in the wall of your stomach: people have died. This warning isn't usually on the label. Compounded boric acid capsules are usually dispensed without a plunger so you're supposed to just poke them up there.

Attending the GP's office and having a swab to test for a problem in the vagina, then going back for results is expensive enough. But, as happened to me the week I wrote this paragraph, being given one prescription for a medication that isn't made any more, and another one 'just in case' that turned out to have an inadequate dosage to eradicate the problem, and having to go to a gynaecologist to get it all explained and sorted, and getting the new medication and wondering how to get it up the top of my vagina without the use of a circus cannon, and swathes of cash out of pocket later, has been almost as irritating as a mysterious vulva.

And I say unto you that it is *pathetic* that women are having to deal with this without well-known, menopause-informed protocols for GPs to diagnose and prescribe the right medication for the right problem. I think you'll find if this happened to most scrotums over the age of 50, we'd all be able to get treatment for free.

How good is your GP at vagina & vulva problems?

Your GP or specialist should be aware of the latest recommendations on diagnosis, dosages and treatments for vaginal infections by the ISSVD, the International Society for the Study of Vulvovaginal Disease (they really shouldn't have put 'disease' in their name because they deal with other conditions, but they did and now they're stuck with it). Doctors should also be aware of the latest info on the website of the Australasian Menopause Society.

Rare, but worth checking for

One cause of an itchy vulva, which sometimes also happens without an itch, is an autoimmune condition that can produce lichen sclerosus or lichen planus. The 'lichen' conditions usually cause a whitening effect, and the appearance of thicker skin patches or scarring, and cracking and bleeding. They need to be treated and monitored by a switched-on GP, gynaecologist or dermatologist with specific steroid creams and medication.

Horror story alert: I know of one woman who went to her GP for 8 years. The doctor never examined her. Each time she reported an itchy vulva she was told it must be thrush and given a prescription for standard treatment. When she finally got fed up and went to a gynaecologist, the extent of the lichen sclerosis had closed over her vagina, poor love: treatment reversed it, but wow, imagine going through that.

Examination is essential to diagnose (very rare) vulval cancer.

Thrush & other yeast infections

If you have recurring vaginal infections and are always told it's thrush, get a swab sent to a pathology lab to make sure you know what you're dealing with. Yeast infections tend to recede in menopause – though not for everyone.

Some GPs also just give medication for thrush every time, without making a definite diagnosis. Medication for thrush doesn't help other yeast-related vaginal infections or other conditions.

Some GPs are giving out old and unhelpful prescriptions for pessaries and creams, suggesting much more infrequent placement of standard pessary treatments, for example three times a week for a week, when every night for three weeks might be needed.

What won't help thrush and other yeast infections: forget yoghurt, cranberry products, tea-tree oil and garlic. They won't help and can be mightily irritating and stinging. Some kinds of probiotic treatment may help thrush, but so far it's not clear which kinds of bacteria, in what sort of dose, stored and delivered in what way actually work, and there's no evidence they help you fix acidity in the long term.

Help to avoid vaginal infections

Sometimes you do everything right and you still get a vaginal infection: it's normal, and not your fault. These things can help:

* A vaginal estrogen cream used twice a week to maintain vaginal bacterial balance.
* Use condoms during sex: sperm can alter pH levels.
* Only use antibiotics if you really need them.
* Don't use any perfumes, soaps, douches or cleansers inside the vagina, which is a self-cleaning part of the body. Many specialists say just using water to clean the vulva is fine, but that's a bridge too far for many of us.
* Very specific doses of a couple of different formulations of 'good bacteria' (not just any probiotic) – ask your doctor which ones have a proven effect.
* After a poo, wipe yourself towards the back, not towards your vagina, to avoid transferring bacteria to where you don't want it.

What helps with an itchy vulva

These things:

- Make sure you have a diagnosis for what's really causing the problem or you'll be treating the wrong thing: take your vulva to a doctor who has seen approximately 900 of them and if necessary get a vaginal swab. Any of various prescription antibacterial, steroid, estrogen creams or other medication may be necessary.
- See the general self-help for itchy skin, earlier in this chapter. Specifically for vulvas: wear cotton, full coverage, non-lacy or scratchy undies, and let your vulva recover completely between a sport or sexual activity that makes it swell or subject to friction.
- Wash yourself and your undies with unscented and non-allergenic soap or non-soap cleanser.
- Some self-help hints say you should soak your vulva in a salt bath twice a day. Gynaecologists say this is unlikely to cure anything on its own; it feels much more like a passed-down remedy that is less effective than what else is now available. Also who has the time or dexterity?
- Sports folk should choose sweat-wicking clothes and padded gear where possible to reduce vulval friction. Chlorine swimmers can get a barrier cream to slather on their vulva before swimming, which will really perk up the change-room chat. Change out of sweaty clothes or wet swimwear ASAP.
- A cool pack is OK (think fridge, not freezer, or protect skin from a frozen pack with layers of tea towel). Never put ice directly on your vulva.
- Ignore 'home remedy' suggestions – don't put bits of garlic up into your vagina, or yoghurt, or kombucha, or Lego. (Furthermore, do not sunbathe your perineum or stick a fork in your toaster.)

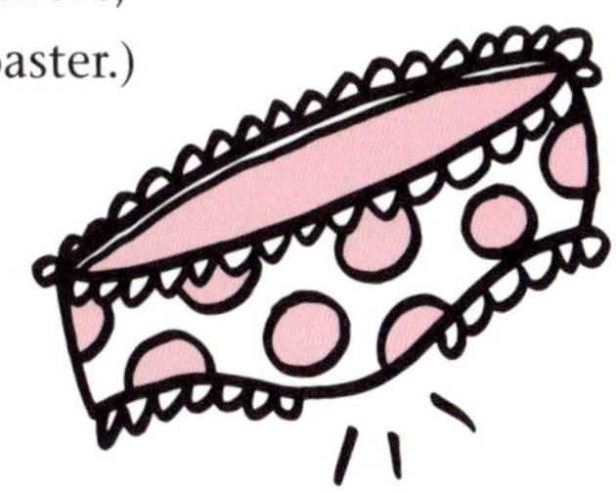

I didn't know 'itchy vulva' was a menopause symptom.
Teri, 50

Why doesn't anything work!!!!???? Bek, 51

What doesn't help with an itchy vulva:

* Avoid all douches, deodorants and any perfumed products on or near your vulva.
* So far nothing reliable suggests probiotics help non-thrush itch conditions, and to help thrush they need to be very specific bacteria flora types, formulations transported in specific conditions, so good luck with that.

MORE INFO on an irritable vulva

betterhealth.vic.gov.au
Search 'vulvar conditions' on this trustworthy state health department site for a fact sheet.

jeanhailes.org.au
Search 'vulval & vaginal irritation' for general vulva info, but remember, peri- and post-menopausal women will need specific diagnosis. There are also fact sheets on lichen sclerosus and other possible culprit conditions.

Your changing vagina

While boys start obsessing about the size of their penis before they're fully steady on toddler feet, women have mostly been encouraged to regard their vagina size only in relation to how a man wants it to feel during sex. Most women otherwise don't care if their vagina is 'tight' or long or short or angled towards the small of their back or straight up and down or turns a slight corner. Only a handful of researchers have even bothered to study it, and even then almost exclusively on small groups of white women.

You will not be astonished to learn that some researchers took it upon themselves to label different vagina shapes as conical, heart-shaped, pumpkin seed and . . . do feel free to join me in wondering idly if they were simply absolute arseholes, 'slug'. Most vaginas minding their own business with nothing inside them are very approximately about 6 cm from the opening up to the cervix, around 3 cm wide inside and about 2.5 cm at the opening in the vulva.

In peri- and menopause the vagina tends to slightly shrink and become drier, and wow are some people using this to try to make millions out of us.

A drier vagina

From the way this is talked about on magazine websites, you'd think the surface of our post-menopausal vagina has the crazy-paving effect of a dry riverbed in a drought or the surface of a pink meringue tapped with spoon. From the advertising of products allegedly to reverse it, you'd be forgiven for imagining your vagina has turned into a dried mango. It becomes marketing-led, medically-unopposed self-diagnosis that is insulting and not even helpful.

All the skin on your body reacts to the fall in estrogen in your body by thinning and this happens to ligaments and other tissues near your bladder, your vagina's inner walls, and the skin on your vulva and perineum, too.

The ludicrously insensitive medical term is vulvovaginal atrophy (VVA), which makes it sound like your vagina shrivels down to a wizened husk like a Twisties packet in the oven. (Do not put a Twisties packet or your vagina into a moderate oven.)

Is there a more romantic and poetic phrase than 'vulvovaginal and urinary tract atrophy'? Hang onto your labia: doctors now use the phrase 'genitourinary syndrome of menopause (GSM)' which they think, Gawd help them, is better. Frankly, I know we have to have medical terms but both phrases can sound to us a bit dehumanising and freaky, when it's a normal problem with some relatively easy solutions.

Treatments for dry vagina

Especially since I've been researching this book and searching menopause products and symptoms, the internet now bombards me day and night with ads for herbal nonsense and cosmetic surgery and impertinent questions. One day I expect to open the front door and there'll be a truck double-parked out the front with a billboard on it, in letters 2 metres tall spelling out 'DRY VAGINA?' Shut UP, I shall mutter and slam the door with élan, if that is also poise, which come to think of it is a brand of incontinence pad.

A standard ongoing fix for dry vagina, regardless of whether you want something to help with your sex life (for that, pop off to Chapter 6, It's Your Sex Life), and which also sorts out your bacteria and acid balance, is an estrogen supplement delivered to the top of the vagina. It's delivered in a cream or pessary, say twice a week, using a plastic plunger, or your finger.

This will provide a better targeted result than using MHT. Lots of women do both, with the usual caveat that MHT isn't suitable for some women with a history of certain medical conditions. In-vagina estrogen is usually considered safe for those with experience of estrogen-related cancers and other conditions but check with your doctor.

Other non-estrogen options good for general use, and some just for when you want more lubrication for sex, can include hyaluronic acid-based creams and non-estrogen steroid medicines known as DHEA, and silicon-based and other sexual lubricants – see Chapter 6, It's Your Sex Life, for details on those. (You don't want to know what DHEA stands for, do you? No you don't. Alright, dehydroepiandrosterone – serves you right.)

Still to this day what's happening in the vagina is taboo, no one talks about the pain of vaginal atrophy and dryness. Camille, 52

[Steroid medication] was awesome for vaginal dryness and sex drive. Regina, 56

Useless, dodgy & inadvisable treatments for dry vagina

Avoid all non-prescription or doctor-unapproved douches, squirters, spritzers, moisturisers, creams or herbal preparations. Your vagina cleans itself and these things are just expensive, unregulated, and in many cases cause itchy and inflamed irritations and intolerances. Dermatologists have them on a list of usual suspects for irritated vulvas and cross vaginas.

Likewise, ignore all non-prescription or doctor-unapproved supplements or creams if they claim any usefulness with vaginal dryness. Including but not restricted to 'French maritime pine bark'; 'alkaline powders', and all those celebrity-marketed powders and pills.

So-called 'laser treatments', and 'wands', and vibrator-looking LED or heat devices, and other devices that look like vibrators and G-spot injections? They. Are. Nonsense. Again, see Chapter 6, It's Your Sex Life, where I get both shouty and shirty about it and help you avoid rip-offs.

Don't even think about vaginal exfoliation products.

Stop it.

The takeaway on your body

Get advice to tackle any body symptoms you need to, from capricious periods to headaches, weeing trouble or an otherwise fickle or furious undercarriage. If perimenopause or menopause might be relevant for you, consider, and insist that your medical advisor considers a possible hormonal reason for any physical health problems.

The relationship with our bodies is usually the longest one we'll ever have. Work with it, not against it. Revel in its every win, and enjoy your body whenever you can (marabou ticklers optional).

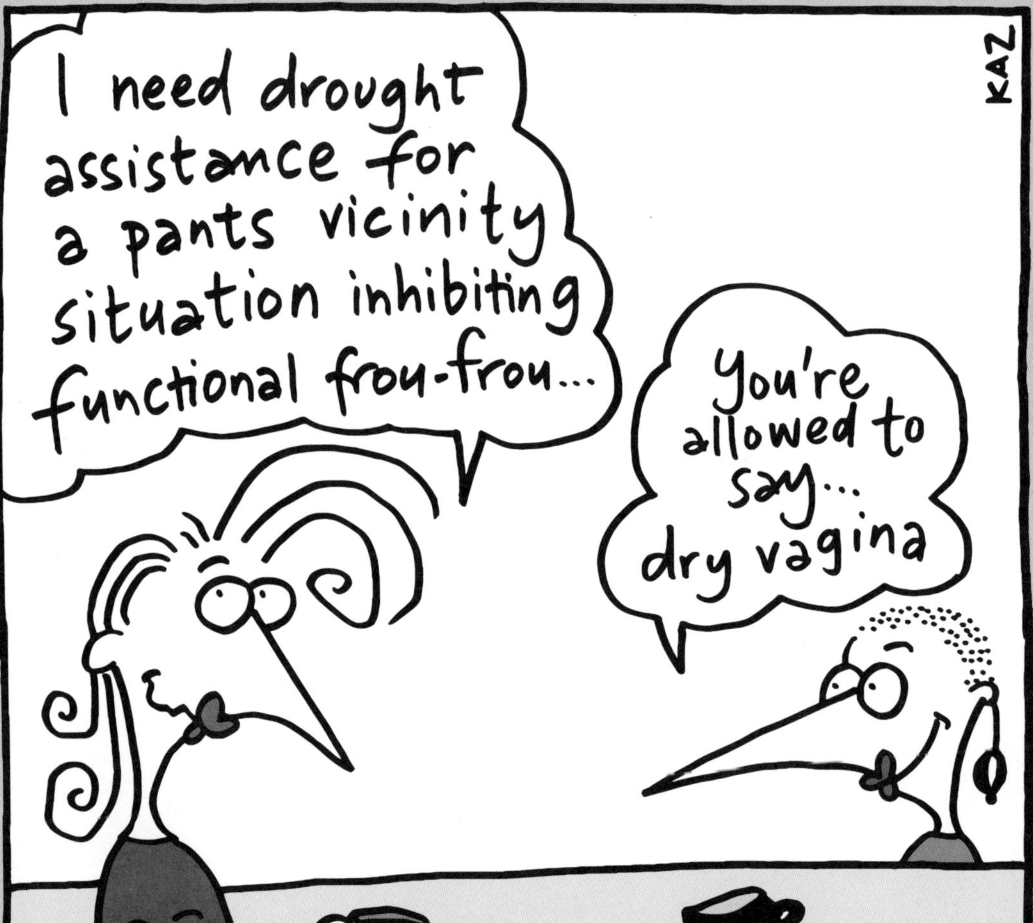
KAZ
I need drought assistance for a pants vicinity situation inhibiting functional frou-frou...
You're allowed to say... dry vagina

6

It's Your Sex Life

I once read a 1962 book for men called *Women A–Z, A Guidebook to the Pursuit and Capture of the Fair Sex*. It was steaming poop but I kept it so I could look up what it says about older women and sex, for research. Surely there'd be some emblematic quote there dismissive of older women (like, over about 27), or perhaps creepily declarative about their sexiness? I tried O for Older (the sole entry under O was Orgies); we weren't under Mature. Or even C for Crone.

Eventually, I found us: under R for Ripeness. It leads off with a quote from a 16th-century French poet: 'I don't like virgins, For they're too green, And I'm not keen on ruins. The one for my taste is a woman who's ripe.' Get stuffed mate, I'm not an air-lifted strawberry.

The author of the book itself, a Jean Jérôme Romanet, added: 'At what age do you go mouldy, ladies? . . . there are so few ripe women who preserve themselves properly . . . they let themselves go to pot.' Romanet seems to have sunk without trace and his translator, Julian Crane . . .

Oh, Kaz, I hear you cry, crossly, *do* stop going down research rabbit holes. Get on with the Sex chapter, woman! Well, have it your way but don't you want to know that Julian Crane was immortalised as the name of a character in the early 2000s US soap opera *Passions*, whose penis is cut off in a crypt and it is sewn back on upside down so if he ever has an erection he will die (Season 9)? Seems fair.

Anyway, where were we? Sex.

One thing that came up again and again in the Menopause Survey for this book is that sex with a drier vagina *hurts*. Thousands of women talked about having their libido affected, but many more talked in terms of not wanting to have sex because of *pain*, not because their desire had otherwise disappeared.

It's often just assumed that all menopausal women lose their libido – their desire for sex evaporates. And yet other women report a surge or a zig-zag of desire in perimenopause, attributed to not having to worry about getting pregnant, or perhaps lower levels of progestogen at different times let higher estrogen and testosterone turn you into a sex-mad fancying machine (not a scientifically proven hypothesis). As usual, we need to allow for individual experiences and effects of hormone carry-on.

We also *really* need to guard against all sorts of absurd products, devices and procedures sold by hucksters, straight-faced believer-nincompoops and the profit-keen who claim it will restore our sexual desire or claim with no evidence that their product will lubricate a drier vagina caused by lower estrogen levels. We shall get to them shortly, at which point I shall go orf like a box of fireworks. Luckily, there are other sensible and proven ways to help.

Has anyone ever investigated whether sex drive actually declines, or is it just because many of us are partnered with middle-aged men. Maybe it's not us, it's them! **Bernadette, 53**

My sex drive went through the roof! Could not get enough. Had to buy a vibrator for the first time in my life! My husband couldn't keep up. Literally! **Mary, 55**

My sex drive has increased. I'm finding and rediscovering myself as a person. **Julianne, 47**

I can't be bothered with sex, I'd rather sort myself out. Five minutes, job done. **Maudy, 56**

Oh God, who wants to have sex? No inclination and dried-out bits! **JS, 55**

I have a completely different body and nothing that worked or felt good before feels good now. My body is foreign to both of us. **Kate, 50**

Sex toys, steamy movies and novels help a LOT. **Liz, 51**

Hormones made me really horny. Took a specialist to sort it for me. It's not something you can tell someone without it sounding like a joke. **Sandi, 55**

What perimenopause does to desire

Many perimenopausal women report lack of interest in sex. But lots say they're interested all right, but the sex they used to like is no fun anymore due to dry vagina situation. Or they're too busy, too annoyed and too tired.

With my husband of almost 30 years . . . my libido hasn't waned but his has. I feel rejected and now sleep in a different bedroom. Christine, 49

Women are now far more likely to have sex into their seventies than they were in the past (or at least, tell anyone about it). We might have assumed it's because they're still enjoying it. But reliable Australian research shows that almost 90 per cent of older women (aged 65 to 79) have low sexual desire, and more sadly, about a third of women who were having sex with a partner were having a horrid – rather than a torrid – time.

Australian women told a reputable 2017 survey that their lack of interest had multiple reasons: a presumed change in hormone levels, but also distress about incontinence, dry vagina problems, feeling depressed, and though it wasn't precisely worded in the survey, I'll add: because they were sick of their partner being a dud in bed.

A lot of women who talk to counsellors and psychiatrists about sex say they feel they have to compete against younger women to keep the interest of their partners. A changing face and body, their shrinking self-esteem and physical and mental symptoms of perimenopause combine to make them feel unworthy and discardable. Discardable may not be a word, but never mind, it's definitely a feeling. In some awful cases, it's actually voiced by a partner on their way out the door.

For many of us, we feel so worried about being undesirable, we forget to ask what *we* might desire. Is it to feel better; to feel worthy; to feel sexy; to feel at peace with not having sex? Like perimenopause symptoms, it's different for everyone.

My sex drive came back. I started experiencing G-spot orgasms. Helen, 62

Fear of intimacy. Forced self to try sex: painful & awful . . . Doc said vaginismus (in my head), but was actually prolapse. Davida, 57

I want to want to have intercourse and don't have to be talked into it. Robyn, 58

I do not feel sexual towards my husband at all and refuse to fake it . . . so if he doesn't want to live like that he needs to do something about it e.g. leave me. . . . I love him and we have a great relationship. Sandra, 56

The stock shortages of the HRT I was prescribed has been complete rubbish. Kirsten, 56

The crazy sex drive at the beginning of perimenopause took me completely by surprise and caused a complete shake-up of my life. Ruth, 54

How can I go from a total hornbag to a complete nun so quickly? When will it end? Mell, 47

Moved into my own bedroom. Love it! Margot, 53

I now get a lot of pain after orgasm, and all the doctor had to advise was ways to AVOID having orgasm. Kate, 58

I just don't want sex. Helen, 56

Years ago an author whose name rhymes with Fettina Barndt who isn't a clinical psychologist wrote a book about interest in sex from interviews with 98 straight couples. One reviewer summed it up by saying 'nine times out of ten it was the male who wanted more sex'. I think the real picture is more complex.

In more than 7000 responses to my survey for the book *Women's Stuff* in the year 2010, there were hundreds of unsolicited quotes from women who wanted more sex with their straight male partners, as well as hundreds saying they couldn't really be bothered with it anymore.

And again, in the Survey for this book, ten or so years later, almost one in five of the respondents said their fall in libido in perimenopause was truly terrible; just under a quarter said it was tough; about 23 per cent said it was sometimes annoying; about 17 per cent said it happened but didn't bother them much, and just under 17 per cent said their desire for sex was unaffected. Nearly half said they were worried about sex-life changes.

Women have identified their reasons for losing interest in sex include feeling more self-conscious about body and face changes caused by time, not enjoying sex and regarding it more as a duty, hating the endless thrusting friction sort of sex that seemed to be wanted by men who took medication for long-lasting erections, having a partner who's not interested or doesn't make them feel wanted, partners who didn't make an effort to find out how to make sex good, and the side effects of medication.

Sex life repair, or don't care?

You might want to lubricate your perimenopausal or menopausal vagina to have sex with a person or a sex toy, or you might rather have a digestive biscuit. If you don't need or want a penetrative sex life (now there's a romantic phrase) and quite sensibly try not to put anything in your vagina unless it's strictly necessary, you might be more comfortable restoring the self-sauciness of your vagina anyway.

A regular application of an in-vagina estrogen cream or pessary, for example, will make the vagina more self-saucing again and contribute to good pelvic floor and bladder function. They can also guard against vaginal infections, which cause itchy vulva and other symptoms, so a vaginal estrogen cream can be a good idea regardless of the state of your sex life (see the 'Lubricants to use during sex' section coming up).

A lot of recommendations about menopause assume you just need vaginal lubrication need to 'keep a man happy'. I don't want to shock anyone to their very core, but some women are having sex with other women, and non-binary and trans people are having sex with each other and also women, and some of us are quite happy to have sex entirely alone.

Perimenopausal and menopausal women experiencing painful or unsatisfactory sex of any kind will also have to assess how much of it can be put down to uncomfortable or painful friction due to a much drier vagina and how much is a failure of communication, and a partner's cluelessness or uncaring attitude. It broke my heart to hear menopause specialists tell me some of their patients want painkillers so they can keep having sex the way a man wants to, especially the ones whose partners take a Viagra and keep an erection for ages.

My slimebag ex had an affair, leaving us for his bikini babe. He told me he didn't want to be saddled with an old woman. He was a year older than me. Kate, 62

I hate that low libido is seen as something I should 'treat'. Maybe many women just wised up to the fact they had a whole lotta sex cos they felt like they should? Welshy, 46

Penetrative sex was painful due to dry vagina. I couldn't care less if my husband left or stayed. He has stuck around and we found a new way of intimacy/sex. He is a keeper. Helen, 52

Shout-out to the clitoris

'Clitoral atrophy' and a decrease in clitoral feeling after menopause is hardly whispered amid the hubbub of chat about perimenopausal dry vaginas and 'vaginal and vulva atrophy'. And yet it's the clitoris that's literally at the centre of women's sexual pleasure and ability to have orgasms. You'd think it might be a nice idea for women to be told, sure, your husband might be interested in a welcoming vagina, but how's your clitoris going?

Your labia may feel smaller and less plump, too, a combination of ageing and hormone changes. (Taking collagen and elastin or something else in a supplement won't change this, but MHT will have some effect.)

Luckily, when it comes to feeling good, size doesn't have to matter at all. After a few years of less estrogen and testosterone, the clitoris may be smaller, but still do the job of helping you get to orgasm. Here is a happy sentence: stimulating your clitoris helps it stay healthy. Giving your clitoris and/or vagina a bit of a regular tickle and tune-up encourages important nerve action and blood flow. Blood flow is helpful, so if anyone goes through your bedside drawer and asks why you secretly bought a 17-speed clitoral suction vibrator online, tell them it's a medical prescription.

After a hysterectomy, some women experience a change in clitoral and especially vaginal sensation, and doctors really don't have much research about why or what to do about it.

What else might you need to get out of the way before being able to concentrate on delightful orgasms?

First, a short round-up of some knowledge you need in your negligee pocket: contraception, sexually transmitted infections
warning signs and food for thought.

I'd like to know if there is anything I can do, given my age now, to be interested in sex.
Gillian, 64

My clitoris shrank so much it was almost gone. It had almost no feeling. When I told a gyno he told me to talk to a therapist. I explained it was a physical thing but he seemed uninterested. Once I saw an endocrinologist and got onto [MHT medication] it improved.
Sue, 64

Contraception

> Perimenopausal symptoms for a couple of years then . . . a baby after my first grandchild was born! Granny, 65

> I'm glad hubby has the snip. Tracey, 48

'Menopause baby' is such a thing they've even invented a phrase for it. Keep taking contraception for 2 years after your last period if you don't want an accidental mid-life baby. Common contraceptive methods for long-term partnerships include the Pill, the Mirena IUD, implant pellet, and condoms. Doctors usually recommend Pill methods for a lesser risk of heart or stroke problems.

Hope, luck, app-tracked periods and the withdrawal method won't do the job. One of the reasons Mirena IUDs are so common in perimenopause is because many people find them effective against heavy periods as well as providing set-and-forget contraception (for 5 years).

Pharmacies stock the emergency contraceptive 'morning-after pill', which can prevent pregnancy if taken a few days after unprotected sex – as early a possible. This is not the 'abortion pill'.

Sexually transmitted infections (STIs)

In general, people having non-condom-protected sex after menopause have rising rates of contracting an STI. Blokes can't presume they don't have to wear a condom anymore just because pregnancy isn't an issue. Women in menopause can and do contract herpes, chlamydia, syphilis, gonorrhoea, and other nasties, some of which are damaging and have sneaky not-noticeable early symptoms.

Bleeding after sex

Any bleeding after penetrative sex must be checked out. It might just be annoying perimenopause bleeding carry-on, but there's a very slender chance it's a sign of cancer. (Statistically, for argument's sake, this may only apply to one in a thousand people, so it's a 0.001 per cent chance.)

The non-dry, dry vagina

Sometimes it feels like your vagina is not dry at all and is running like a tap, but this might be due to hormonal changes messing up the balance of good and bad bacteria in there. This sort of wetness happens regardless of whether you're aroused or not, is otherwise known as a discharge, and is not helpful for lubrication during sex. Check out the 'Mysteriously Irritable Vulva' section in Chapter 5, It's Your Body.

Communication

Told my hubby how old it made me feel and he is beautiful and reassured me. Ali, 49

Talking about what you want, what you care about, what you like, what you don't want, asking questions; libido has always had more to do with the brain than anything else. As a woman once said to me at work drinks, 'My clitoris is in my ear'. I had to rearrange my facial expression.

Talking at length to my partner about menopause and conveying what I needed to be able to participate in sex. Slowly, gently, slowly, gently – while nowhere near as regular as it once was, is still OK. Anna, 58

I've tried talking to my partner, but he's very dismissive and thinks it's all just an excuse not to have sex. Mandy, 44

Sex life & satisfaction

Two of the main factors in sexual satisfaction are libido and vaginal dryness. We'll look at them in that order.

What might boost libido

These things:

* Not being so bloody tired.
* Being mainly healthy.
* Not drinking more than healthy levels of alcohol.
* Maybe estrogen or testosterone supplements.
* Shared household chores and responsibilities between partners.

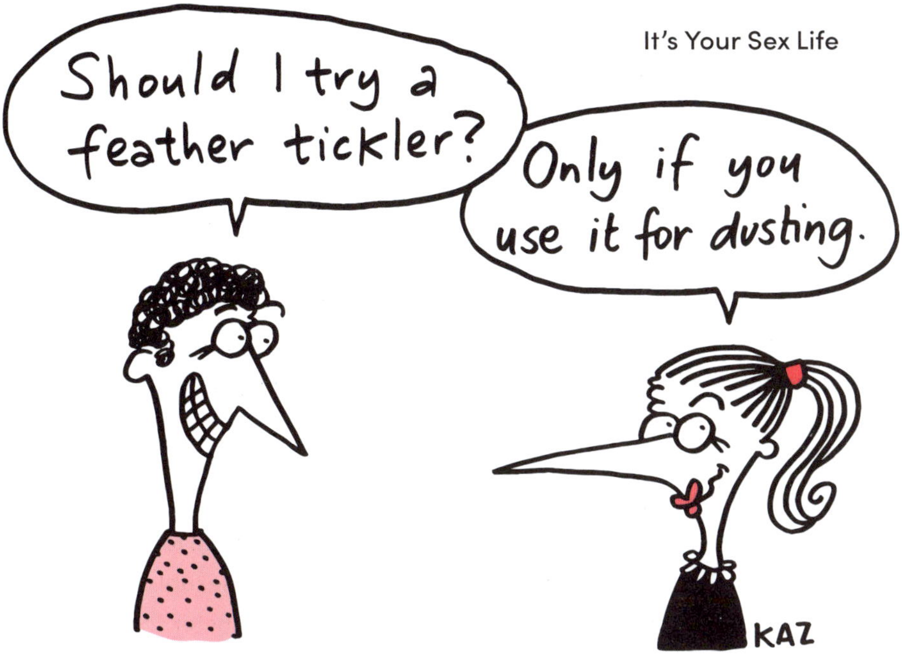
Should I try a feather tickler?
Only if you use it for dusting.
KAZ

What doesn't do anything significant to libido

This stuff:

- Despite rumours, you could eat dates, ginger, chillies and oysters all day and you'd be much more likely to feel sick than automatically want to have sex.
- Unproven 'natural' supplements.
- In-vagina digital or app-related devices.
- Non-testosterone medical attempts at changing a woman's libido are mostly in pill form and sometimes oddly referred to as 'women's Viagra'. Generally, they've caused side effects that include vomiting, or a contraindication with alcohol, or they've proved no better than a placebo in trial studies.

What lowers libido

A combination, often, of:

- Depression and anxiety.
- Being responsible for two or three generations of family stuff.
- The synthetic progestins in most kinds of the Pill, and some MHT, are suspected of mood-flattening, which can affect libido.
- Side effects of some other medications.

Apart from vaginal dryness I feel pretty good. My sex life is getting better and I've been educating my husband a lot about it. He's embracing the 'second spring' concept that is used in Asia to describe this time in life. **Kellie, 49**

Testosterone & libido

Testosterone has been suggested as a libido cure, but the problem is, it doesn't work like that: you can't just take some testosterone medication and turn into a sexual raver. Some women say a boost of testosterone, using a prescribed approved cream delivering a calibrated amount every day, has helped them feel more desirous of sex and less anxious about it; others say it makes no difference, and that instead, getting their estrogen level up again really helped.

Others say they're so bored with what their partner is doing to them they could scream, and no amount of her taking testosterone has made him (it's a him in all the quotes of the Survey) be any more inventive or attentive.

According to current best practice, testosterone isn't useful for your sex life unless you are diagnosed with something called hypoactive sexual desire disorder. And if you do get that diagnosis and use testosterone, your doctor should tell you there are no studies yet on its long-term use. So far, there's no evidence that taking testosterone does anything to help most women who have a standard uninterest in sex they're quite happy with. There's no evidence it helps any of the mental symptoms, bone density or muscle strength.

One leading researcher found that 50 per cent of women given a placebo instead of testosterone in a clinical trial said it had improved their libido.

Doctors doing research to assess alleged libido-affecting products, or treatments for menopause-related sex problems, often use the Female Sexual Function Index and/or an agreed revision of the Female Sexual Distress Scale, questionnaires which rate a woman's feelings and physical reactions. They'll often get women to fill in the questionnaires before and after a treatment (say, testosterone or a lubricant or doing cognitive behaviour therapy) to judge whether something seemed to help.

Before getting a prescription of testosterone, have a talk with your doctor (or yourself) about whether you have a diagnosed case of 'female sexual dysfunction,' or if you're happy to decide you're ready to give up much in the way of penetrative sex anymore – or something in between.

A prescribed, regulated skin patch or cream with testosterone is the preferred delivery method.

Estrogen & libido

The jury is out on whether the extra estrogen in MHT or otherwise affects libido. Some women say yes, some say no.

'Natural' supplements for libido

> 38-year marriage ended, went straight into new relationship and found my inner sex goddess! Sadly menopause hit one year in . . . at least I had a year of decent sex. Annie, 58

Non-medical so-called libido supplements are also unproven, which is doctor-speak for doesn't work, otherwise somebody would have proved that it does. Libido supplements and aphrodisiacs range from rumours about oysters, or maca root, or fenugreek, or saffron to standard vitamins in coy floral packaging to endorsements and slang labels on celebrity-branded 'herbal' products – marketeer Gwyneth Paltrow called hers DTF (Down To Fuck).

The only proven known consistent change that has an effect on women's interest in sex is shown in study after study: when men do more housework and share more of the emotional and family organisational burden, the couple has more sex. In other words, a man doing housework boosts a straight woman's libido.

There's no evidence for any herbal or vitamin supplement or food that boosts a woman's libido. There's no evidence for any rumoured aphrodisiac (except maybe romance novels and sexy talk, and a partner who's done the dishes and wiped down the benches, but nobody's done that specific study as far as I know).

Weapons in the libido-based marketing arsenal include labels that mention the word libido, website and social media-based influencer marketing, and uncritical journalism based on sponsorship or free samples, testimonials (recommendations from members of the public), and claims in provided press releases.

Claims often centre around the idea that the product will 'support blood flow' (well, it won't kill you, which would stop blood flow), or help people get to sleep, or deliver nutrients. Vague claims are made about 'energy levels' and 'stabilising' and 'balancing', and 'said to help with'. In other words,

> My partner just ended her relationship with me because I no longer want sex. I respect this but it's also very sad. PJ, 44

> My sex drive has gotten intermittent – comes and goes for a week or two, and when it's on, it's ON. Tracey, 52

I feel lumpy and unattractive and a bit invisible on dating sites. Jordana, 52

Sex drive increased to the point it became overwhelming, could think of nothing but sex for weeks. Made some bad choices during this time. Kez, 46

Bummer about not wanting sex, my partner still sulks about it but finally got the 'don't even try' message. But I'd still like him to want to do other activities with me, like take me out for dinner. Gillian, 50

HRT now for 4 years and I felt like a new woman. My husband could come back upstairs to be with me again. Kerri, 58

I have absolutely NO interest in sex. George Clooney could do a striptease in front of me and I could not raise the enthusiasm. Cathryn, 58

I have friends who have been left by their partner as their sex life wasn't good due to effects of menopause. Jacqui, 57

I'm worried my husband is trapped with me. I've tried what feels like everything. Is it terrible to wish your husband would leave you, because you are letting him down? Kylie, 42

I worry about finding a partner at my age, and ending up alone for the rest of my life: I can't be bothered doing anything about it. Hilary, 50

I am amazed at how common it is to stop having sex, and never have the intention or inclination to ever have sex again. Suzie, 57

My mother and both my sisters sailed through with zero symptoms. I assumed I would too! I was so very wrong. Catherine, 60

I am a sweaty, depressed, overweight tired nurse with anger issues. Now if that's not sexy, I don't know what is . . . Sacha, 51

they claim they help the body do normal stuff, with no proof of an effect on libido. Usually they contain various safe-sounding plant ingredients such as green tea, and broccoli, and might include standard vitamins or minerals like iron, magnesium and zinc.

Some online go further, claiming 'clinically shown to promote a woman's sexual vitality'. How the blazing bollocks is that measured? This claim was made because one ingredient in a supplement contained saponins, which may create a weak estrogenic effect in the body: but not enough to change any of your hormone levels or recreate a pre-menopause state. It's so tenuous as to be in different postcode zones.

Articles and supporting stuff for the products can range from the unproven to the nonsensical, including the idea that toxins cause a lowered libido and sniffing basil raises it.

One study wheeled out to support a supplement claimed it had a beneficial effect on sleep and sexual desire, but found no difference in the average hormone levels between those taking it and those not taking it. I guess the claimed effect must be magic.

It takes some chutzpah to sell a so-called libido supplement if you're getting enough general vitamins, because there is no known extra 'natural' ingredient they can sell you that will definitely or even probably change your libido.

I masturbate to orgasm every week on a set day, regardless of what other liaisons I might have. I treat it as a health and resilience tool. Jennifer, 55

Less interest in sex . . . feels like an upside and a relief. Carolyn, 50

I didn't mourn the loss of my fertility, but the loss of my identity as a sexy babe. That's been hard. Liz, 57

What helps is a kind partner and cuddles. Beryl, 67

MORE INFO on libido & sex

Desire is linked to mood, and mental health. (See Chapter 4, It's Your Mind, for more.)

menopause.org.au
Search 'Sexual difficulties in the menopause' on the Australian Menopause Society site.

Your drier vagina & sex

> The physician at the women's health centre was quite brusque and talked about potential atrophy. Atrophy – what a word for a teary, anxious menopausal woman to hear!
> Robyn, 59

Probably, possibly, we're guessing (can we get some more research over here?), half to most peri- and menopausal women have trouble with vaginal and vulval dryness and irritation, rudely termed 'vaginal atrophy'. It can make our sex life, and confidence, take a dive.

Doctors and the inelegantly-named International Society for the Study of Vulvovaginal Disease (ISSVD) – which is all over the vagina-vulva situation, disease or no disease – are more likely to use terms like genitourinary syndrome of menopause. Well, it's marginally better than 'atrophy', if you squint and have had a sherry.

Many so-called treatments for dry vagina are hard-sell, unhelpful nonsense. Nothing rejuvenates or makes a vagina younger, despite marketing terms. All vaginal atrophy really means is that we become less of a self-saucing pudding, and need to add the sauce ourselves if we want to have sex without painful, dry friction.

In the Survey for this book, more than 4000 women answered a question about using a lubricant during sex: more than half thought it helped.

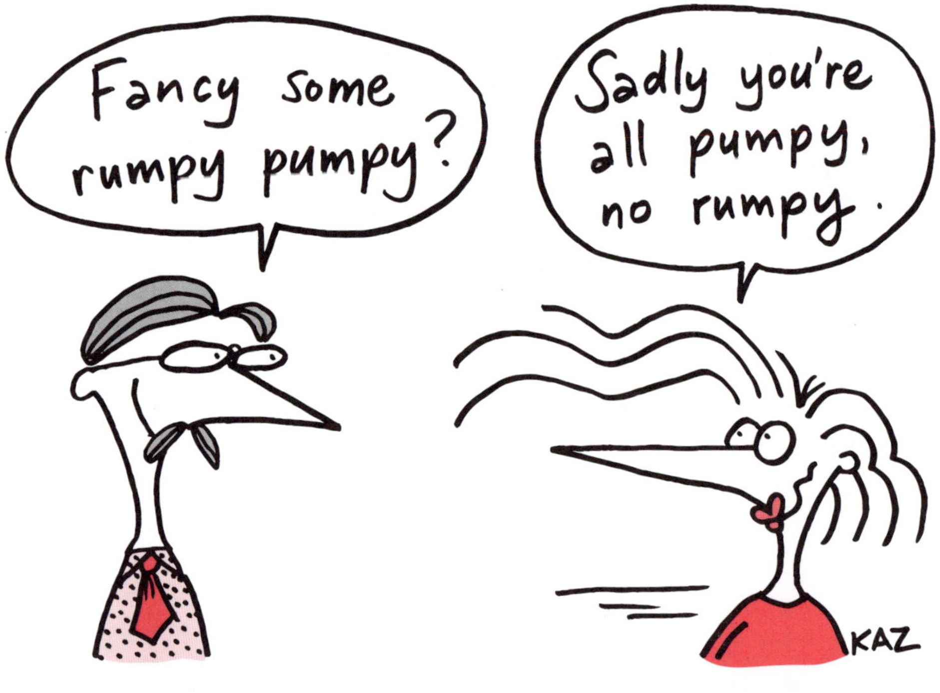
Fancy some rumpy pumpy?
Sadly you're all pumpy, no rumpy.
KAZ

Painful sex

Painful sex caused by vaginal dryness or by something else, is known by doctors as dyspareunia, which quite honestly sounds like a species of geranium.

A huge majority of women who answered the Menopause Survey questions about sex for this book – about 65 per cent – said that they experienced a dry vagina as a peri-menopause and menopause symptom; and about 50 per cent said perimenopausal sex really hurt.

What can we do if have searing, knife-like pain during sexual intercourse? Does estrogen cream help? I don't know enough about any solutions but live in avoidance and fear. Olivia, 55

I have always wanted to know about treatments for making sex less painful. Maybe a topical cream that numbs and helps stop the stinging. Mitch, 62

One male gynaecologist told me to 'stop having rough sex'. I'd been single for years . . . Anne, 60

Sex hurt and I ended up with friction burns so badly that I was blistered and the GP tested me for herpes three times!!! It took three negative results for them to concede it was vaginal atrophy. Stressful and invasive. Kylie, 42

Sexual contact is razor-blades painful. Jan, 54

What helps general vaginal dryness

See the 'Your changing vagina' section over in Chapter 5, It's Your Body (or use the Index), but in short there are two main ways to treat vaginal dryness that's affecting your sex life: using an estrogen product, which will also help balance the microbiome (good and bad natural bacteria) in your vagina; or use a lubricant during sex. So:

* An estrogen-based cream or pessary can be placed high up in your vagina a couple of times a week using a self-basting little device.
* MHT helps, maybe.

Vaginal dryness extended to the whole general fanny area, and my skin was so dry I got little tears in places. I was prescribed a moisturiser and was told to lather it on generously daily. It was messy and I had to wear pads, but it worked. Kaz, 54

* Research continues into non-estrogen vaginal moisturisers and some non-estrogen products are already available. They don't do double duty like estrogen creams, which also balance your vaginal bacteria and help strengthen pelvic floor function.

Vaginal dryness has been avoided so far by acquiring a much younger companion. Erica, 50

In-vagina estrogen

Women who are taking topical estrogen cream or pessaries in the vagina, or a non-hormonal vaginal moisturiser two or three times a week, will have a more moisturised vagina, and boost their pelvic floor health, but they might still need lubricants during sex, as do many pre-perimenopausal women.

Prescribed in-vagina estrogen products are generally considered safe for women who can't take oral estrogen following cancer diagnosis, because they don't get any estrogen near breasts or the uterus, nor raise the risk of stroke, but ask your oncologist, gynaecologist, endocrinologist or GP.

I was prescribed an estrogen cream for topical use on my inner thigh. Based on my not being permitted to use HRT I was too afraid to try the cream. Catherine, 45

Vaginal moisturisers

There's a lot of big money put into ads for dry-vagina products, focusing on sexy and empowering imagery for older women, using models and the language of independence, and freedom. When it comes to menopause marketing, avoiding a man's sexual dissatisfaction is often implied.

No doubt they'll soon be using everything in the marketing arsenal: comedians, glamour, fancy names to do with queens, goddesses, various incarnations of the word feminine, icons of historical womanhood (I'm waiting for the Joan of Arc pessary), as well as 'you're worth it' pampering ideas, mature-age heart-throb silver foxes smouldering at the camera and the ye olde icon for selling women anything – the transformational butterfly.

Some commercial vaginal moisturisers might provide a temporary moisturising effect, but be careful of irritations, depending on the ingredients. In general the studies for them are not conclusive, based on their exact ingredients and dose.

> An expensive vaginal moisturiser does help somewhat but it can't be taken anywhere near when you want to have sex – my partner says it feels like I've put Vicks up there. ROFL.
> Cathie, 53

Don't buy a 'douche' or 'vaginal hygiene' product. You don't need to wash inside your vagina, and many of these products are responsible for irritation, and even infections, especially in perimenopause and beyond when your skin is thinner.

Ask a pharmacist rather than buying online or at a supermarket. As mentioned, non-hormone vaginal moisturising products don't efficiently help balance your vaginal pH as an estrogen cream does (see the 'Your changing vagina' and 'Mysteriously Irritable Vulva' sections in Chapter 5, It's Your Body).

Sellers of non-estrogenic vaginal lubricants say suggestive things like their product will have no adverse effect on a penis, as if estrogen cream does. It doesn't, because the estrogenic vaginal cream makes the vagina no more estrogen-ish than it used to be before the menopause. Penises can breathe easy (if the penis is breathing, please see a doctor).

What doesn't help general vaginal dryness

* So-called vaginal 'rejuvenation' surgery and laser procedures – see the argghhh-making details coming up.
* Pelvic floor (Kegel) exercises.
* Douches or other so-called cleansers.
* Non-prescription hormonal vaginal products often advertised as bio-identical hormones. Please check with your doctor. These products are not more 'natural' or better for you, and may not be registered and regulated for safety and doses.
* So-called phytoestrogen products based on red clover, black cohosh and soy (no evidence so far, and black cohosh can cause liver damage).

> I tried an over-the-counter vaginal cream from the chemist that felt like burning, and it was extremely embarrassing to have to go to the doctor about it on a Sunday morning.
> Lisa, 55

> OMG. Vaginal lubricants have saved my sanity.
> Adrienne, 52

> I went on a clinical trial because sex suddenly didn't enter my head, completely lost interest. Was shocked to discover that it was only about lubrication.
> **Hel, 53**

* Anything in the grab-bag of perfumed or coloured vaginal moisturisers, so-called G-spot or other vaginal injections, vaginal exfoliators (Good Lord and a half, NO), and luuuuuudicrous products promising to promote in-vagina collagen production.
* Any of those non-prescription dinky devices that look like little vibrators or wands that you put up your vagina (see 'Wands & other in-vagina devices' on page 294).

Lubricants to use during sex

In recent years, some social media happily ran ads for erection-help products, but routinely blocked ads for women's vaginal lubricants. Obviously we've known since the 1400s that women's bodies are way more dangerously disgusting than men's, and more sexual, and what comes out of our vagina can poison fruit trees and must not be mentioned (makes the sign of the cross). (See my book *You're Doing It Wrong: A History of Bad & Bonkers Advice to Women.*)

It's not wise to pop anything non-prescription up into your vagina except standard plant-based oils and water-based commercial sex lubricants, some of which have their own issues and irritants. (More on that coming up.)

> In the last 2 years I have had two different lovers, both younger than me and the sex has been awesome. I've needed no help with lube. **Libby, 51**

> HRT was key – my dry, chafing sore vagina has returned to something like its old self. Sex can still be painful, however.
> **Marion, 51**

While a vaginal moisturiser should give you relief from dry friction and itchiness, you'll still probably need a lubricant during the actual sex. Many companies now make sex lubricants – intimate or personal are usually the euphemisms used.

Lubricants should be clearly labelled as to whether they are water-, oil- or silicone-based. Preservative added is a good thing; in this case, you don't want to be shoving something that's gorn off up between your sensitive wonderwalls.

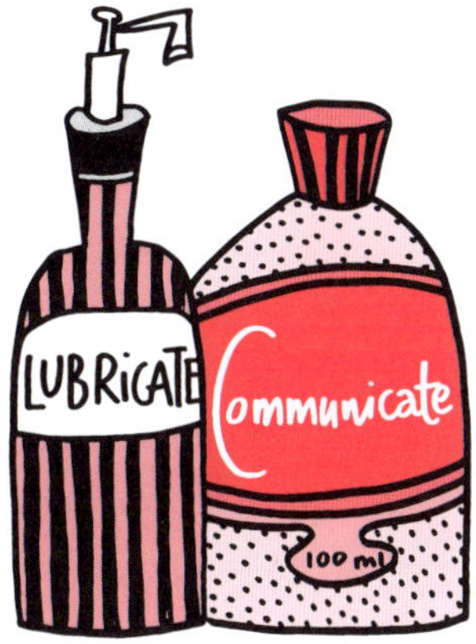

An increasingly common ingredient is CBD (cannabis oil): it doesn't make you high but sellers claim it relaxes muscles. The jury's still so far out on that, it's over the horizon.

Stuff to know:

* Look for a product designed to be a sex lubricant, one with no fragrance, alcohol or flavours or extra colouring.
* Any product may cause irritation for you.
* Avoid parabens and sulphates (common irritants).
* Go for a water-based lubricant although they do tend to wear off and need to be reapplied. Water-based lubricants are best to use with sex toys as some silicone-based ones can damage the surface of silicone toys, but it probably doesn't matter that much. Silicone lubricant is the hardest to wash off and more expensive.
* The glyceride in hyaluronic acid-based general vaginal moisturisers damages condoms.
* Oil-based lubricants also break down latex condom surfaces, a diaphragm or other latex products. Oils are harder to wash off people and sheets.
* DIY vegetable and other food oils can increase risk of vaginal infection, and some smell weird or cause stinging, especially on the thinner skin inside a menopausal vagina. Common recommendations are coconut oil, and purpose-made aloe vera sex lubricants or pure aloe oil, but do a rash test.
* There's no good reason to use any of the following as a sexual lubricant: powder, yoghurt, butter, margarine, Vaseline, baby oil, spit, conditioner or shampoo, body moisturiser, honey, Vegemite, marmalade (stand down, Lady Marmalade, *voulez-vous coucher avec* something else *ce soir*).

The multiple lube thing is really helpful – the balm is thick and protects the thin skin, the water-based feels like what my body produces naturally, and the silicone stuff is mostly on toys or my partner, and it lasts forever. Kate, 55

Husband prefers not to use lubricant – have to insist, otherwise I am in pain for days. Sarah, 51

(Sarah, I think I speak for us all when I say please ditch your bloody husband.)

Sex toys for the menopause

There's a boom in the sale of vibrators for older women; for those who enjoy a spot of alone sex or those who often have an accomplice. Quite a few companies now specialise in bendy silicone-covered dildos with a softer surface and some 'give', rather than hard plastic or glass dildos which have about the same comfort level as a sawn-off chair leg. Other vibrator products leave the vagina alone and concentrate on Orgasm Central, the clitoris.

> That new vibrator that does the suction thing on your clit. Woo hoo. Told by doctor at least two self-pleasuring orgasms per week required for vaginal health.
> Therese, 57

Beware of vibrators with apps that control them, or collect data. Might be best if only you know when you're using them and whether it's on a turbo setting.

You might consider vibrator must-have elements include medical-grade silicone (usually less-allergy-ruffling than latex), waterproof, USB charging (no batteries so better for the environment), a non-lifelike skin colour of any shade to avoid the ick factor, and a range of speeds that do not escalate to a punishing thumping. But you do you.

Other allegedly vagina-moisturising stuff you might want to totally avoid

I'd ignore these things if I were you:

Wands & other in-vagina devices

Devices which have an LED light, vibrate, claim to be magnetic, and/or 'emit gentle heat' and claim to increase vaginal blood flow, whether or not it sends data to an app plus you pay extra for a gel to allegedly enhance any for-heaven's-sake-that's-not-going-to-happen effect and little wands promising magnetic pulses, or, come off it, bi polar radiofrequency that 'improves your vagina's appearance'. WHAT? IT IS INSIDE YOU AND NOBODY CAN SEE IN THERE AND THIS IS UTTER RUBBISH AND IT MAKES ME WANT TO SMASH SOME WINDSCREENS WITH A TOFFEE HAMMER.

Anyway, they do not moisturise your vagina, they do not make it tighter, they do nothing useful and cost hundreds of dollars. I've seen online so-called journalists recommending them, saying 'real science is behind it', on sites that 'receive a portion of sales from products purchased from this article'. I will fight them on the school oval.

Vaginal laser procedures

Do. Not. Do. This.

That's my advice. Some gynaecologists and even GPs around the world are heavily advertising or suggesting to clients a laser procedure called 'vaginal rejuvenation', aka other silly phrases such as the 'MonaLisa Touch'. Specialists who don't make money from doing this tell me they said no to renting a laser machine equipment for $150,000 to $200,000 a year, which would have meant they had to hustle for enough clients to cover the cost of something that doesn't work. The lease cost is why the 'procedure' costs many hundreds, or even thousands of dollars. There's no Medicare benefit payable (and neither there should be) and each doctor invents their own price.

There's no such officially recognised gynaecology qualification as a 'vaginal laser specialist': usually the only training provided is how to use the machine and promote the procedure. Australian health regulators don't recognise it as a treatment to combat vaginal dryness; there's no central regulation of it and no public health data collected on who's doing it.

The 'treatment' uses heat created by laser beams to deliberately cause limited burn damage to the inside surface of the vagina, which according to people who have done it, produces varying degrees of pain. In cases where something goes wrong, severe burns have been inflicted. As the vagina tries to heal itself, the skin swells temporarily, feeling spongier because it produces new cells and mucous to try to protect itself from the injury.

This swelling inside the vagina has prompted advertisers to claim wrongly that the treatment makes the vagina 'tighter'. It does not. Because the amazing self-cleaning recovering vagina heals over a few days or weeks and gets back to its own normal, it is then deemed to be too dry again and a new laser 'treatment' is recommended.

Some women have reported feeling significant pain during and after the procedure, others say afterwards it's like having your insides sunburned. American regulators and anecdotal evidence in Australia says that women have suffered burns, scarring, the walls of their vagina sticking together while healing, and recurring and chronic pain.

While vaginal laser-wielders say there should be at least three treatments, and more after 18 months for a 'top-up,' there's no known scientifically reliable study to say why. No study exists on long-term effects. There's no acceptable research to back newer claims that it helps with pelvic floor problems or leaky wee, and specialists say they can't see how it could. Overseas, the treatment is often said to improve long-term sexual satisfaction, and simulate proof of 'virginity'. Eurghh.

Most of the people doing laser treatments also prescribe women topical and/or other estrogen treatments at the same time, which would improve lubrication, that may then be attributed to the laser. Of 2900 women who answered the question in the Menopause Survey about their experience with the vaginal laser, 98 per cent said they don't know if it helped.

MonaLisa Touch. Useless for me; uncomfortable and expensive.
Jane, 57

No claimed effect from vaginal lasers was produced in the first independent, randomised, double-blind study in which people didn't know if they were getting the laser treatment or a pretend one. No uptick in vaginal moistness, no help with an itchy vulva, no better urinary function nor anything else significant. If women have this treatment and think it's helped them, specialists believe they're experiencing a placebo effect: possibly more powerful if you're spent hundreds or thousands of dollars on something. Few of us want to admit we've been somehow scammed, or pressured into presuming a benefit when there really wasn't one.

I paid a fair amount for vaginal laser procedures and they really did not do much at all.
Sharon, 50

None of the gynaecologists that I consider the top specialists in Australia do this procedure. Many are scathing about it, even sweary.

The most recent available statement from the peak professional body of gynaecologists, the Royal Australia and New Zealand College of Obstetricians and Gynaecologists says there's no evidence that vaginal laser procedures are useful or effective and risks include scarring, damage to the vaginal walls, disfigurement, infection and painful sex.

Vaginal & clitoral injections

Do. Not. Do. This. Either.

Even if it's a qualified doctor offering a 'G-shot' or 'O-shot', both injection titles patented for marketing use by doctors in the US and also going by other names. And don't get an injection of your own harvested blood platelets or stem cells into the wall of your vagina: there's no independent evidence whatsoever for any orgasmic benefit recognised by vagina experts, or that doesn't come from people making money out of it.

I would absolutely not trust claims by doctors who say it improves sexual arousal by, say, 87 per cent (but of course not 86), or the claim that it does anything at all to help incontinence problems. People who've had the injection describe intense pain even with numbing cream. Yeah, because they're basically injecting right into different hidden parts of your clitoris structure, through your vaginal wall.

For me this is the quintessential classic of the genre 'Just because it can be done, doesn't mean you should do it'.

Vaginal injections are wackily expensive, and introduce an element of risk where there is no need. Ask a gynaecologist or endocrinologist with a menopause specialty who does not make money from these 'services' and I bet you they say don't waste your money and make an unbecoming, snorty sort of a noise.

The takeaway on your sex life

Give everything dubious a long hard stare and possibly run away instead of putting it in your vagina – that goes for douches and cleansers, dodgy moisturisers, so-called wellness or 'rejuvenation' devices, and any part of a man who has a waxed ringmaster moustache (IMO).

Straight or gay, if it gets in the way, get help. You don't have to have a sex life at all, but don't put up with a bad one. There's no point addressing your libido if any resulting sex is going to hurt or bore you insensible.

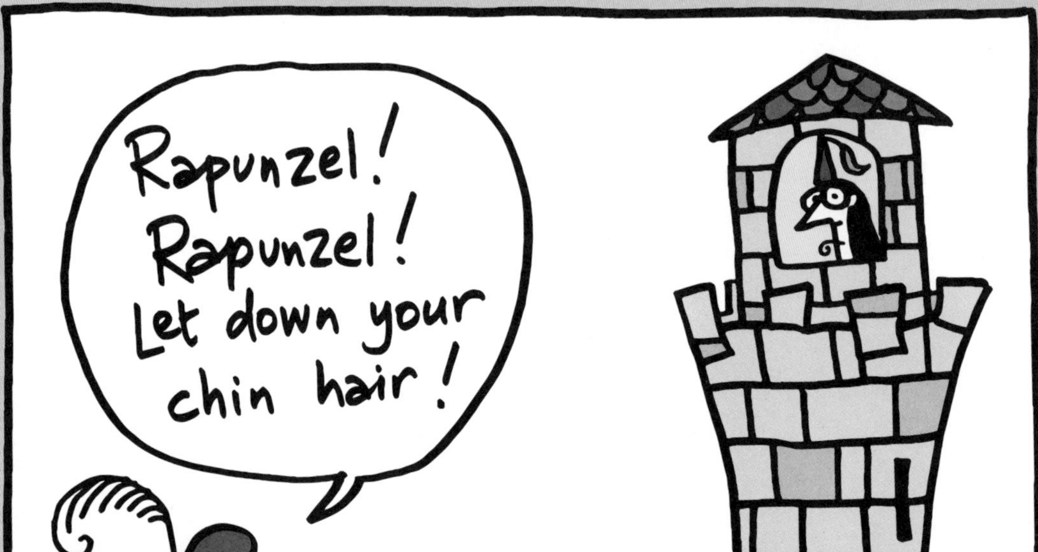
Rapunzel! Rapunzel! Let down your chin hair!
KAZ

7

It's How You Look

When the Witch of the West in the musical *Wicked*, Elphaba, sings that she's 'defying gravity', she isn't talking about menopausal bosoms, or a real face.

Women in peri- or in menopause are still told how to act by a society with impossible standards about everything from how we speak to what we wear, and whether our face looks as old as the rest of us. We're told to 'grow old gracefully', which is to say, not at all. Women are mocked for looking older and mocked for looking like they've 'had work'. Can't win that one.

I always thought the retro-cult hit 1980s TV show *The Golden Girls* was about elderly women in a retirement village of some kind, but over the 8-year-long course of the series Rose is meant to be aged 55 to 62 (though she pretended to be 47 at the start), and Blanche and Dorothy's characters aged from 53 to 60. When I think back to my nanna's generation, they didn't dye their hair much past the age of 55, or do much to themselves except for the occasional swipe of Apricot Coral lippy and a slather of Nivea from an industrial-sized jar.

As Judith Lucy says,
'You can age naturally or you can look weird.' I prefer the former!
Bee, 48
(This is outrageous, but since my dear friend Jude always credited me when she said this on stage, I shall overlook the matter.)

Looking older and going grey aren't symptoms of menopause in the way we understand hormonal carry-on, although hormones contribute. And these effects of being older are sometimes the ones we feel most challenged by, or, if they don't annoy us, seem to annoy other people, for whom looking older is considered a fate worse than . . . well, death.

I feel like I've been trying to write reassuring and practical things about the bombardment of the unfair and unrealistic 'body and beauty' culture/marketing/worldview almost all my life. But here we go again. (See Chapter 3, It's Your Approach, for the 'Exercise' and 'Eating & weight' sections.)

You can't keep your face. The older you get, the more your choice is probably between looking older or weirder. People who use fillers and paralysing injections will be cross about this, and some will say hotly, 'I don't look weird'. What they mean is, 'I could look a lot weirder'. They're right.

But they don't look young or frozen in time. Eventually, they just look like somebody who's had paralysing injections and fillers, just as others will look like they're older. Depending on the friendship group or profession you're in, cosmetic procedures might feel compulsory, normalised, done in secret, or (ha) frowned upon.

One choice is not more moral than another; but one is more expensive and carries much more risk. As usual, women are condemned by others whichever route they take. A series of disabling and disfiguring injectables, and botched filler and filler-removal scandals, in recent years has shown that under-regulated, under-qualified doctors and nurses in the cosmetic industry took their toll. I believe one of the reasons it took so long for these investigative stories to break is that in the past, male-dominated newsrooms considered cosmetic procedures as vain, and therefore trivial.

How are we to simultaneously grow old gracefully, embrace the body we're in, go make-up free, look decades younger than we are, not dye our hair because it's vain, dye our hair because natural grey is more likely to look like steel wool than a luxurious ironed mane of silver, embrace the natural look but don't actually look natural, and find more time for yourself, pay for fillers,

I just don't have the energy to put on a sparkly lip and be fabulous anymore like I'm told it will make me feel better.
Al, 49

Botox, lasers, skin treatment, and expensive anti-ageing cosmetics which are not anti-ageing? (That's a trick question.)

The internet knows how old you are and what you've searched online, hence the endless, unsolicited ads in your social media feed for wrinkles, so-called bloating (aka having a stomach and the ineluctable hormonal re-distribution of weight), and more. My algorithm sends me a steady stream of self-loathery; I've managed to confuse it further by searching for heavy meta-skateboard memes and Eastern European fish species.

In the Survey, more than 6200 women indicated what they worried about when it comes to their appearance: more than a third said facial wrinkles; about a third said thinning hair, and another third said, well, they worried about . . . kind of . . . everything.

Lots of women mentioned unexpected skin changes that gave them the irrits as they got older, including enduring pimples, and rosacea, a red rash or blotches that can flare up on their own, especially from drinking alcohol, exercise or being in the sun.

I recently read one of those 'Five essential make-up tips for older women' articles, which flounces out with the usual stricty-pants rules based on some pitiless marketeer's prompts: use reflective make-up foundation, match your lipstick to your gum colour, don't tattoo your brows in case they go wrong, don't wear any eye shadow and conceal the dark marks under your eyes (try a velvet curtain). Likewise, women are told to dress carefully so as not to 'age themselves' as if ageing was a matter of forgetfulness, not chronology.

I don't like society's obsession with looking younger than you are.
Dimity, 55

Didn't think I was vain but maybe I am. Feeling a tad anxious about this, never used to feel anxiety about my looks.
Pamela, 49

The hands at the end of my arms look so old.
Lizza, 58

I have to draw my eyebrows on with a bloody pencil. **Esmerelda, 52**

None of us like losing our looks.
Steph, 53

There are hairs in places I don't want them, my boobs are bigger than ever before & gravity is a cruel thing! My hair is thinner & going grey, my skin is not as it was. **Jan, 60**

Take me as I am.
Petta, 49

My face is my story.
Fiona, 61

May I be impertinent enough to suggest:

- Leave the pitiless lighting to hotel, car, shop and aeroplane toilets, not your home.
- Do an occasional check to make sure you don't have broccoli on your teeth or lipstick or an eyebrow.
- Use mirrors for glancing, not inspecting, except for regular checks (once every month, or February 29th in a leap year), using turned-up lighting or a dreaded magnifying mirror to admire/pluck any stray chin hairs or tiny scissors to arrest the more tendrilish nose hairs.

If you want to; otherwise let the fluffening run free.

I'm always reminded of the eventual, hilarious transformation of Dame Barbara Cartland, to whom it never occurred that her eyesight was worse. This resulted in her startling make-up choices in her 80s and 90s: false eyelashes the size of tarantulas, iridescent blue eyeshadow up to the drawn-in eyebrows and giant plate-sized circles of hot pink rouge. Best of all, because she couldn't see her wrinkles anymore, she firmly explained that they'd been erased by the honey made in bees' heads, normally fed to larval queen bees in the hive.

We'll get onto hair (grey hair, thinning hair and the hair that migrates from your legs to your upper lip) but first, let's talk skin.

Skin changes

Dry skin in general is in Chapter 5, It's Your Body, and how a dry vagina affects hotsi-totsiness is in Chapter 6, It's Your Sex Life. But now . . . back to gravity.

I look like a perfect combination of my parents, complete with thinning hair (thanks, Mum) and sagging jowls (thanks, Dad). Di, 54

My anti-ageing remedies are natural. Corporations targeting the fears of women can go fuck themselves, as far as I'm concerned. Lisa, 51

I jump on Instagram and see flawless filtered faces (sometimes of people I know) and it erodes my self-esteem. Barbara, 48

Wrinkles & gravity

> Freedom not to be so concerned with aesthetics! I feel I've earned my wrinkles and I'm not ashamed of them.
> **Irene, 61**

You know how you do that thing when you look at a crowded kindergarten class photo and try and pick out the face that belonged to an adult you know? Or those 'Which celebrity is this?' childhood photos online? It's because we have at least three or four phases of face in our lives: little kid, teen, adult, and old. We have the adult version of our face, if we're lucky, for a few decades.

If you look at a very old woman's face, and then immediately at her kindergarten pic, you might be lucky to spot any telltale features that have survived, except perhaps a twinkle in the eye. The much older face is relaxed and folded into myriad wrinkles, with pouches, and droops caused by gravity and depletion of self-made collagen and elastin.

In perimenopause we're not there yet. But we're all on our way. After the age of 50 the jawline softens, and eyelids drape down. We get thinner lips and upper lip lines, and our hands and necks will look as old as we are. Places we used sunscreen on will look years, maybe decades, younger.

Eyebrows start to disappear, the fat padding around the eyes and cheekbones takes its leave, and previous lines that only appeared during a particular facial expression begin to be etched faintly, then assertively stay put, even when you don't frown or smile.

> My facial skin has really suddenly lost all elasticity and I'm sick of people asking me if I'm tired because my face looks like an empty bag.
> **Sam, 50**

Or as my daughter once said fondly when she was a child running a little forefinger down my forehead: 'Mummy, you have a barcode.'

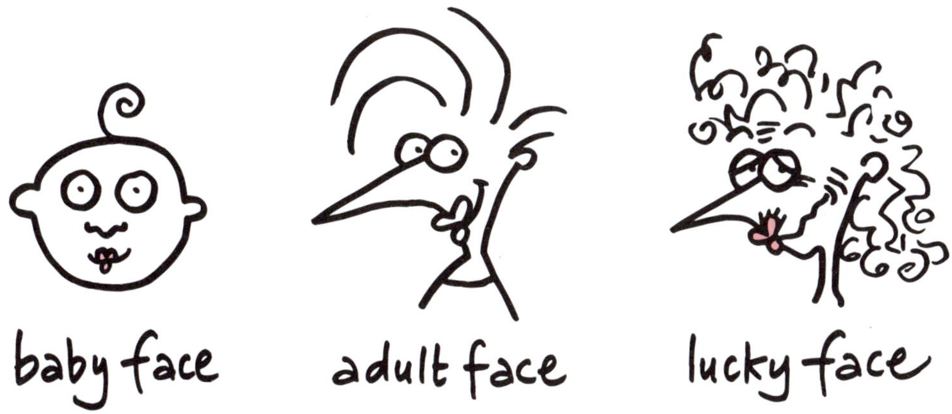

> Looking old terrifies me. I think it's because the outside doesn't match the inside and it just feels so weird and wrong. Also I think society sees old women as ridiculous. Like you lose your credibility. Ali, 49

> I'm always looking at other people's wrinkles. I think mine are worse, Lee 52

> My face is my face. I like it. Annette, 53

It seems just as we get used to our adult face, it starts morphing into a middle-aged face, and then an elderly one. As changes seem to accelerate, it can feel like we're losing the 'comfortable in your own skin' feeling because when we look in the mirror, it seems to be not us at all, but our mothers, or an older version of ourselves that doesn't match how we feel as our middle-aged face gently scrumples into our old one. Statistically we're living longer, and that means we're going to look older, because we are.

In the Survey, about four in five women said they use 'anti-ageing' creams. One in five had tried face peels; about 18 per cent used Botox or similar products.

Word alert

To make women feel worse about themselves, cosmetic surgeons and salon marketing have popularised certain cruel or self-loathing language: back fat, marionette lines, stringy neck, unacceptable nose, breast atrophy. Breast enlargement is always referred to as the more approving 'enhancement' or 'augmentation'. 'Tubular breast correction' means making breasts less pointy. Other words are used to minimise the procedure and possible gruesome side effects, including 'tummy tuck', refresh, 'little lift'. Don't start me on 'vaginal rejuvenation' (too late, see Chapter 6, It's Your Sex Life, for more than you bargained on what that nonsense actually means).

When words mean nothing

None of these terms opposite used in ads for cosmetics mean anything, really. They're all things that women want, which sellers say they can deliver. They certainly don't guarantee the product will do what you think it will do, or what they're implying it will do. Even if they say it in French. Look out for marketing about 'studies prove' or 'clinically proven'. Something that made five mice livers look younger in a Finnish laboratory petri dish or a survey of five women who got free samples is not proof of anything.

Here are some marketing words to consider disbelieving or scoffing at, that might have been made up to match what you're worried about:

Magic impossibilities
Anti-ageing
Chemical free
Homeopathic

Sciencey
Technology
-ceuticals
Cellular health
Science-based
Bio-
Micro-
Phyto-
Nutri-
Medi-
Pharma-
Clinically proven
Proven
Formula
Shown to

We know you want it
Age-defying
Anti-wrinkle
Minimiser
Day cream
Night cream
Eye cream
Neck cream
Filler
Plumper
Deep

Pretendy surgery
Lifting
Sculpting

Meaningless
Supports
Encourages
Helps
Helps support
Approved
Improving
Improves the appearance of

Rooly rooly good
Potent
Super
Rapid
Multi-effect
Supreme
Essential
Advanced

Lantern-like
Radiance
Glow
Light
Brighten
Luminous

Fancypants
Ultimate
Luxury

Wellnessy
Clean eating
Natural
Green
Healthy

Time-travelling
Youth
Young
Replenish
Renew
Repair
Restore
Recover
Reverse
Regeneration
Corrector
Resilience

Warlike strength
Salon formula
Triple-effect
Wrinkle-fighting
Combats
Extra/maximum strength
Defence
Restorative

Doesn't do anything of the sort
Firming

Kindness
Nurturing
Care

Could mean anything
Visible
Award-winning
Smoothing
Active

Extra points to Dior for coming right out and calling one of its face creams 'Prestige'. And to Clinique for getting away with the product name that sounds like a drunken tirade about weaponry: 'Repairwear Laser Focus Night'.

> I don't buy into any of them (I am a scientist). I use a moisturiser on my face and body, that's the extent of my care regime. Louise, 52

> Was really annoyed when I was about 40 and having a facial. The young woman doing it said I had a lot of wrinkles around my eyes and mouth. Der! Dinah, 59

Why does your face change?

We look older because:

- our skin is less plumped out by fat padding where it used to be (cheeks, lips, breasts).
- our skin droops due to gravity and much less elastin and the protein collagen in our skin
- skin changes make for a less uniform colour and texture: spots and patches appear. These changes can come quicker or be more noticeable if you've spent time in the sun, ever smoked, or have been exposed to heavy air pollution.

Prinkles

During perimenopause it's quite normal to get pimples on wrinkles: prinkles. Yes. It is preposterous. That is all.

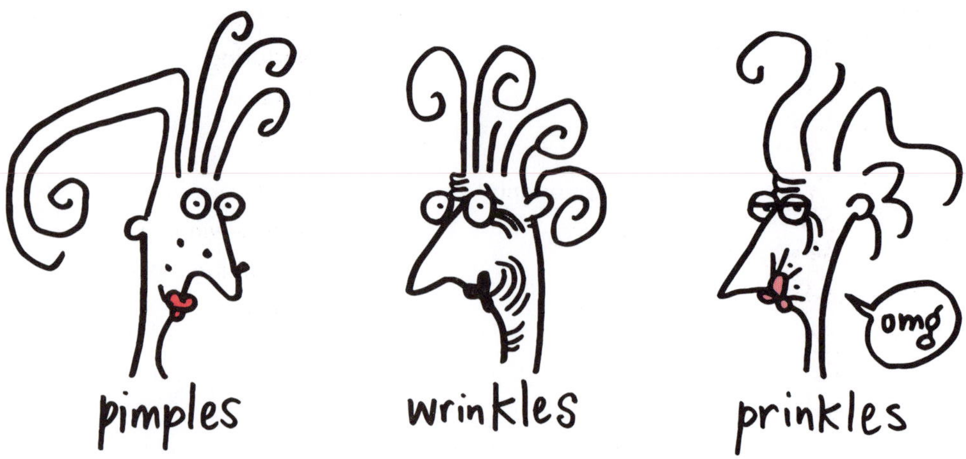

Things that can change or affect your skin

I'm not recommending these, just saying they can do something to your skin. None are free of side effects, risks, costs and emotional impacts:

* An estrogen supplement will help reverse some of the effects of thinner, drier skin and eyes, in general, and help keep some collagen production going, although it doesn't prevent or reverse any effects of skin ageing. MHT is not a good treatment if you just want cosmetic results.
* High levels of vitamin A can affect the skin in different ways. (Very high levels of vitamin A can cause birth defects: consult a doctor.)
* Some pharmaceutical and cosmetic products include acids and exfoliants and take off the top layer of skin, causing temporary plumping and pinking on pale skin due to inflammation; the skin resurfaces itself looking 'newer'.
* Moisturisers, sunscreens and barrier creams protect skin.
* Cosmetic or corrective surgery can excise or hoist skin, but further changes in your own levels of elastin and collagen, and gravity, will again create sagging.

> Anti-ageing is a made up term. You can't anti-age, we're all ageing. Emily, 47

> I hate myself for this vanity. Michelle, 54

What causes wrinkles

Over time, these things cause lines:

* moving your face
* natural reduction in body-made collagen and elastin
* staying alive
* smoking
* the effects of sunlight
* a low humidity, winter or summer environment.

> I fell for anti-ageing products in my 30s. No longer bothered. Cecile, 47

> I like my wrinkles. They show I have lived and have an expressive face. Margot, 53

> I worked hard to get all my wrinkles and laugh lines. Leigh, 49

What helps reduce wrinkles

Inclusion in this list should not be mistaken for a recommendation:

* Any moisturiser will 'reduce the appearance of fine lines' while it's on, as it softens the top layer of skin.
* Medical-grade injected paralysing toxins will create a temporary effect, preventing you from exercising muscles.
* Don't ever form facial expressions which may reveal a line; also avoid thoughts, which can lead to facial expressions.
* Live underground.

What doesn't change, reverse or prevent wrinkles

These things:

* moisturisers, with or without special ingredients
* injected fillers
* ingestible and topical products containing collagen
* facial exercises
* electrical currents
* skin-heating devices
* radio waves
* puncturing the skin, including acupuncture and 'vampire facials'
* tiny rollers made of jade, plastic, marble, rubber, cheese or anything else
* anything claimed to 'better deliver' or get moisturiser deeper into your skin
* alleged 'superfoods', supplements in the form of powders, tinctures, pills, green powders, marine oil, fish oil, crude oil or oil paint
* any so-called cellulite 'treatment' that is rubbed extra-vigorously will cause low-level swelling and redness, which may temporarily mask the look of cellulite dimples.

It's hard to see your body deteriorating and watching yourself turn into your mother. Jeannie, 59

Do we ever know if face cream really makes a difference? But we still use them. Mel, 57

All these products don't work but we keep buying them in hope. Leanne, 56

I want to be able to celebrate who I am, and what I can do, rather than focus on physical traits. This is not an easy journey in today's world. Justine, 52

Collagen

As you get older your body makes less collagen to plump out your skin. You can't replace it by injecting collagen into your skin as it won't do the job in the same way as body-made collagen, or have the same effect.

Collagen molecules are too big to be absorbed into the skin from the outside to do anything useful: think of it as trying to fit a chair down a plughole. It doesn't work and there's no point. Dermatologists who don't sell collagen-containing products generally don't think ingesting collagen can help much or at all, including cow, pig or marine collagen products in food, powders or pills.

'Vegan' collagen is not actually collagen, and any marketing that says a cream or pill 'supports collagen' or 'supports elastin' or is 'scientifically proven' almost certainly means nothing for your skin.

A new sensitivity

Many women in the Survey reported greater sensitivity to products, and having to deal with unfamiliar rashes in perimenopause. You may need to experiment with very plain, non-perfumed products with few ingredients.

All my skin products started producing itchy, red reactions. Months of dermatitis. Only one very cheap moisturiser doesn't upset my face. Angela, 53

Facial peels, abrasions, blading & exfoliation

There's a long history of removing the top layer of your skin for 'newer', glowing (red and irritated) skin to grow back, recover and resurface, going all the way back to the ghastly results wrought with sulphuric acid in the 19th century.

Now, chemical peels, lasers and scrubs have varying degrees of depth and effect. Older skin may not recover in the way younger skin did, so even if done by a professional, risks can include scarring, pigmentation changes and infection. I'm afraid you'll have to 'do your own research' before that leap of faith. Please do see the 'Who's Who in skin & hair doctors' box, on page 319.

I feel more myself. Being invisible means you can do what you like! Imelda, 65

I finally don't allow myself to feel judged by other because of my appearance. I finally own my big bum. Lisa, 54

Botox & fillers

As loooong ago as 2016, the membership organisation covering non-surgical cosmetic procedures (mainly paralysing injections and fillers) estimated that more than a billion dollars is spent by Australians each year on laser hair removal, chemical peels and injections, with $350 million going to paralysing injections such as Botox (there's no way of verifying those figures, which just keep being repeated in online stories).

Some women spend hundreds of dollars, perhaps thousands, each year to get Botox and plumping filler injections, whether or not they want to look like someone on a Housewives franchise reality show. It's common to start in their 20s.

Feminists now will say, 'Oh, I just do it so I don't look tired'. And I get it. We don't want to feel tired, look tired, feel our faces slipping away from us. You're damned if you don't (she's let herself go, let's cast someone younger, that's not the image we want in this company) and damned if you do (she's vain, she looks weird, who even is she, she can't move her face).

Botox and other paralysing agents are now normalised to the point that it's considered a woman's choice to spend hundreds of dollars a year on it, and the fact the active ingredient is a toxin isn't worth mentioning in online articles about it. (For the record, the amount of toxin in one unit of Botox is the measurement that's enough to kill a mouse, but obviously it doesn't have the same effect on a human.)

I find it so hard to look in the mirror and see wrinkles and jowls. I had assumed I would meet ageing with grace and peace, but I don't at all . . . I meet it with panic and despair. **Elizabeth, 48**

I don't judge others for it – I understand the pressure women are under. I just don't think it is right in society overall. **Amanda, 49**

I feel embarrassed that I've had Botox five times, and haven't told anyone! **Natasha, 46**

Botox was not useful. I think I am happy with my face now. **Stix, 59**

I only did it a few times but loved it. I found I felt so good about myself after that, I didn't go back! **Lisa, 51**

I think about my deteriorating 'beauty' and what a great mother I am to my 19-year-old daughter - she tells me all the time that I am so important to her and she appreciates my love and wisdom. **Marian, 61**

Had Botox once and won't again – it looks weird and I'd rather spend money on adventures. **JJ, 64**

Paralysing and filler injections usually are absorbed into the body over time, but a rise in botched jobs and lasting effects, especially by unqualified 'practitioners', has seriously alarmed health regulators. Injections to allegedly 'remove' or dissolve fillers have themselves caused infections and disfigurement.

I don't wear a bra after realising I had achieved age-induced invisibility. I discovered this at a Coles deli counter. Becky, 69

Do it disgracefully. Lee, 58

Age gracefully. Whether that means doing nothing or doing everything possible to pretend it's not happening. It doesn't matter what anyone else thinks or does. Kylie, 57

'Ageing gracefully'

Variously interpreted as a senior version of sit down and shoosh, or an exhortation not to slack off your grooming for a nanosecond.

Celebrity 40, celebrity 50, and celebrity 60

If I see one more stupid magazine or social media photo of a celebrity with a face as smooth and white as a boiled egg, and a heading like '50 is the new 30' I shall scream. No it isn't. 50 is fucking 50, and that's okay. That's an achievement, damnit.

When you see a photo of a 60-year-old celebrity who looks like they're in their 20s, you're seeing genes, and artifice, and probably cosmetic surgery and injections, and the work of a couple of hours of make-up and more of hair, and professional lighting and then a whole lot of digital alteration.

We're compared to celebrities who lie about their age and lie about how they got their body to look like that. If you're going to compare yourself to a digitally altered Elle Macpherson in a bikini or Jennifer Lopez pole-dancing, you may as well compare yourself to a meerkat for all it has to do with you.

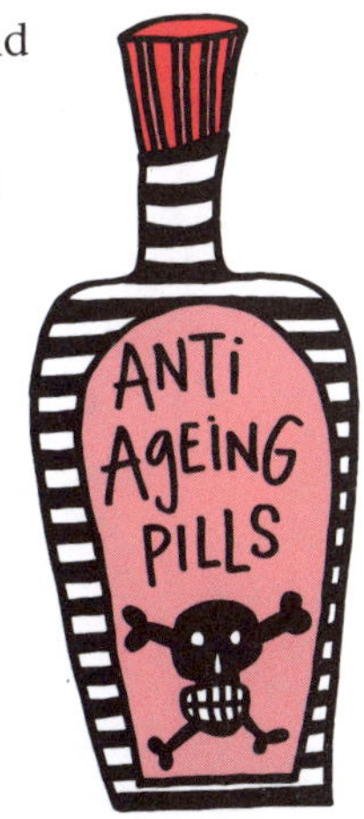

I swear by my Korean snail mucin (a face cream with snail mucus)! Keeps me dewy. Rachel, 50

Wearing a bikini in your 50s is not an achievement, it's either just going for a swim, or a performance. Looking at social media about grey hair, it's always older models with the same sort of figure, with professionally just-done hair. Find yourself looking at articles on 'mid-life' or 'middle-age' embaubled by altered photos of celebrities in their 60s or even 70s who look like robots upholstered in Laminex? Close the browser window, burn the newspaper magazine section, or audibly taunt it. I *know* you know this but I'm telling you again because we need to chant to ourselves: 'That's not real.'

I'm not opposed to more tweakments . . . I sometimes worry that I should put my money to better use (such as topping up my super).
Anna, 45

Women should be allowed to age naturally. Fuck the patriarchy.
Katie, 61

Adjusting compliments

'You don't look it' is meant to be a compliment when you tell someone your age (although they may well mean that when you're 52 you look like a sprightly octogenarian). In my mother's generation, 'well-preserved' was a compliment, as if women were prize pickles. We can truthfully say to our friends, 'You look gorgeous', or 'You look great' or 'Where did you get those fabulous shoes?'. We don't have to say, 'You look young'. We *don't* look young.

And conversely, there should be no insult in 'She's looking her age' or 'She seems every bit of her 50-plus years'. Damn right she does, she bloody earned it.

Every line is a badge of honour. Ageing is a privilege not afforded to everyone.
Wendy, 53

All the women on my mum's side eventually have eyelids obscuring part of their vision. I'm going to get mine fixed.
Liz, 60

I earned these winkles and am happy to wear them. Ruthie, 60

Crow's feet – a sign of a life well laughed!
Kerri-Ann, 61

I'm me. I don't need to look like anyone else.
Jen, 70

Who's Who in cosmetic practitioners

(See also the 'Who's Who in skin & hair doctors' box on page 319.)

The past ineffectiveness or inability of medical regulatory bodies to police the cosmetic procedures industry in a meaningful way has led to some terrible outcomes for patients or clients. Mostly, you're on your own to decide whether a practitioner is safe or compliant, or appropriately experienced and skilled.

Some devices and/or procedures they're used for are unregistered with health authorities and therefore unregulated and uncontrolled. No cosmetic injection, laser or other service is risk-free. The federal government recently required state and territory health ministers to begin talks on reforming the rules on who can call themselves a cosmetic surgeon or physician, and to ban 'patient testimonials' as marketing.

Plastic surgeons

Australian plastic surgeons are doctors who do basic medical training (a 4–6 year degree, followed by a year of training in a hospital), at least two more years in surgical training, then five more years in the Plastic and Reconstructive Surgery training program of the Royal Australasian College of Surgeons, with extra study, exams and training, including observing, assisting and performing thousands of surgeries in total. This is the only qualification in plastic or cosmetic surgery recognised by the Australian Government. Qualified doctors have these letters after their name: FRACS–Plast.

You need the FRACS-Plast qualification to be a member of the Australian Society of Plastic Surgeons (ASPS), which has a subgroup of members who belong to the Australasian Society of Aesthetic Plastic Surgeons (ASAPS), meaning they have a special interest in cosmetic work, and/or the Australian Academy of Facial Plastic Surgery (AAFPS), whose members are ear, nose and throat surgeons with a special interest in facial cosmetic surgery. These letters don't indicate an extra qualification but show their field of expertise or special interest.

Having a properly qualified plastic surgeon doesn't mean your procedure or surgery is guaranteed to be a success. Things can still go wrong – mistakes, unavoidable complications, and infections. Even when a surgeon is satisfied with their job, you might have expected different results.

The Australian Society of Plastic Surgeons site **plasticsurgery.org.au** has lots of info on risks and results, and FAQs about surgery, diagrams showing how procedures work. (Infoline 1300 367 446)

'Cosmetic surgeon', 'cosmetic doctor', 'aesthetic physician'
Several clinics advertise the fact that work is done by 'cosmetic doctors' or 'specialists'. This can mean a GP who's seen a training video or attended a two-day course and then added letters after their name. You cannot legally call yourself a plastic surgeon unless you've successfully completed all the training and experience (see page 313).

Laws are under review but at the time of writing in several places in Australia you can call yourself a 'cosmetic surgeon', 'cosmetic doctor' or 'cosmetic specialist' if you have a standard GP level of training.

A cosmetic doctor who isn't a plastic surgeon may have extensive experience in doing a certain sort of procedure and be good at it, or might not be good at it. They may be a GP who has never performed even the most basic surgeries by themselves, nor be qualified as a member of the Royal Australasian College of Surgeons (RACS). Words like 'Cosmetic Institute' or 'Cosmetic Clinic' don't indicate anything except it's a business name given to a clinic by the person who owns it. Currently, two organisations represent members who are cosmetic doctors, but there's no accepted nationally recognised specialty qualification of cosmetic surgery.

The Australasian College of Cosmetic Surgery: the letters MACCS after a doctor's name mean that he or she is a member, but don't relate to any qualifications. This can mean they're a GP who has made cosmetic procedures, their specialty. Many of these doctors use a seal or logo on advertisements and in clinics. The College conducts training, has a voluntary code of practice, and runs an in-house complaints panel with no legal powers.

The Cosmetic Physicians Society of Australasia: members are mainly GPs who do non-surgical cosmetic procedures such as filler and paralysing injections. Membership is indicated by the letters CPSA after a doctor's name (unrelated to qualifications), or a seal or logo on advertisements and in clinics.

medicalboard.gov.au
The site of the federal government's Medical Board of Australia. Choose 'Look up a practitioner' for your doctor's qualifications and registration status or special requirements. You can check if your doctor has ever been deregistered or has special regulatory conditions imposed on their practice.

Aestheticians, technicians & beauty therapists

Any of these can point a laser or other cosmetic device at you or conduct a chemical peel of your skin. I could, if I felt like it. Anybody can legally operate an ultrasound machine or a laser they've hired or bought, for cosmetic reasons. They may have just watched a video on how to use the equipment. Some workplaces require more training and experience.

There are myriad private college diplomas and certificates for cosmetic workers. Some therapists are members of the Association of Professional Aestheticians of Australia (APAA) or its subset, the Australian Medical and Clinical Laser Professionals (AMCLP). Those letters indicate membership of the group, not specialist qualifications.

If your skin is going to be pierced or peeled away or abraded, or if 'waves' of any kind or a heat device is involved, it's safest to make sure your treatment is administered by a doctor with the highest relevant qualifications, such as a dermatologist.

Salons that call themselves a 'clinic' or 'institute' and talk of 'patients', put staff in white coats, and use terms such as 'serums' and 'cosmeceutical', may not have a single medically qualified person on staff. I don't think anyone should be breaking your skin or using a medical device on you unless they have medical or extremely high-standard science-based qualifications. Ask what each treatment really means and if a doctor is involved, then check qualifications.

Nurses

Qualified 'theatre' nurses will assist in operations in registered hospitals. In clinics doing only cosmetic operations, check the qualifications of the nurses. A nurse 'under a doctor's supervision' (usually meaning a doctor has seen you first and prescribed the 'treatment') can inject paralysers and fillers into your face, and assist during other procedures and surgical operations, and recovery time.

The letters after a nurse's name should include RN for Registered Nurse (with the Nursing and Midwifery Board of Australia) or EN (for enrolled nurse, an official, lesser nursing qualification).

There are no extra qualifications for nurses doing cosmetic work recognised by the Australian Government's medical authorities, and you'll have to make your own assessment of their training, experience and skill level.

nursingmidwiferyboard.gov.au

To check if a nurse is registered with the federal government's Nursing and Midwifery Board of Australia, choose 'Look up a practitioner'.

> I just try to remember my body has done its very best to house this spirit of mine. In my younger years I was not always appreciative of the way it looked and I did not treat it in the way it deserved.
> **Lisa, 51**

The impact on my appearance has been the worst aspect of menopause for me. I had no idea that everything can change. Nicole, 55

I think women should do what they want. I used to be judgemental of others doing stuff, but I have changed my mind. After all, I do a lot to enhance my appearance in other ways, and I certainly care about how I look. Dimity, 51

A combination of poverty and feminism rules out surgery. Marlo, 54

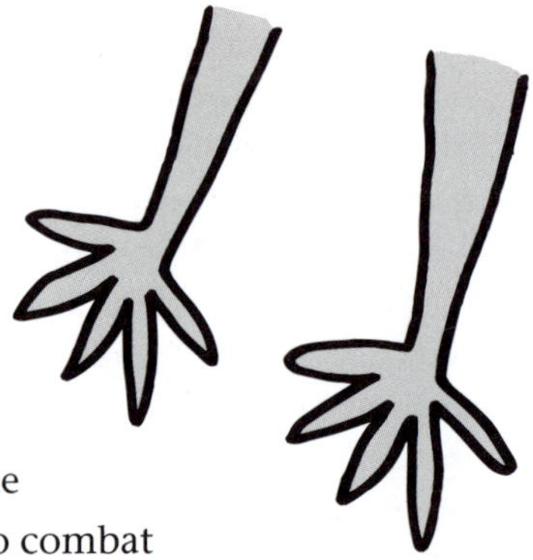

Hands

Women who have facelifts, paralysing injections and fillers are warned that their hands 'give them away' as it's harder to hide the effects of age there. My mother gave me a pair of white cotton 'driving gloves' when I turned 40 to combat age-spots forming on my hands from UV damage. (I didn't wear them.)

No exfoliator, moisturisers, acid treatment, collagen pills or plumping injections will reverse the ageing look of your hands, or reverse your larger knuckles, or prevent you from developing arthritis when you're older. Think about everything you've been able to do with your hands, and what you might use them for: crocheting a feminist doily, fondling a lover, or taking up archery with flaming arrows. And painting your nails with glitter polish and little stickers of daisies: in fact, you may as well do this to your knees, too, or you might be accused of growing old gracefully.

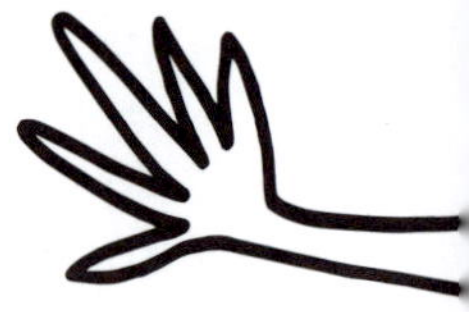

Brittle nails

'Don't break my nails, my flaky, breaky nails,' goes the well-known song. At least doctors call this brittle nail syndrome and not 'deficient crone-claws' or something equally mean. There's not enough research, but lack of estrogen has a role. Brittle nails can be made worse by dehydrated hands (use a hand moisturiser) or hands that are in water very often; and some nail polishes and especially gel manicure products also make it worse.

Hangnails, splitting nails and ingrown toenails can damage the thinning skin around them and cause little infections. Brittle nails (and thinning hair) can also be caused by a hypothyroid condition which has other symptoms that can look like perimenopause, such as weight gain and feeling exhausted. Iron deficiency may also be a culprit, so you might want to check this out. (Blood tests can be ordered by your GP.)

About 60 per cent of the respondents to the Survey experienced brittle nails from the time of perimenopause.

Things that will help your nails

Buy a yacht and insist servants do all the housework, garden work and craft work, and only use your hands for imperious gesturing. Also:

* You can paint nails with a protective, non-damaging, easily removable polish that might help splitting.
* Correct any protein deficiency with what you eat, and get enough B vitamins and iron.
* Moisturise your hands and in the crevices around nails.
* Protect your hands from hot water with rubber gloves.
* Use non-soap cleanser on hands, wash in lukewarm water.
* A special nail-strengthening polish will help make a fingernail or toenail stronger while it's on.
* If you can afford them or find time to DIY, attention from a podiatrist (foot specialist) and pedicures can maintain toenails to help avoid ingrown or breakage problems.

What won't help make stronger nails

No health-shop or non-prescription pharmacy supplement powder or pill, regardless of alleged miracle or useful ingredients, is known to make any difference to nail growth or strength. These things don't help:

* Artificial nails glued on.
* Long nails that catch on things.
* Acetone nail remover.

Lastly, do something fun with your body's end bits rather than just look at them . . . all right, I just wanted to say it: put your hands in the air like you just don't care.

Neck

> If I'd woken up 15 years ago with the face I have now, I would have screamed the house down. Me

Nora Ephron's book title *I Feel Bad About My Neck* was instantly recognisable to most women of a certain age and baffled men, who if they ever think about their neck at all, it's about whether it's too hot or too cold, and not what it looks like. You're stuck with your neck because sadly it attaches your head.

Lack of estrogen means thinning skin, and the combination of gravity and less elastin and collagen, and a lifetime of putting sunscreen only down to the jawline often means a neck can look wrinklier than the face. Like many white women I have a condition called poikiloderma, red neck marks caused by sun damage – this is where the phrase rednecks came from.

> Not wrinkles so much but the chook neck upsets me . . .
> Sue, 70

> My brother once told me he loved his wife like she was 25. She's still the same girl, she's just got an older face. I love that.
> Andrea, 51

Gums & teeth

Thinner, drier skin and less estrogen in the body can contribute to gums receding more, and bleeding. Teeth can also start to misbehave as you get older. If you can afford it, go see your dentist regularly to make sure none of this develops into a problem.

> I just try to remember my body has done its very best to house this spirit of mine. In my younger years I was not always appreciative of the way it looked and I did not treat it in the way it deserved.
> Lisa, 51

> It's fantastic not thinking about how I look and feeling the pressure of the male gaze. It's also difficult losing the male gaze.
> Nicola, 56

> I think about my deteriorating 'beauty' and think about what a great mother I am to my 19-year-old daughter – she tells me all the time that I am so important to her and she appreciates my love and wisdom.
> Marian, 61

Who's who in skin & hair doctors

See also 'Who's Who in cosmetic practitioners' on page 313.

GP A general practitioner has 4–6 years of university medical study, intern experience in a hospital, passed the exam and may have extra specialties or training. They can help with diagnosis, do a mole check and deal with many standard skin condition diagnoses. It's not legally required but a GP will need to formally refer you to a dermatologist if you want a Medicare rebate. Your GP will be advised of diagnosis and ongoing care recommendations and can reissue new prescriptions.

A **medical dermatologist** is a doctor who has the 4–6 year medical degree, followed by a year of hospital residency and/or research experience, then another 4–5 years of specialist dermatology study and experience to become an expert on skin, nails and hair. Letters after their name are FACD for Fellow of the Australasian College of Dermatologists.

A **cosmetic dermatologist** is a fully qualified medical dermatologist but one who specialises in cosmetic treatments including fillers, paralysing chemicals, and laser procedures. A cosmetic dermatologist's waiting room, office and website is often full of posters and brochures.

Trichologist Anyone can call themselves a trichologist, said to be a 'hair expert'; they're not doctors and don't have a recognised university-level qualification. Some private organisations conduct online and other courses. Trichologists work in hair-replacement companies or independently with private clients and set their own fees. Dermatologists have expressed concern that products, supplements and treatments have no acceptable scientific evidence to back their use.

* MORE INFO on skin & hair practitioners

Complaints about beauty therapists or similar services can be made to the Health Care Complaints Commission or equivalent in your state or territory.

dermcoll.asn.au
The Australasian College of Dermatologists has info on qualified doctors, plus fact sheets on various skin conditions.

Cellulite

As skin is thinner in menopausal women, veins and normal fat, including some on the thighs, can become easier to spot. Cellulite is not a medical term but a name invented by a French marketing person in the 1920s. The end. So-called firming cream will do nothing, and scrubbing just creates a low-level swelling which can make the skin look less bumpy for a very short time.

Eyes

There isn't anything special about eye cream, no matter what so-called beauty experts tell you. They take their information from product sellers, not independent dermatologists: sometimes they just regurgitate bits of press releases. They say the skin around the eyes is more delicate than the rest of your face, and possibly more sensitive. All that means is, don't use a face moisturiser that stings around your eyes. Use one that doesn't: it doesn't have to be a specific eye cream. You might feel that dabbing on a thick and pricey cream very pattingly with one finger is more ritualistic, but please don't fool yourself that there's any special effect.

Hair changes

Not long ago a supposedly progressive old-man-commentator with a big following on Twitter used a photo of a politician fronting a press conference, declaring that she needed a better hairdresser. If I really stare at the picture, I can see that she has visible flyaway and broken hair along her part, and is very slightly receding and greying at the temples. The commentator, who is bald with a face like a bowl of spiced nuts, was branding her dishevelled and unkempt, one of the traditional slurs against a woman. If we were still in the 19th century, he might have called her a slovenly chit.

What he was sneering at is menopausal hair.

When I was young, I think I also presumed that the coarser, flyaway broken hairs and phouffy front bits and messy buns of older women was because they were too busy or didn't care about doing their hair. I didn't realise that their hair itself had changed.

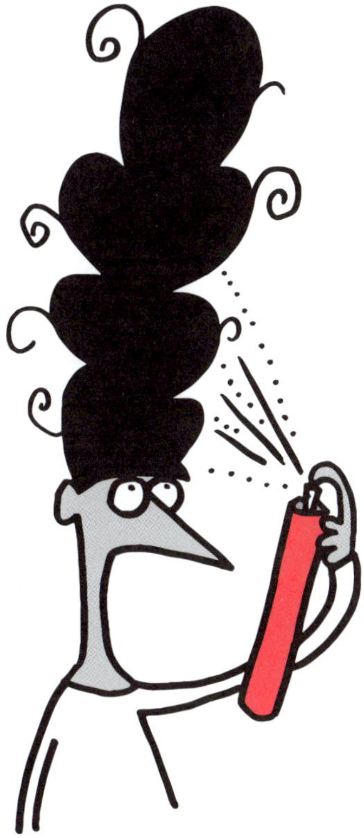

Coarser, breaky, flyaway hair that seems to grow out at odd angles for no bloody reason at all, and thinning hair occur around perimenopause and the first years of menopause. This means you can use a coating shampoo and conditioner and brush your hair and still look like you fought a possum.

So I started noticing that most celebrities over 50 that we see, including women on TV, have just had their hair done by a professional hairdresser who has smoothed and sprayed their hair. Older women politicians and executives, fronting a doorstep interview or a press conference in the middle of the day, have two kinds of hair. Either an expensive hairdo, especially independently wealthy city-based conservative politicians. Or – if they're standing in a stiff breeze or have daylight behind them or a podium at their workplace – they might have flyaway, broken hair that looks like it hasn't been brushed.

The older women in positions of power with bizarre, immoveable hair-helmets crop-dusted with half a can of hairspray are also mocked for messy-looking hair. Damned if they do, damned if they don't. I bet it's also why post-menopausal women of my grandmother's generation put their hair into then-fashionable tight curlers and setting lotion: aiming for more control and a curlier, bald-spot-disguising style.

Menopausal hair is lying in wait for most of us, another imposition of something used to castigate us, something we can't control without time and money and effort that men in the public eye, with their almost universal standard short hair or baldness, can safely dodge.

This section talks about all the hair changes associated with perimenopause and menopause: grey hair, hair loss, and disappearing body hair in some places turning up elsewhere. Do your eyebrows really emigrate to your top lip? Why are your nipples trying to grow a goatee?

We'll start with body hair and move on up. See 'More info on skin & hair practitioners', on page 319.

Yeah, I started dyeing my hair, but not to look natural or younger. I dyed it hot, hot pink, because I don't care what anyone else thinks anymore. **Briony, 52**

Need to shave almost every day. Too embarrassed to see someone about it. CD, 49

Body & facial hair

To simplify things a lot, when your body stops making as much estrogen as it used to, the androgen hormones including testosterone have a greater effect on you because they're no longer opposed, or balanced, by estrogen levels.

To put things a bit too baldly (oh dear):

* Having enough estrogen tends to allow more luxuriant, robust hair to grow on your legs, eyebrows, underarms, head (scalp) and pubic area. When estrogen declines, the growth of these hairs declines.
* Androgen hormones such as testosterone put hair on our upper lip, chin and maybe sideburns. When androgens are not as opposed, these hairs can multiply.

I now have an eyebrow on my chin. Helen, 57

I have more hairs on my chin than front bottom. Rebecca, 58

This means that in perimenopause and then menopause – regardless of whether you're taking MHT – there'll be changes in your body hair. Generally, people feel their leg hair and underarm hair disappears and turns up on their chin and upper lip.

Of more than 7000 respondents to questions about hair in the Survey, almost 34 per cent didn't develop more facial hair in perimenopause and menopause, whereas about two-thirds did, and about one in five found it tough or terrible. About a third of women noticed they had less body hair.

If you're worried about facial hair you can wax or pluck it, using a magnifying mirror and a good light (or grow a jaunty circus ringmaster's moustache). Or you can pay to be waxed or threaded.

You can dye eyebrows yourself using salon products bought online but do take care. I did this the other day, forgot I had it on, and during a spirited phone conversation with my editor, wiped it all over my forehead and my left ear, and looked like a dazed mud-wrestler for somewhat longer than necessary.

If I became incapacitated I would have a full beard and THIS SCARES ME MORE THAN ANYTHING ELSE. Debbie, 58

And no-one EVER talks about chin hair!! CHIN HAIR! For the longest time, I thought it was something weird about me. Amanda, 49

Head hair loss

Various studies and surveys reckon two-thirds of menopausal women have hair loss, a third of women over 70 have hair loss, and all women will eventually 'go' grey or white. I don't suppose such statistics really matter, though, do they? The most important thing is to help the people who are distressed by their own head hair loss.

Estrogen loss contributes to head hair changes but the other effects of natural ageing contribute a lot too. Individual hair follicles can get smaller and/or stop growing a hair; as you get older your hair-replacement cycle slows and isn't as efficient. Hair can also be affected by stress, and some medical conditions and their treatments.

Getting older causes some or all of this characteristic carry-on:

* thinner individual hairs, so less bouffy hair
* fewer hairs on the scalp overall, so it feels like your ponytail's shrinking
* hair loss causing a receding effect at the temples
* brittle hairs breaking, causing a flyaway, phouffy effect
* the appearance of much thinner or 'bald' spots
* more falling-out hair than was normal for you before.

Reading medical stuff about hair loss is exhausting, lots of talk of lateral and vertex and temporal region and vellus hair ratio. What's known as typical 'male pattern hair loss' usually refers to a receding front hairline and most noticeable hair loss at the temples, plus a possible bald spot in the middle top of the head, then often usual spread to wider or complete baldness.

Characteristic 'female pattern hair loss' is the one caused by hormone changes, aka androgenic alopecia (pronounced and-roh-jenick allo-pee-shar), described as hair loss and scalp peek-a-booing, especially along the central parting sort of area. It's my sorrowful duty to report that a doctor may eventually also say 'senile alopecia', and if so, you may shriek.

A receding hairline of sorts is also common in older women, including the menopausal phouff on the temples caused by thinning and broken hair. Another, rarer thing is called frontal fibrosing alopecia, which is losing hair at the temples and all along the front hairline. What matters is how you see your own individual situation and not whether the 'pattern' is called male or female. The main thing is, if you have distressing hair loss, be off to a dermatologist for a diagnosis.

Just under half of the respondents to the Survey registered hair loss and just over half noticed head hair changes after they entered perimenopause, though most found it not too confronting.

Even when we understand, especially after age 55, that this is normal and natural, it's fair enough not to like it. Changes or loss of control over what your hair looks like can be more confronting for many women than other physical changes. (And yes, I can hear and appreciate a ladylike snort from those who lost all their hair, and eyebrows, during chemotherapy or radiation therapy, which didn't grow back the same and perhaps never quite behaved itself again. And I salute you with a raised glass of a dear little cocktail and a well-formed biscuit.)

Through rather complicated mechanisms, stress is known to cause greying or thinning hair, especially sudden and extreme periods of grief or intense anxiety, sometimes temporarily. But because trauma isn't something you'd actively ask for, or be able to easily control, saying 'be less stressed' isn't so much a handy hint as a sentence that will incite at least one reader to bite someone, and fair enough. Hair loss caused by traction damage from pulling on your hair, tight styling, extensions or weaves can often be reversed.

Some prescription medications can help retain or regrow hair or oppose androgen hormones, which cause hair loss. Some GPs can be reluctant to prescribe them because they're unsure what dose to use for hair loss. Don't self-prescribe or take anyone else's hair medication because some side effects or medication combinations can be dangerous. For medication, you may need a dermatologist's expertise in prescribing; then you can have a GP reissue prescriptions.

Doctors will be reluctant to prescribe MHT if the only thing you want to deal with is hair loss, because it's not an efficient treatment for that. There are better frontline solutions.

Things that can help hair loss

These:

- With your GP, rule out an underlying medical condition causing hair loss, including a thyroid condition.
- Address any deficiencies of protein, iron and vitamin B in your diet.

Never expected to have a bald patch in my pubic hair. Spoken to other ladies who have a bald patch in the same area. Rose, 57

The hair breakage is off the charts. Lisa, 49

- Discuss medication with your GP, and perhaps a dermatologist as the first prescriber.
- Confide your worries in a good hairdresser. Clever style changes can help. Very dark hair and severe styles tend to make baldier spots more noticeable.
- Hats and wraps can disguise hair problems, and protect your scalp from sunburn, which can damage hair follicles.
- Some women wear 'halos', wiglets and other hair products for a bit of extra volume.
- Some products will coat the hair and make it easier to style and stop phouffing so much.

> It is harder to make your hair stylish when it has thinned and there is less to work with. But I am happy with the colour changing as I get older.
> Caryn, 59

Things that don't help with hair loss

These:

- No topical product will change your hair's own consistency, thickness or the way it grows: not conditioner, shampoo, pastes, serums and the like, with or without protein, keratin, collagen, crushed diamonds or other non-pharmaceutical ingredients.
- Some shampoos and other products can strip hair of any remaining moisture or coating, causing more flyaways.
- Some conditioners and 'volumising' products put a thin coating on each hair, which can make it seem thicker, but can also weigh it down.
- The fewer products, washes and styling you can get away with the better.
- Post-wash mousses, spray, or styling gloop can smooth flyaway hair but they can't replace or reconstitute hair itself.
- Supplements, such as powders and vitamin pills, don't help unless the hair loss is caused by a deficiency, which is rare. None are known to create new hair growth or slow thinning.
- Non-pharmaceutical products advertised as 'supporting' hair growth, or hair 'health' will not change your hair growth or thickness.

The jury's out on some hair treatments

Clinical trials continue to refine non-pharmaceutical plant-ingredient hair growth supplements with promising results in respectable studies, but so far no proof of the best formulation is obvious. Many of these studies are being funded by would-be sellers of the product. Look for brands with the backing of respected universities or similar studies with placebo and double-blind study elements. It's impossible for a non-scientist to be able to evaluate talk of nutraceutical bio-optimised phytoactivity faff.

There are also experiments with injecting your own platelet-rich plasma into your scalp. It's expensive (thousands of dollars), a palaver and there is not yet any proof it works. It's just a theory: practitioners who do it usually suggest re-jabs every few months which costs even more. Most of this is done on men. Women already have more platelets than men.

Grey hair

The last 10 years has seen a greyzillion photos of models aged anywhere from 25 to 60 with smooth faces and deliciously supple, silver hair; usually bouncey, straight, subtly silver-highlighted cloudlike halo. Sometimes the model is even older, described as a *former* model even though she is, clearly, still modelling the idea of unattainable ageing. Usually this model will be whippet-thin and have fish-knife cheekbones with her wrinkles digitally removed so her face looks like it's been resurfaced with marzipan icing – perhaps a few artful smile lines around the eyes will be allowed to stand.

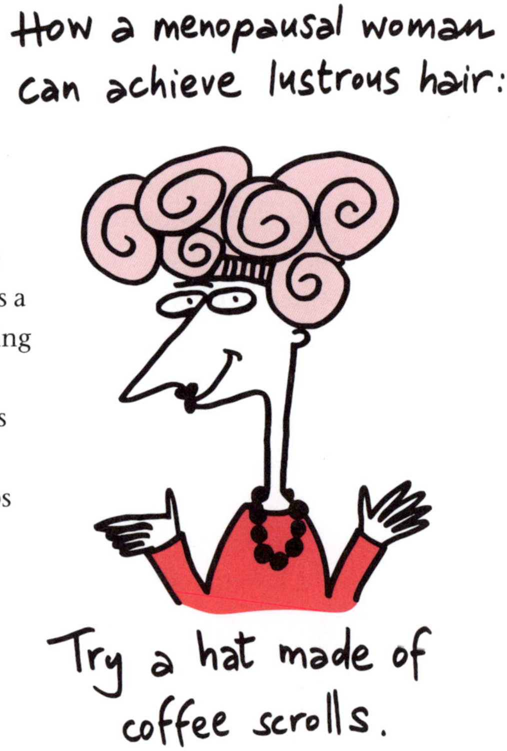
How a menopausal woman can achieve lustrous hair:
Try a hat made of coffee scrolls.

I am now 70 per cent grey. I am perhaps early with grey hair but I have really enjoyed embracing my age and the changes that come with it. Mary, 47

I don't mind about my face, I do care about my hair. Maggie, 57

I love the changes in my hair. The grey streak makes me look intelligent (I tell myself). Mari, 42

Real, free-range grey hair is not like that at all. Shiny, thick grey hair that lies flat and smooth costs a lot of money and weekly or daily attentions from a hairdresser to behave like that. Or it's a wig. Professionally untended grey hair is coarser, patchier, drier, more brittle and breaking, and fall-y-outier, and subject to the command of genetic heritage, hormonal and age-related changes.

In the past, it was normal for women over time to have 'salt and pepper', and eventually, white hair as the natural pigments in hair stopped being produced. Certainly, through most of my grandmother's and mother's generation and circumstances, having your own money to spend on yourself, or doing it, was considered indefensible or impossible.

I didn't ever dye my hair,
am a Silvery Crone; absolutely
a woman of power now.
Ciel, 64

I have changed my look
and gone more bold. A peroxide
blonde pixie and colourful clothes.
I will not fade into the background.
Emily, 47

I don't mind having old
hair but I don't want an old face.
Mars, 49

Now, it's normal for most women over 40 to dye their hair. Collectively we spend billions more every year than our grandmothers did on home and salon dye and products to mitigate the menopausal effects on hair. It can come as a real 'Oh my GOD, of course!' moment to realise that your eyebrows, underarm and pubic hair is going grey, too. It's normal, just not quite as common, for some women to get their first grey head hairs or a streak of grey in their 20s and 30s.

There was a huge response to the questions in my Survey about grey hair. Although greying hair is not only a simple response caused by hormone changes, it tends to happen around the same time as other perimenopause symptoms such as thinning hair, and so comes as part of the deal.

The reasons for women dyeing their grey hair are many: we want to look younger, or to retain our sense of self, to try to decide how we want to look. We represent the first couple of generations who take for granted that we should do everything we can to control how we look, rather than letting it take its own course. And we live in a world where hair choices are judged by bosses, partners, friends and even strangers.

In the Survey, just over half of women who answered the question said they dyed their hair to cover grey.

For many people, letting themselves go completely grey was a bridge too far: it made them feel they looked older than they felt; it didn't match 'who I am'; other people reacted to it in disapproving or discriminatory or patronising ways. Some women knew their friends or children would see grey hair as old, or would otherwise disapprove; some felt their husbands (it was always a husband in these answers) would find them less attractive

One representative respondent said, 'It's been empowering to embrace the grey, but it shits me when I get asked if I have a seniors card – I'm 49, FFS!'

A comment of 'Oh, you're so brave to go grey' has many possible hidden meanings: I'd never do that, you're an idiot; I wish I was brave enough to do that; I'm going to do that, too, and how do you afford hundreds of dollars professionally skilled salon folderol? It's considered brave or foolhardy in the workplace to 'look your age', and be dismissed – perhaps literally – for it.

But there are now many influencers and online magazine articles about 'going grey gracefully' and 'embracing the greys'.

If you want to go grey

You'll find that your everyday grey hair won't look like the pictures of models with grey hair. If you can afford it, find a good hairdresser to help you make the transition.

If you don't want to go grey

You'll probably need to spend serious money, or have a friend who's a hairdresser, to look like you haven't done anything. Shampoo, conditioner and other styling products can't change your hair, only coat it.

Who to listen to about grey hair

Ask yourself who is telling you something and what are they trying to sell you, even if it's their own mindset, not a shampoo and conditioner set. A friend I know was told by one of her childhood gang to start dyeing her hair again because 'Everyone knows we're the same age and I don't want anyone to know I'm old enough to go grey like you'.

> I was such a crashing bore about it for 2 years: should I, shouldn't I, how could I, do I regret it.
> Gina, 58, on going grey

I saw a magazine article about a grey-mopped model icon only to read that she believed her hair was changed by mysterious injections given by her doctor, and that she had grown a new, younger face after it was chemically abraded when she was 37. I wouldn't even ask her directions to the corner shop if I were you.

The only thing I find confronting is finding grey eyebrows and grey pubes! Lol!! Those buggers are so wiry!! Gail, 58

Age & style

Brace yourself for lots of articles and ads on your ageing appearance (the 107 signs of ageing), especially the ones with sentences such as 'Ageing is optional' (well, you could hurl yourself into a sea trench instead). You'll be told you have to have a young attitude, a spring in your step (these articles are a filo pastry of clichés; always another layer), stay flexible, have a magic immune system, do face yoga, breathe properly, sit up straight, stand on your head for lymphatic drainage purposes (this is particularly tawdry nonsense, by the way), do swing dancing in rubber thigh-boots, and dress 'appropriately'.

Dressing your age

Depending on a magazine site writer's own fears and biases, or whatever they're trying to sell you, you'll be told to look elegant and understated in pleated skirts and argyle jumpers, or dress like you're about to kayak round an island, or in four layers of paper-bag-coloured linen awnings, or it's compulsory to wear high-vis fluorescent chartreuse and giant raspberry-lolly-coloured glasses frames.

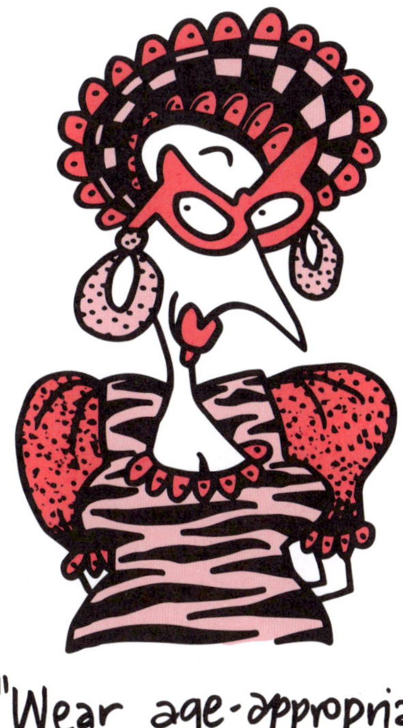

"Wear age-appropriate clothes."

Ugh, 'dress your age'. What does that even mean? Your age varies, and so can your clothes, if you want them to. You can settle into your own style or start experimenting at the op-shop; you don't need an article to tell you that.

While I'm on the subject, as I said in my book *You're Doing It Wrong: A History of Bad & Bonkers Advice to Women*, an insult often wielded against older women was originally a compliment.

I go to the pool and walk around in my bathers and don't care that I have lumpy thighs and a fat stomach – because I'm invisible! Finally.
Jo, 56

I get to wear cowboy boots to work and I don't care what people think!
Fiona, 45

I like to wear nice clothes and keep my appearance up for me, no one else.
Vanessa, 53

I can wear white pants without fear!
Lou, 53

I'm more prepared to dress comfortably and wear what I feel like . . . I wasted so much time when I was younger trying to force myself to become socially acceptable.
Rachel, 48

Wearing whatever I want – stripes, fruit patterns, colours, silly shoes, etc and not caring. **Jenna, 50**

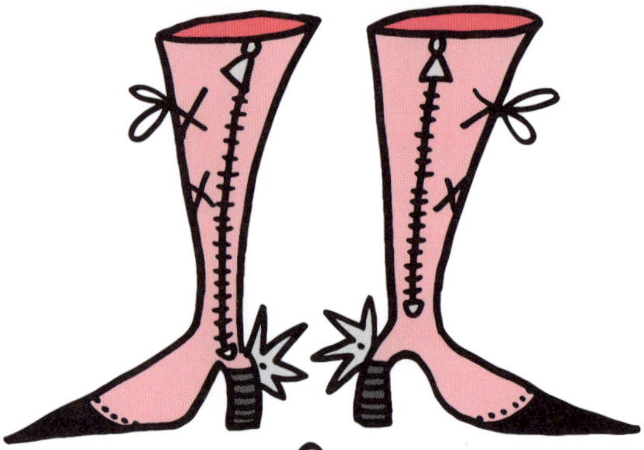

Let yourself go-go boots

'Mutton dressed as lamb' was once an approving nod to a mature woman who managed her budget well enough to follow fashion.

We're warned that a bobby pin with a bow on a young woman is insouciant; on an older woman it says I can't find my hairnet and I found this in Lost Property. A floral ankle-length prairie dress on a young woman is an adorable retro whim; on an older woman it's a repurposed couch cover. If our eye shadow goes all the way up to the eyebrow it isn't fashion-forward, it's evidence of a nervous breakdown. Away with the lot of them.

I think at this age we probably know how we want to dress ourselves, thank yorr. (There's a point at which wearing high heels seems less sensible than wearing a flaming paper-mâché banana on your head, but when you cross that line is up to you.)

Partly due to hormonal changes as we age and partly due to comfort-leisure wear, as we get older, men, women and non-binary people tend to look more like each other, as we stop using so many coded hair, make-up and clothes signifiers to indicate 'feminine' or 'masculine'. Somehow, being older for many people means no longer performing so much as one gender or the other, and just being 'you'.

Frankly, Rod Stewart in his later years looks like nothing so much as a retired netball coach called Lorraine. One day a bigot is going to challenge somebody's Aunty Pam in her comfortable sneakers and sensible fleece vest and try to order them out of the toilets. Aunty Pam is going to give them the rounds of the kitchen and rightly so.

The takeaway on how you look

Maybe it's time to start being an appreciator of beauty, not a tormented marketing pushover. Behold, in the faces of friends, in clouds, in flowers, in sunrises (okay, sure, sleep in if possible – you can get away with sunsets), at free galleries and museums, in small moments and big favours, and kindlier mirrors.

If miracle anti-ageing products and procedures really worked, most influencers would have anti-aged themselves back to toddlerhood.

It's okay that you look your age. And if you feel like it, act your shoe size.

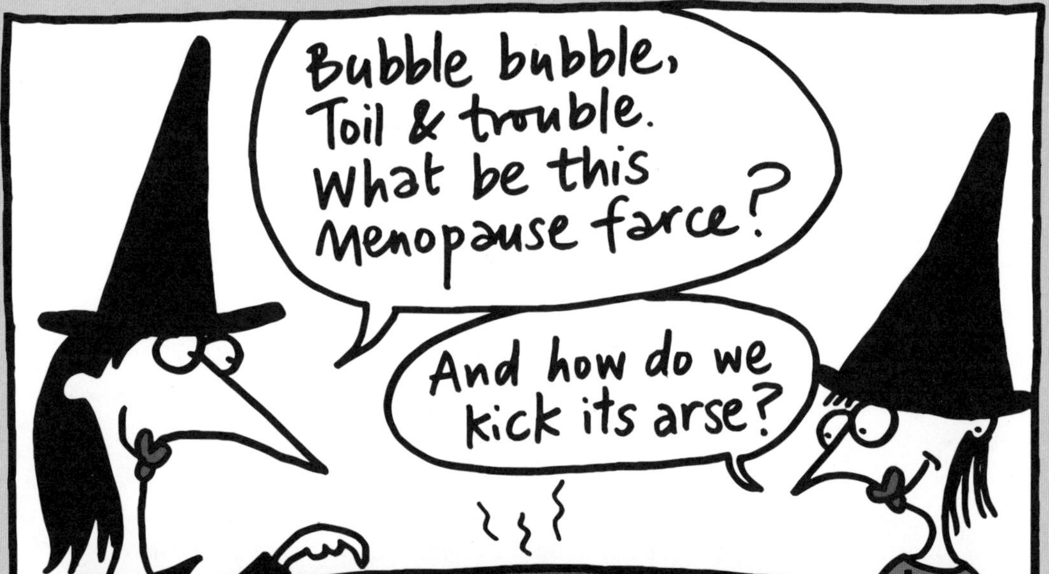
Bubble bubble, Toil & trouble. What be this Menopause farce?
And how do we kick its arse?

8

It's Your Future

You will be as peeved as I am, I bet, about the perimenopause and menopause advice that tells you to cheer up and start freedom-frolicking. I'm not saying ALL you need is a positive attitude, so please don't strike me with your aforementioned moisturising spatula. I'm no fan of the blithe assumption that all perimenopausal and older women have oodles of superannuation, paid-off housing and a Hollywood life, cavorting about in a greige-coloured linen caftan and patio-pants on a yacht in the vicinity of Portugal doing kissy-faces at the deckhands. No, indeed.

But.

We do get only one life (I think). And many of us will be perimenopausal for years, and 'in menopause' for decades. So it's not a bad time to re-evaluate, do a life inventory, find a way to feel optimistic. If you want to.

Do you feel like evaluating your life? Or just having a cup of tea? Do you want to chill? Do you want to have adventures? Do you want to renovate your relationships? Do you want to have a financial plan, or reach out for help because you don't have enough finances for a plan? Do you want to switch careers, retire early, get shit done or back right off? With limited time left, compared to when you were 20, what books do you want to read, what trails do you want to explore? What uncomfortable high heels do you want to burn? What makes your life worth living and how do you get more of that?

Far be it for me to shriek into your face that you're in the last half or third of your life, but TAKE A LONG HARD LOOK AT YOURSELF. No, not your outfit (you look amazing, move on). Have a squizz within. Not that I'm suggesting you have sex in the front yard with a passer-by, or embezzle enough money to buy a small crimson Corvette. But give yourself a little space and time to think about what makes you calm, happy.

Don't think about what you 'should' do. If you knew that you had only 2 years left, what would you do with yourself?

Finding peace and energy after menopause is a subversive act. Freedom from the gaze and the harassment. Finding new purpose and deciding what's important and keeping healthy and happier for as long as possible. Making connections and lives or deciding what to keep from old life. How to assert yourself in a family or society. How to avoid advocating only for yourself, and how to be part of a community and advocate for those who could do with your amplifying voice.

I always liked this quote from Heather Havrilesky in *New York* magazine, which made me think of older women. (Older than, say, 32.) 'You do it however *you* want to do it, and God bless, but I'm going to follow my most audacious and inappropriate whims wherever they lead.'

So I also asked some of the thousands of respondents to the Survey for this book for the benefit of their perimenopause and menopause experiences. Do they, perhaps, have advice or mottoes or advice for everyone else? Did they ever. Along with many fears of being financially bereft, with no secure housing or income prospects, there were thousands of emblematic positive thoughts to share.

Alison, Genevieve, and about a gerzillion others say that talking and laughing with friends is the most important thing for them. Carolyn says she and her friends are hilarious together and anyone who doesn't think so can fuck off.

Myrto reckons she wasted too many years caring what other people thought about her, and now she's no longer scared to speak up about whatever she want to. Donna relishes being a 'difficult woman'.

So many women encouraged a variation of what 'Cleopatra' suggests: she wants you to 'care much, much less about what people think of you . . . I have a better appreciation of what's important to me: family, friends, love and adventure.' Rebecca adds, 'Wisdom, Experience. Survival.' Jodie says she's let go of a lot of stuff, and realised 'it's OK to ask for help'.

Mei speaks for a lot of us when she says, 'I've become invisible to some of the usual abusers and harassers of women.' Shirlie wants to recommend yoga, meditation and mindfulness.

'What are the good things?' asks Rachael. 'Everything, my lovely. Freedom, the love of old old friends, the ability to be a rock for little ones coming into adulthood, the gravitas I can bring to my job. Sure, I'm not the babe I once was, but I actually enjoy the disintegration of my looks. I like watching it, I sigh and accept its day is done.' Stacey is relieved she's given up chasing an unrealistic body shape for her.

Katherina tries to do something new every year (so far: cold water swimming, salsa dancing, the drums). Rowena's started a university degree for the first time. Mona is 76 now, and she's joined an exercise class, done French online and followed a creative writing course by publishing a murder mystery.

Marianne says she's overlooked, so she says and does whatever she likes and has moved away from toxic friends. Cecile is relieved she doesn't have to pack school lunches or go to school sports days any more. Lily's trying hard to find anything positive. Sita says she's had so many ups and downs she now has a heightened appreciation for the good stuff.

Bella and Leesa reckon they're wiser. Fiona's braver. (Liz jokes she's mostly just wider.) Grace says she's done with 'tolerating foolery and entitlement'. Kate yells at men if they're being rude or stupid. Nessa got help to force an abuser from her house. Mack is rapt that the younger generation of women are ever-bolder. Bronwyn eats desserts now. Eliza got a dog.

Gail urges you to throw out your clothes that became too tight round the middle. Marti says don't stop there and gives away everything she can. Ayisha says she laughs longer and more heartily these days. 'Moo' and lots of others say they're mentoring younger people, if they ask. Cass says she has sex 'all the time and I don't worry about getting pregnant'. Anita says she has menstruated on many continents and speaks for so many more in being thrilled she'll never have another period.

Ginni's thinking about personal boundaries and where she wants to put them. Elke says she's grateful she doesn't feel naïve any more. Jay liked letting go of the fantasy of what life should be and wants to appreciate what is. Sal says she's so much cooler than she was in her 20s but nobody's noticed. Narelle says she knows now to be kinder to people because you never know what they've been through.

Nicky points out, 'I'm a leader and a role model when I'm not going insane'. Jackie says a bonus part of ageing is bigger underpants.

Rebecca's never felt better. Di announced that if you eat orange vegetables you can alter the age you go through menopause (Oh, Di.) Loulou says to 'ask the experts, not the snake oil salespeople'. Shazza says to keep the pressure on the medical profession; if more women ask for guidance and advice there will surely be more answers. Trish says to surround yourself with nature and friends.

Tiffany used to disparage old ladyish pursuits but is now perfectly thrilled to be knitting, spinning, reading and feeding the magpies. Kathy says new generations of older women are rising up; we're strong, mature, intelligent, and powerful. Our minds sharp and our bodies mighty. Sharrow agrees: when you come out the other side, you feel powerful and bold.

Tracey reminds you that you have decades of knowledge and life experience. Tamara puts it this way: 'I am a crone. I deserve respect.' Tania advises to envelop yourself in whatever gives you joy. Beth explains, 'I am out the other side wiser, more compassionate and more authentic. I am both stronger and softer'.

'Find the girl you were at age 9,' says Trudy. 'She's in there. Buried beneath a pile of life. The world deserves YOU.'

Everyone has their own idea of what to add to a recipe for their future in their own imaginary cauldron: throw in your witchy dreams, plans and ideas. Some eye of newt and self-esteem affirmations, maybe, because if others don't value us we must value ourselves. A list of things that make you happy. Compliments received. Maybe some medication, maybe not. A touch of attitude. Achievements, knowledge, a dash of humility and curiosity. A soupçon of useful, righteous anger. A way to advocate for and help others. The kindness of friends. Family. Community. Red shoes. Singing. Dancing. Laughing. A public library card.

Definitely fold in some freedom from the judgement of others. A metaphorical leaf, for nature. The memories of things that broke you and the ones that made you stronger and wiser. Sprinkle over some pulverised, chopped-up 'shoulds', to taste. Stir in the ashes of the concept of perfection.

Boil, baby, boil.

Kaz x

Acknowledgements

The women

I thank the 9000 or so brave women who clicked on my Menopause Survey conducted for this book, all over Australia. Not all of you answered every question, of course, but there were 76,000 questions answered with the written word. It was phenomenal, and the statistical results, but especially your voices, informed every single page of this book. I read every one of the replies, written by you in solidarity, in bewilderment, in anger, in hope. Thank you for helping me, and thank you for trusting me.

I hope this book gives you some answers and you can feel my respect and appreciation. The quotes are scattered throughout as a conversation: many respondents chose their own false name, many wanted their own first name used; I have edited or punctuated some quotes where needed for the sense of them. Occasionally I changed a pseudonym, especially if I thought it revealed something the respondent wouldn't want known.

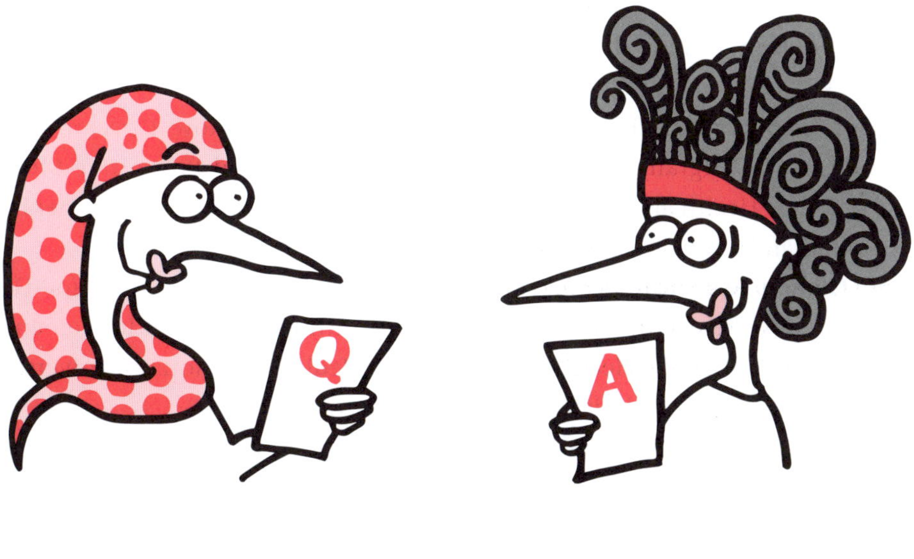

The survey maven

Carolyn Whyte was the survey researcher, online wrangler, results administrator and collator-analyst. I could not have extracted and drawn some conclusions from all this amazing information without her hard work, technical skills and insights.

The doctors

I'm always so grateful for the kind help of so many doctors and other medical experts (including scientific researchers) who help inform my books, help check draft manuscripts for mistakes, omissions, or things that have changed. Not all the medical experts have seen all the chapters or finished ones, so any errors are down to me, despite my best efforts.

I've omitted from the names of the stellar medical consultants on this book their extensive list of acronyms, their boxfuls of extra medical qualifications, and their senior membership of many peak specialist bodies and important medical organisations, and their national official honours such as Orders of Australia, for their service to medicine and scientific research. Rest assured, many of them have so many qualifications and awards that there are scrambled alphabets after their names. Their titles and positions were the ones held at the time of researching and writing the book.

For important interviews before I started writing, about perimenopause and menopause in general, or specific sections, a huge thank you in no particular order to:

Dr Sonia Davison, head of the Australasian Menopause Society, endocrinologist at the Jean Hailes Women's Health organisation.

Professor Susan Davis, NHMRC Senior Principal Research Fellow: Director, Women's Health Research Program Department of Epidemiology and Preventive Medicine, School of Public Health and Preventive Medicine at Monash University, former head of the Australasian Menopause Society.

Adjunct Clinical Associate Professor Amanda Vincent, endocrinologist and Head of Early Menopause Research, Monash Centre for Health Research and Implementation (MCHRI), School of Public Health and Preventive Medicine at Monash University and past president of the Australasian Menopause Society.

Associate Professor Len Kliman, consultant gynaecologist and obstetrician.

Dr Vijay Roach, obstetrician and gynaecologist at North Shore Private Hospital and past president of RANZCOG.

Dr Colleen MacMillan, Agriculture and Food, plant chemist and senior research scientist at the Commonwealth Scientific and Industrial Research Organisation (CSIRO). And person who can say molecular biology of gibberellin synthesis with a proper straight face.

Professor Jayashri Kulkarni, women's specialist psychiatrist, Director of the Monash Alfred Psychiatry Research Centre and Head Central Clinical School Department of Psychiatry.

Dr Shalini Arunogiri, specialist psychiatrist in addiction studies, senior lecturer, Deputy Head of Department at the Alfred Psychiatry Research Centre.

Dr Sandra Elmer, urological surgeon.

Associate Professor Dr Ada Cheung, endocrinologist NHMRC & Dame Kate Campbell Research Fellow and Head of Trans Health Research Group, Melbourne University.

Tamara Wraith, specialist physiotherapist.

Michael Buckley, pharmacist and hormone product manufacturer.

For above & beyond checking sometimes unreasonably large parts of the manuscript, these absolute tippety-top expert legends:

Dr Vijay Roach.

Associate Professor Len Kliman.

Professor Jayashri Kulkarni.

Dr Shalini Arunogiri.

Associate Professor Dr Ada Cheung.

Dr Audrey Wang, urological surgeon at Westmead Hospital NSW; spokesperson for Urological Society of Australia and New Zealand.

Dr Jo-Ann See, consultant dermatologist, Australasian College of Dermatologists.

Elizabeth Hewett, accredited specialist exercise physiologist, Pilates teacher and strength and conditioning coach.

Associate Professor Caroline Gurvich, Clinical Neuropsychologist Head, Cognition and Hormones Group, Department of Psychiatry and brain fog researcher, Monash University.

Big thanks to even more people & organisations who facilitated or provided help:

The Royal Australian and New Zealand College of Obstetricians and Gynaecologists (RANZCOG); Andre Khoury.

The Royal Australian College of General Practitioners (RACGP); Ally Francis, who provided checkers of GP qualification requirements.

Jean Hailes for Women's Health: medical staff and Jo Roberts.

Associate Professor Alison M. Downham Moore, History and Medical Humanities Department, Associate Dean of Research for the School of Humanities and Communication Arts, Western Sydney University; in particular her book, *The French Invention of Menopause and the Medicalisation of Women's Ageing: A History*, Oxford University Press, 2022.

Julia Nurse's 2022 article on the Wellcome Collection website about menopause treatments and medical opinions since medieval times.

Professor Kathleen Riach, Professor of Organization Studies, Responsible and Sustainable Management Lead, University of Glasgow Adam Smith Business School.

I acknowledge information from research studies, and where used prominently in the text, they include:

Research analysis presented by Professor Rod Baber at the RANZCOG conference in 2021, and other reported comments of his about studies on cancer risk and estrogen, including historical information in the article 'Medical Management of the Menopause' in *Obstetrics & Gynaecology Magazine*, 2017.

Menopause Primer by Susan Davis, Irene Lambrinoudaki, Maryann Lumsden, Gita Mishra, Lubna Pal, Margaret Rees, Nanette Santoro and Tommaso Simoncini, 2015 and other research led by Susan Davis.

Premature Ovarian Insufficiency: an International Menopause Society White Paper, by N. Panay, R. Anderson, R. Nappi, A. Vincent, S. Vujovic, L. Webber and W. Wolfman, 2020.

Moderate Alcohol Intake and Cancer Incidence in Women, by Naomi E. Allen, Valerie Beral, Delphine Casabonne, Sau Wan Kan, Gillian K. Reeves, Anna Brown, Jane Green on behalf of the Million Women Study collaborators, 2009.

And

Two anonymous compounding pharmacists.
The Continence Foundation of Australia; Victoria Hooper.
Australian Commission on Safety and Quality in Health Care; Tommy Jessop.
Business journalist Richard Gluyas; ASIC Media National Manager Gervase Greene, and staffer Angela Friend.
CSIRO communications; Kate Langford.
Australian College of Dermatologists; Ally Chandler.
Clinical Professor Peter Dwyer, gynaecologist and urogynaecologist, director of Urogynaecology at the Mercy Hospital for Women, Melbourne; University of Melbourne.
I did not interview him, but I'd also like to acknowledge the medical ethics activist and public health doctor Honorary Adjunct Associate Professor Dr Ken Harvey, for his body of work in exposing unproven 'wellness' supplements and so-called diet products, and identifying unsupported advertising claims for pharmaceutical and 'natural' products.

Publishing

My publisher–editor and structural engineer Brandon VanOver – my comrade-in-words, who never blinks, even when the heading is Mysteriously Irritable Vulva; and my long-time indispensible collaborator, this book's designer and Big 5 suite-of-books designer, Adam Laszczuk.
Kalhari Jayaweera for a fabulously helpful set of copyedit checks.
The proofreader: Cristina Briones.
The typesetters: Julian Mole and Ann Wilson at Post Pre-press.
For getting the Menopause Survey out there and newsletter wrangling: Marketeers Heidi Camilleri, Tessa Robinson; Mel Boudib and digital designer Rowena Sy. Thanks to publicist Anyez Lindop.

My folk

Thank you to my pandemic-writing-bubble-buddy, Carolyn Fraser; Annie, Gaily, Gina and Jude; VMCL; Glenda Fell Jones, Philippa Hawker and my Reading Group members, perpetual encouragers all; to Kai Howells for keeping the computer going and making sure I didn't lose whole chapters in the abyss.

And a salute to my shields and spears, Claire Harrison at Creative Representation and Kevin Whyte, the Token Group.

Getting safe

Women can be at risk of controlling, belittling, abusive and violent relationships at any time of their lives. Perimenopause and menopause can be times where they feel extra-precarious and unsure of themselves. Please reach out for help in planning to get to a safe emotional and physical place. There are ways to hide visits to websites and phone surveillance, so if this is an issue, use a friend's phone to get your first advice.

1800respect.org.au
Helpline: 1800 737 732
aka: 1800 RESPECT
Phone and online chat and help; you can be totally anonymous. Plus step-by-step advice for safety planning, for when you're ready. Has escape bag hints and checklist.

Other websites with handy info and reality checks about what a healthy relationship is:

relationshipsaustralia.org.au
Peak Australian body with services to help.

betterhealth.vic.gov.au/health/healthyliving/relationship-support-services
Ridiculously long site name, but useful info.

sayitoutloud.org.au
Info for LGBTIQ+ folk.

joinonelove.org
Aimed at US young people but useful about good versus bad relationships.
The emergency number in Australia is 000.
The emergency number in New Zealand is 111.

Index

n

o

p

r

s

t

u

THINGS to SEE

Places to go

Lists

Notes

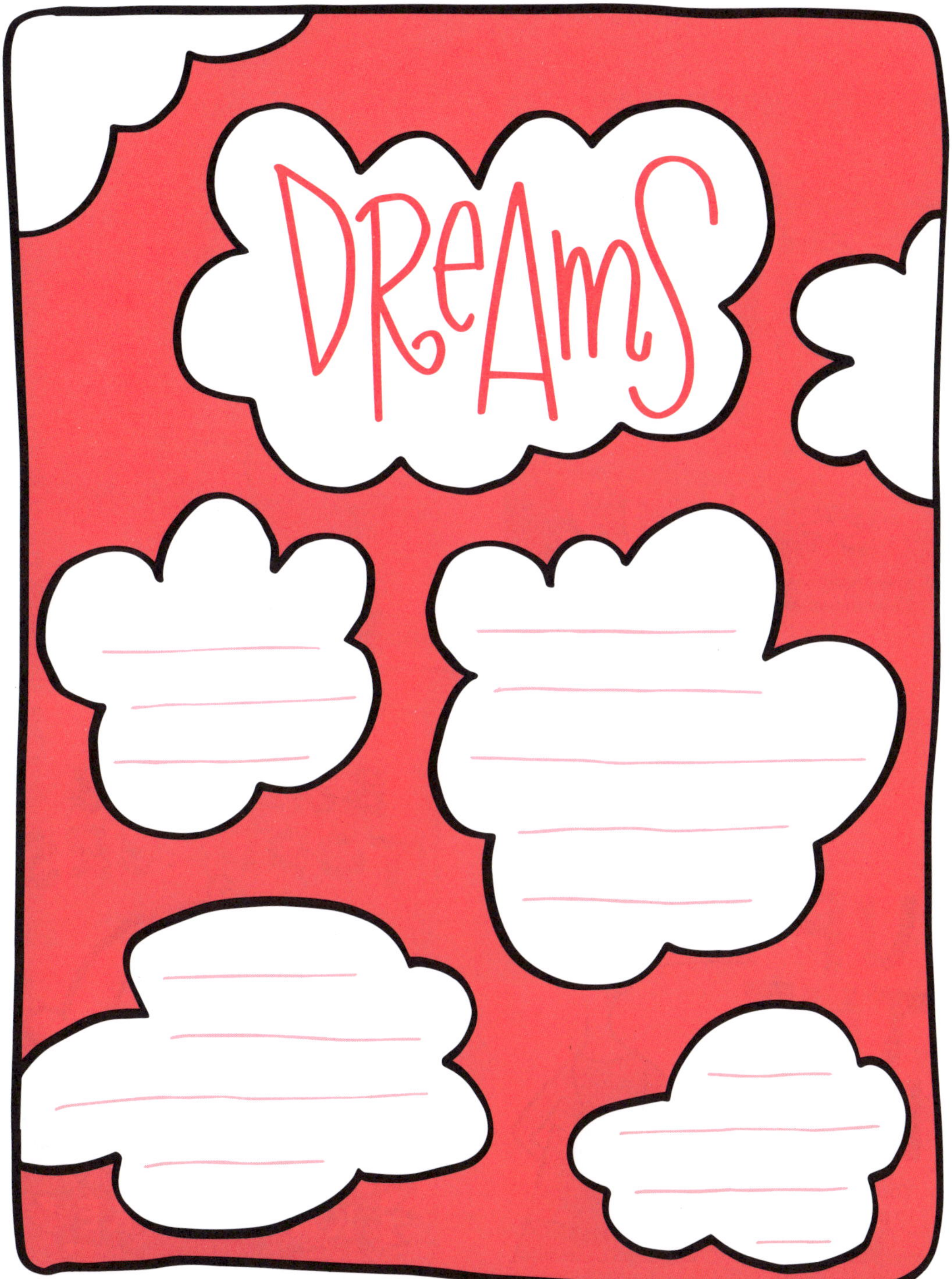
DREAMS

more books from kaz

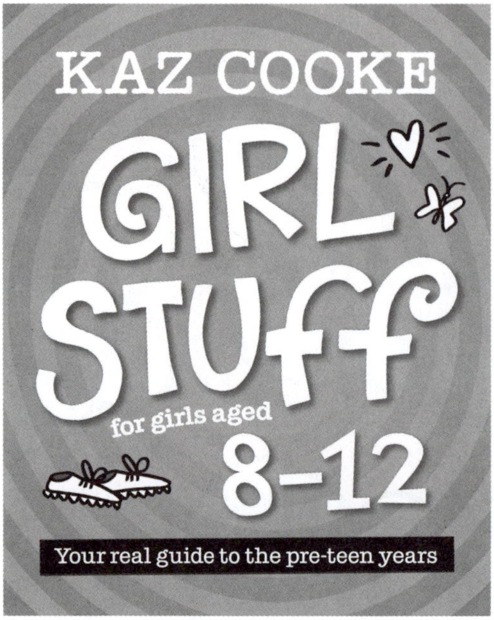

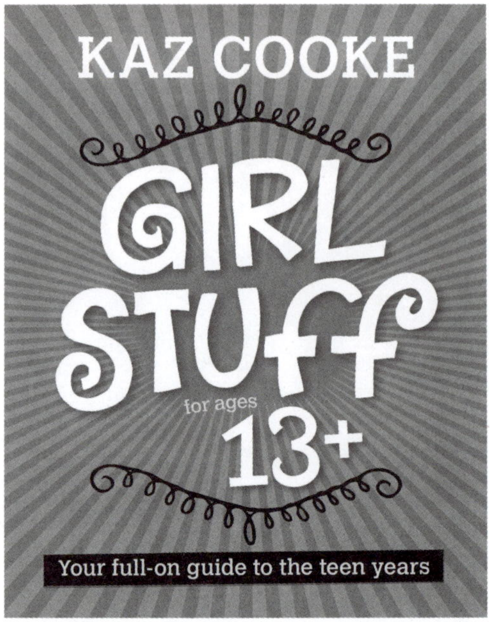

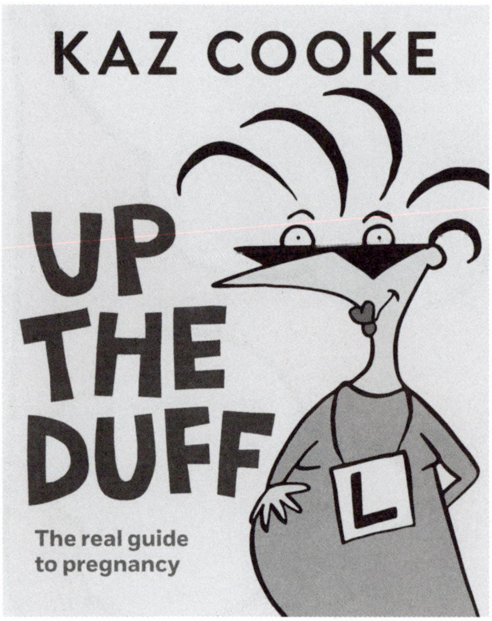

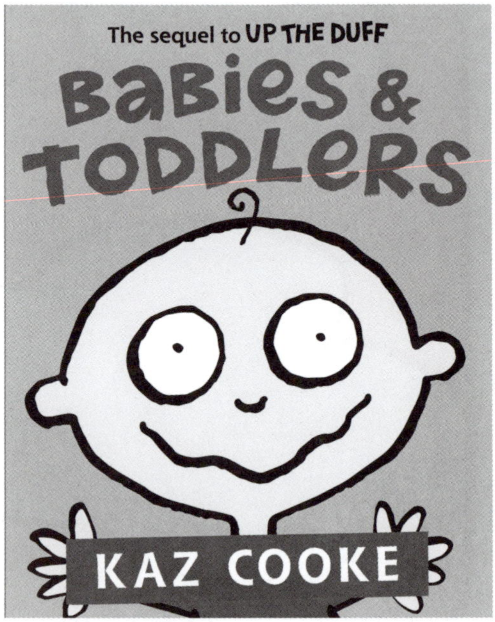

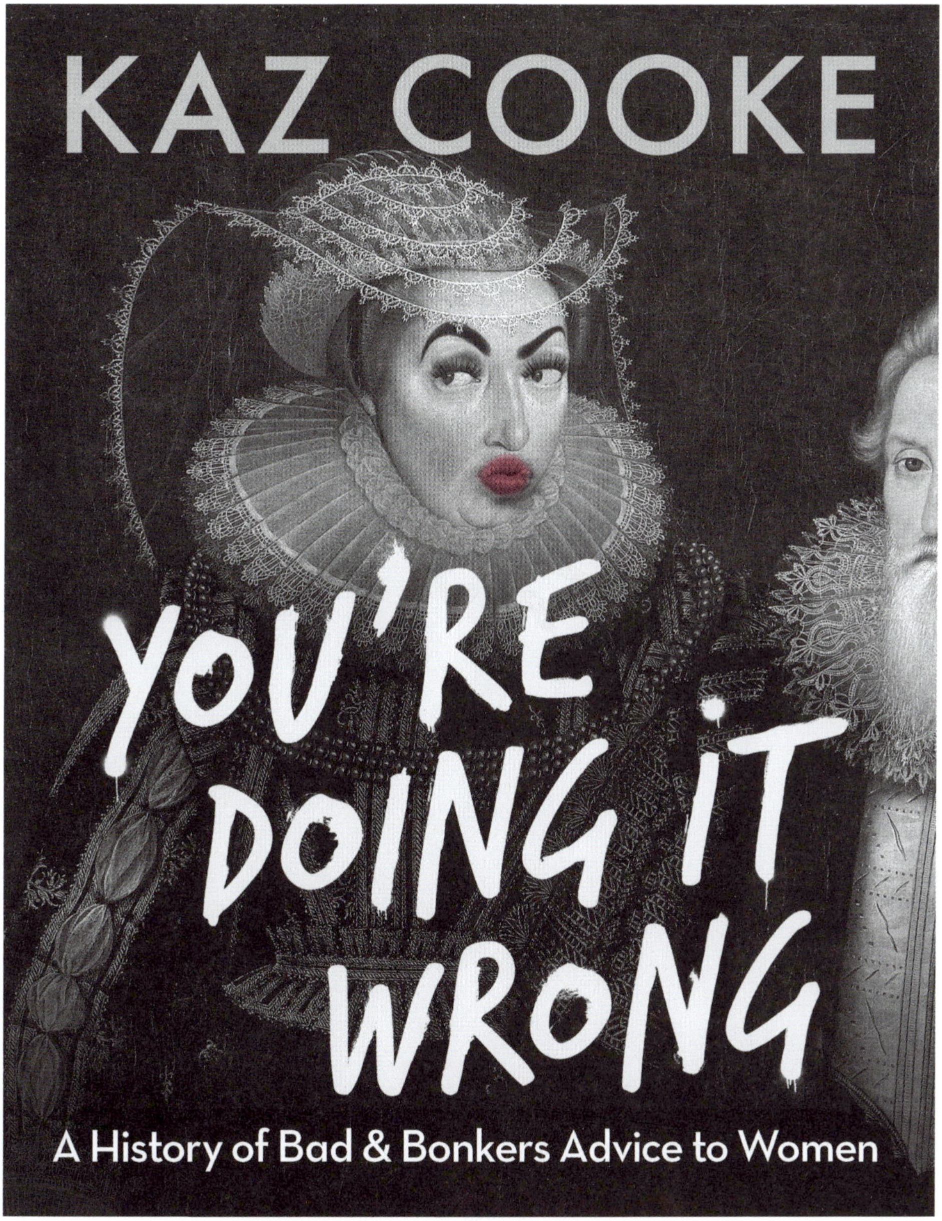
KAZ COOKE
YOU'RE DOING IT WRONG
A History of Bad & Bonkers Advice to Women

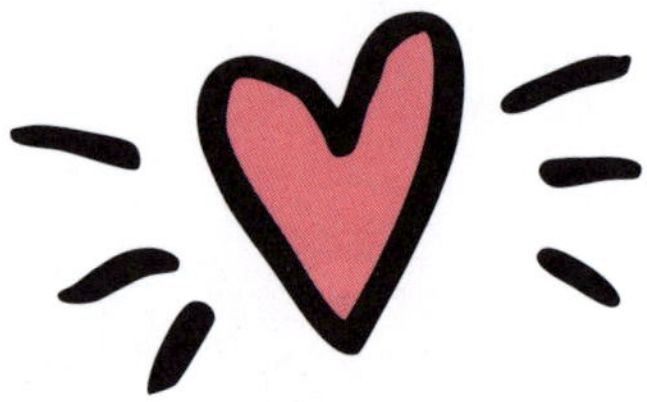

IMPORTANT NOTE

You should make sure you have the latest edition or reprint of this book to maximise medical update information. While best efforts have been made to be accurate and factual, none of the information in this book should take the place of individual consultation, diagnosis and treatment advice from a medical professional. Medical advice changes over time and varies according to different patients and their circumstances.

VIKING

UK | USA | Canada | Ireland | Australia
India | New Zealand | South Africa | China

Viking is part of the Penguin Random House group of companies
whose addresses can be found at global.penguinrandomhouse.com.

Penguin
Random House
Australia

First published by Viking in 2023

Cover design by Kaz Cooke and Adam Laszczuk © Penguin Random House Australia Pty Ltd
Text design by Adam Laszczuk © Penguin Random House Australia Pty Ltd
Illustrations by Kaz Cooke
Typeset in 9.5/15 pt ITC Stone Serif by Post Pre-press, Brisbane, Queensland
Printed and bound in China by 1010 Printing International Ltd.

NATIONAL LIBRARY OF AUSTRALIA
A catalogue record for this book is available from the National Library of Australia

978 1 76089 696 6

penguin.com.au

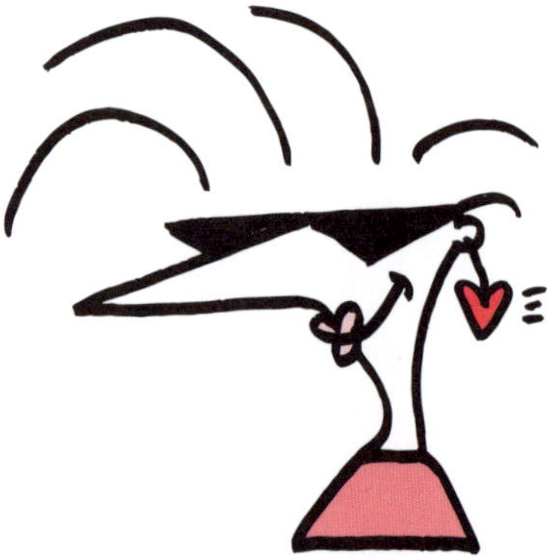

Kaz Cooke is a former journalist, a writer and cartoonist, and the author of bestselling books including *The Modern Girl's Guide to Everything*; *Real Gorgeous*; *Girl Stuff 8–12*; *Girl Stuff 13+*; *Up The Duff*; *Babies and Toddlers*; and *You're Doing It Wrong: A History of Bad & Bonkers Advice to Women*.

kazcooke.com.au